# Orthodontic-Surgical Partnership i
and Palate Treatment

Samuel Berkowitz

# Orthodontic-Surgical Partnership in Cleft Lip and Palate Treatment

Achieving Good Occlusion, Facial Aesthetics, Speech and Psychosocial Development

Springer

Samuel Berkowitz
Coral Gables, FL
USA

ISBN 978-3-030-54302-0     ISBN 978-3-030-54300-6  (eBook)
https://doi.org/10.1007/978-3-030-54300-6

© Springer Nature Switzerland AG 2022
This work is subject to copyright. All rights are reserved by the Publisher, whether the whole or part of the material is concerned, specifically the rights of translation, reprinting, reuse of illustrations, recitation, broadcasting, reproduction on microfilms or in any other physical way, and transmission or information storage and retrieval, electronic adaptation, computer software, or by similar or dissimilar methodology now known or hereafter developed.
The use of general descriptive names, registered names, trademarks, service marks, etc. in this publication does not imply, even in the absence of a specific statement, that such names are exempt from the relevant protective laws and regulations and therefore free for general use.
The publisher, the authors, and the editors are safe to assume that the advice and information in this book are believed to be true and accurate at the date of publication. Neither the publisher nor the authors or the editors give a warranty, expressed or implied, with respect to the material contained herein or for any errors or omissions that may have been made. The publisher remains neutral with regard to jurisdictional claims in published maps and institutional affiliations.

This Springer imprint is published by the registered company Springer Nature Switzerland AG
The registered company address is: Gewerbestrasse 11, 6330 Cham, Switzerland

# Foreword

| | |
|---|---|
| 1959 | Orthodontics Specialty—University of Illinois College of Dentistry |
| | M.S. Thesis: Serial Cephalometric Study of Eight Complete Bilateral Cleft Lip and Palate Patients From Birth To Eight Years of Age |
| 1959 | Orthodontist—Cleft Palate Team, Miami Children's Hospital |
| 1963–2000 | Clinical Professor of Surgery and Pediatrics, University of Miami Miller School of Medicine |
| 1963–2000 | South Florida Cleft Palate-Craniofacial Program, Mailman Center, University of Miami Miller School of Medicine |
| Present | University of Illinois College of Dentistry, Orthodontic Department- Adjunct Professor in Craniofacial Anomalies |

**Memberships**
- American Cleft Palate Craniofacial Association
- American Association of Orthodontics
- American Dental Association
- International College of Dentists
- Florida Dental Association
- Florida Cleft Palate Association

**Achievements**
- **American Cleft Palate Craniofacial Association—2016 Honors of the Association**—for a lifetime of research and care toward improving the treatment of children born with cleft lip and palate and other craniofacial anomalies.
- **Milo Hellman Award of Special Merit**. This award was based on a 3-D Study of serial cleft palate casts using a digitizer created by NASA specifically for this study.
- **Honoree**—Edward Angle Society of Orthodontists
- **Honoree**—International Cleft Palate Foundation—First World Meeting (Zurich)
- **Adjunct Professor of Orthodontics**—Nova Southeastern University Dental School Lecturer on Cleft Palate Treatment
- **Adjunct Professor of Orthodontics**—University of Illinois School of Dentistry – Lecturer on Cleft Palate Treatment.
- **Past President**—American Cleft Palate Association Educational Foundation
- **Past President**—Florida Cleft Palate Association
- **National Museum of Health and Medicine** at the Institute of Pathology—Walter Reed Hospital, Washington D.C. has over 900 of my cases consisting of serial records of cephalographs, dental casts, intraoral and extraoral photographs of all cleft lip and palate types including digital records of all treatment records with their treatment histories.
- **Clinical Director of Research** at the University of Miami School of Medicine Cleft Palate Program. The project was to study the long-term treatment effects on facial and palatal development. The results of these studies are also in storage and available for us.
- Since 1960 attended every American Cleft Palate-Craniofacial Association Annual Meeting, Florida Cleft Palate Association meetings as well as all International Cleft Palate Congress meetings held in different countries every four years.

- Asked to debate in England, Dr. William Shaw, Manchester University Cleft Palate Program on the ethical issue of using "trials" to determine the "best" facial/palatal surgical treatment.
- Lectures in Rome and Bologna, Italy on cleft palate treatment.

**Articles**
- Berkowitz S. (1959) Facial growth in BCLP from birth to eight years of age – Master Thesis, University of Illinois
- Berkowitz S, Pruzansky S. (1969) Stereophotogrammetry of serial casts of cleft palate. Angle Orthod. 38: 136-149.
- Berkowitz S. (1971) Stereophotogrammetric analysis of casts of normal and abnormal palates. Am J of Orthod. Vol. 60: 1-18.
- Berkowitz S, Krischner J, Pruzansky S. Quantitative analysis of cleft palate casts. (1974) CPJ, 11:2, 134-160.
- Berkowitz S, (1977) Section III Orofacial growth and dentistry: State of the art report on neonatal maxillary orthopedics. CPJ: 14: 288-301.
- Berkowitz S, Cuzzi J. (1977) Biostereometric analysis of surgically corrected abnormal faces. Am J Orthod. 12:5, 526-538.
- Berkowitz S, (1978) State of the art in cleft palate, orofacial growth. Am J Orthod: 74:5, 564-576.
- Berkowitz S, Gonzalez G, Nghiem-Phu . (1982) An optical profilometer – A new instrument for the three dimensional measurement of cleft palate casts. CPJ 19:2. 129-138.
- Berkowitz S. (1985) Timing cleft palate closure – Age should not be the sole determinant. J Craniofacial Genet Devel Biol; (Supple.) 1:69-83.
- Berkowitz S. (1990) Complete unilateral cleft lip and palate: Serial three dimensional studies of excellent growth. In Bardach J, Morris H.L. Multidisciplinary Management of Cleft Lip and Palate. WB Saunders Co., Philadelphia, 456-473,
- Berkowitz S. (1995) Ethical issues in the case of surgical repair of cleft palate. CPCJ 32:4. 271-281.
- Berkowitz S. (1996) A comparison of treatment results in complete bilateral cleft lip and palate using a conservative approach versus Millard-Latham PSOT procedure. In: Sadowsky P.L. (Ed). Seminars in Orthodontics Cleft Lip and Palate. Saunders Co. Philadelphia 169-184.
- Berkowitz S. (1998) Prerandomization of clinical trials: A more ethical way for performing cleft palate research. Plast Recons Surg. 1724-1728.
- Berkowitz S, Millard D.R., Latham R.A, Wolfe S.A. (1998) A discussion of presurgical orthodontics in patients with clefts. Cleft Pal J. 25:4.
- Berkowitz S, Lestrel P.E, Takahashi. (1999) Shape changes in the cleft palate maxilla: a longitudinal study. Cleft Palate-Craniofacial J. 76:4: 292-30
- Berkowitz S. (1999) Treatment of congenital craniofacial anomalies: Team management with concern for the whole child. Int. Ped. 14:2; 77-82.
- Berkowitz S, Mejia M, Bystrik A. (2004) A comparison of the effects of the Latham-Millard procedure with those of a conservative treatment approach for dental occlusion and facial aesthetics in unilateral and bilateral complete cleft lip and palate: Part 1. Dental occlusion. Plast Reconst Surg: 113:1-18.
- Berkowitz S, Duncan R, Evans C, Friede H, Kuijpers-Jagtman A, Prahl-Anderson B, Rosenstein S. (2005) Timing of cleft palate closure should be based on the ratio of the area of the cleft to that of the palatal segments and not on age alone. Plast Reconst Surg. 115:6: 1483-1499.
- Berkowitz S. (2006) Timing of cleft palate closure should be based on the ratio of the area of the cleft to that of the palatal segments and not on age alone. Ch. 17 in: Berkowitz S (ed) Cleft Lip and Palate: Diagnosis and Management; 2nd Ed. Springer Verlag, Heidelberg-Berlin.

- Berkowitz S. (2009) Gingivoperiosteoplasty as well as early palatal cleft closure is unproductive. J. Cran Surg 20:8: 1-9
- Berkowitz S. (2010) The need to establish an on-line cleft palate teaching program for orthodontic residents and practicing orthodontists. Letter to the Editor. AJO-DO. 137:5:p577
- Berkowitz S. (2014) The present state of treatment in cleft palate: What still needs to be done. Cleft Palate J.
- Berkowitz, S. (2014) The Need for Differential Diagnosis in Cleft Palate Treatment Planning. Dentistry. 4:218.DOI: 10.4172/2161-1122.1000218
- Berkowitz, S. (2015) A Review of the Cleft Lip/Palate Literature Reveals That Differential Diagnosis of the Facial Skeleton and Musculature is Essential to Achieve all Treatment Goals. J of Craniofacial Surgery. 26:4
- Berkowitz S. (2015) The need to establish a cleft palate teaching program for residents and practicing orthodontists (An on-line cleft palate teaching program). Dent. Oral. Craniofac Res. 1(4): 114-115
- Berkowitz S. (2016) The facial growth pattern and the amount of palatal bone deficiency relative to cleft size should be considered in cleft lip and palate treatment planning. (Plast Reconstr Surg Glob Open 2016;4:e705; doi 10:1097/GOX.0000000000000629. May 6, 2016
- Berkowitz S. (2016) Letter To The Editor. Cleft Pal J. Response to Article: Allareddy V. et al, Operative and immediate postoperative outcomes of using a Latham-type dentomaxillary appliance in patients with unilateral complete cleft lip and palate. Cleft Pal Craniofac J. 2015:42:405-410 (May 2016 pp 377-377)
- Berkowitz S. (2017) Letter to the Editor. Cleft Pal Craniofac J. Response to Article: Meazzuni MC. et al. 'Long-term follow-up of UCLP patients: Surgical and orthodontic burden of care during growth and final orthognathic surgery need. Cleft Pal Craniofac J. Jul 2017: 54-4 pp 489-490
- Berkowitz S. (2017) Letter to the Editor. Cleft Pal Craniofacial J. Response to Article Vyas PM et al. 'Primary Premaxillary Setback and Repair of Bilateral Complete Cleft Lip: Indications. Techniques, and Outcomes' Cleft Pal Craniofac J. July 2017: 54-4 pp 493-493
- Berkowitz. S. (2019) Letter to the Editor. Cleft Pal Craniofacial J. Why Hasn't Cutting and Grayson Done a Longitudinal Study to Show Why Nasoalveolar Molding Should Not Be Used. Cleft Pal Craniofac J. Jan 2019: 56. 1, pp 141

**Books**
- For Professionals
  - Cleft Lip and Palate in Plastic Surgery of the Facial Skeleton, Eds. Wolfe S.A, Berkowitz S. (1989) Little Brown, Boston
  - Cleft Lip and Palate and Craniofacial Anomalies: Perspectives in Management. Singular Publishing, San Diego. (1996)
  - Cleft Lip and Palate: Diagnosis and Management – Edition 2. Springer-Verlag, Heidelberg, Berlin, New York (2006)
  - Cleft Lip and Palate: Diagnosis and Management – Edition 3. Springer Verlag, Heidelberg, Berlin, New York (2013)
- For Parents
  - The Cleft Palate Story (1994) Quintessence Publishing, Carol Stream, IL
  - The Cleft Palate Story (Revised) (2006) Slack Inc. Thorofare, NJ.
- Pamphlets
  - Steps in Habilitation: Feeding your Baby. (1972) for Mead Johnson, Bristol Myers Co. Evanston, IL

- The Road to Normalcy – for the Cleft Lip and Palate Child. (1972) for Mead Johnson Nutritional Division.
- Web Sites
  - Cleftlippalate.org
  - Cleftlippalateaudiovisuallecture.org
  - Cleftlippalatetreatment.org

Coral Gables, FL, USA                                      Samuel Berkowitz

# The Proper Mindset

*In assessing failure in facial and palate growth most surgeons focus on the surgical skills and/or surgical protocols involved. This leaves other possible explanations still unexplored.*

*Cleft lip and palate does not represent a simple fixed entity [that can be] subject to generalizations and classification and last of all to rigid therapeutic formulas.*—Pruzansky, "Description Classification…", 1953

# Facial-Palatal Problem Statement

Cleft lip and palate is one of the most frequent congenital anomalies. The incidence of clefting of some kind in the Caucasian population is approximately 1 in 600 births. It is higher in the Oriental groups and lower in the black groups.

Not all clefts are alike. Clefts can involve only the lip and alveolar ridge (primary palate), only the hard and soft palate (secondary palate), or both the primary and secondary palates. Clefts involving the primary palate, the secondary palate, or both vary in severity. Clefts of the lip may not extend to the floor of the nostril, may not involve all of the primary palate or secondary palate, and may occur on one or both sides. Considering the heterogeneous nature of clefting, treatment needs to be planned in accordance with the specific problems and needs of each patient.

Although the treatment of cleft lip and cleft palate has progressed markedly in the last 25 years, there is still a great need for improvement in diagnosis and treatment planning. However, to accomplish this goal our current diagnostic categories may need to be revised, and the possibility that clefts that are similarly classified may react differently to the same surgical procedure must be examined. The ultimate aim of the study was to provide a better objective understanding of the reasons, form, and the characteristics of these differing outcomes… and by so doing provide a broader and more informative knowledge base for making diagnostic and treatment decisions concerning cleft lip and cleft palate.

At present in the realm of cleft lip and palate therapy, much of the planning for treatment is at best an "educated art." Clinical reports of various treatment protocols, emanating from the many and widely separated cleft lip and plate treatment centers, are usually anecdotal and understandably supportive of the clinic's own treatment concepts. Although the protocols may differ significantly, the surgeons tend to be satisfied with their own results.

Certain questions inevitably arise. Do several different surgical procedures yield universally acceptable results which allow for normal palatal development? Are the outcome reports self-serving or can there indeed be a variety of effective surgical procedures? In those cases that undeniably failed, what were the errors, if any, in diagnosis and treatment planning? In assessing the failure, most surgeons focus on the purely surgical skills and/or surgical protocols involved but this leaves other possible explanations still unexplored. In recent years, it has been suggested that variations in the physical characteristics of the deformity—the geometric relationship of the palatal segments to each other at birth and the size of the cleft space relative to the amount of available soft tissue used to close the cleft space—may have an impact on treatment outcome. The importance of three-dimensional measurements is highlighted, and it is urged that the arch form and size of the cleft space at the time of surgery be taken into consideration in the treatment of infants with complete clefts of the lip and palate.

# Preface

These findings show that within certain defined limits, the success or failure of the surgical procedure depends on the initial state and the variables inherent in the maneuver. Subtle differences among patients will be prognostic of the subsequent state and the differences between surgeons. No matter what type of treatment surgeons have favored, they have not been able to explain why their surgical method of choice, when performed on similar clefts at the same age, often yielded different results. Why some cases appear to show "catch-up growth" resulting in good facial and palatal form and functional dental occlusion, whereas others show poor facial and palatial development.

If we assume that qualified surgeons within a given institution or region, practicing a specific series of techniques over a given period of time, represent a constant, the difference in success or failure should reside in the initial state, the geometric and size relationship of the palatal segments to the size and shape of the cleft space which reflects the degree of palatal-skeletal relationship to cleft size.

Coral Gables, FL, USA                                                                                          Samuel Berkowitz

# Qualifications of Cleft Team Members: To Be Trained and Experienced

The paramount interest of both the Bureau of Maternal and Child Health and the American Cleft Palate-Craniofacial Association is the quality of care for patients. It is thus essential that all team members be trained and experienced in the care of patients with craniofacial anomalies.

## Surgery and Orthodontics

Reconstruction in facial cleft surgery and orthodontics aims to establish normality in form and function, by moving normal tissues into normal position at appropriate ages. If necessary, it involves replacing what is missing with like tissue, such as bone grafts for large bony areas. Surgery begins in early childhood to provide normal muscle function to provide an environment for normal palatal and facial growth.

## Orthodontics

Orthodontists are involved with the study and guidance of the growth and development of the face and dentition of the child with a cleft or craniofacial anomaly from birth to adolescence.

As a result of special training to become a Developmental Anatomist, their role includes recording the changing facial morphology and jaw function as a result of surgery and growth.

They provide orthodontic/orthopedic treatment if necessary and general expertise for consultation with all of the other members of the cleft and craniofacial team. Orthodontists are involved in one way or another with virtually all of the treatment procedures provided by all of the team's specialists.

Since palatal clefts vary in the extent of osteogenic and muscular deficiencies, surgeons should recognize that all clefts, although similarly classified, are not the same, and therefore, each case requires differential diagnosis and treatment planning. What may be the treatment of choice for one patient may be totally different for another, even with the same cleft type at birth.

# Acknowledgments

I would like to thank the following for influencing, assembling, and producing this material:
- Colleagues in the American Cleft Palate-Craniofacial Association
- Attendees of ACPA's international conferences who have influenced my thinking
- Lynn, my wife of 50+ years, who has continually encouraged me in my profession and this project
- Beth Jo and Debra Lee, my daughters, and their families
- Gillian Kelley for her masterful production coordination
- David Berkowitz Sklar for his production effort

*In Memory of Samuel Pruzansky, D.D.S., who started me on this trip to Cleft Palate Land*

# Contents

1 **The Normal Face**.................................................. 1
   1.1 Balanced Muscle Forces ...................................... 2
   1.2 Normal Facial Musculature ................................... 3
   1.3 BCLP ...................................................... 3
   1.4 UCLP ...................................................... 3

2 **Causes of Clefts of the Secondary Palate** ............................ 5
   2.1 Migration of Undifferentiated Mesenchymal Cells
       to Various Parts of the Face .................................. 5
   2.2 Various Problems that Can Arise .............................. 6
   2.3 Neural Crest ................................................ 7
   2.4 Lip Areas of Cell Penetration.................................. 7

3 **Embryoparthenogenesis**............................................ 9
   3.1 Facial Development Between 5½ Weeks and 8 Weeks ............ 9
   3.2 7½ Week Embryo........................................... 10
   3.3 10 Week Embryo ........................................... 10
   3.4 Pattern of Palatal Fusion .................................... 11
       3.4.1 7½ Week Embryo.................................... 11
   3.5 Causes of Clefting .......................................... 12
   3.6 Palatal Osteodeficiency is Usually Found in ALL Cleft Types ..... 12
   3.7 Example of Severe Osteogenic Palatal Deficiency ............... 13
   3.8 Variations in Submucous Cleft Palate ......................... 14
   3.9 Obtuse CB ................................................. 17
   3.10 Acute CB .................................................. 17
   3.11 Nasopharyngeal Space....................................... 18
   3.12 Variations in Facial Growth Patterns .......................... 19
   3.13 In Both CBCLP and CUCLP the Facial Growth Pattern Determines
       the Final Facial Profile....................................... 19
   3.14 Velopharyngeal Closure Patterns.............................. 20
   3.15 Lateral Cephs Before and After Surgery To Lengthen the Soft Palate ........ 25

4 **Variation in Cleft Types** ........................................... 27
   4.1 Isolated Cleft Palate......................................... 27
   4.2 Variations in Anterior-Posterior Length of the Two Segments
       in Unilateral Cleft Lip and Palate ............................. 28
   4.3 Effect of Lip and Palatal Clefting on Maxillary Segments ........ 29
   4.4 Variations in Bilateral Cleft Lip and Palate Types................ 29
   4.5 Review of the Literature...................................... 31
       4.5.1 Surgical Procedure (Type and Timing) ................. 31

# 5 Surgery ... 35
5.1 The Vomer Flap: Good or Bad? ... 35
5.2 Von Langenbeck (Simple Closure) ... 36
    5.2.1 Palatoplasty ... 36
5.3 V-Y Lengthening Veau-Wardill-Kilner Procedure ... 37
5.4 Double-Reversing Z-Plasty (Furlow Procedure) ... 38
5.5 Palatal Surgery ... 39
    5.5.1 Procedure ... 39
    5.5.2 What Should Not Be Done ... 39
5.6 Osteotomies: To Close the Cleft Space—Not Acceptable ... 40

# 6 Orthodontics ... 43
6.1 Speech Aid Appliances ... 45

# 7 Complete Unilateral Cleft Lip and Palate Conservative Treatment (Non-presurgical Orthopedics) ... 51
7.1 The Neonatal Palatal Form in Complete Clefts of the Lip and Palate: The Effect of Muscle Forces ... 51
7.2 The Influence of Surgery on Palatal Form and Growth ... 51
7.3 Complete Unilateral Cleft Lip and Palate ... 53
7.4 Complete Unilateral Cleft Lip and Palate ... 54
7.5 Two Cases Which Show Severe Overlap of Palatal Segments with Closure of the Cleft Space ... 55
7.6 CASE SM XX-53 ... 57
    7.6.1 Serial Cases Show Changes in Palatal Relationships ... 57
7.7 Complete Unilateral Cleft Lip and Palate ... 62
7.8 Molding Geometric Relationships ... 63
7.9 Berkowitz Palatal Growth Analysis ... 67
7.10 Rapid Closure of the Palatal Cleft Space ... 68
7.11 Rolf Tindlund Bergen Norway ... 69
7.12 Complete Unilateral Cleft Lip and Palate ... 79
    7.12.1 Minor Orthodontics ... 79
    7.12.2 Failure of Advancing Teeth with Protraction Facial Mask ... 83
7.13 Complete Unilateral Cleft Lip and Palate ... 84
7.14 Various Facial Growth Patterns Coben Analysis: Basion Horizontal ... 90
7.15 Complete Unilateral Cleft Lip/Palate ... 91
7.16 Median Cleft of the Premaxilla ... 95
    7.16.1 Cleft of the Alveolus only with Missing Central and Lateral Incisors ... 95

# 8 Protraction Facial Mask ... 97
8.1 Protraction Facial Mask Orthopedics ... 97
8.2 Distraction Osteogenesis ... 98
    8.2.1 The Rigid External Distraction (RED II) System: Polley and Figuroa ... 98
    8.2.2 Before and After: Results of Using the Rigid External Distraction (RED II) System ... 100
8.3 Distraction Osteogenesis to the Mandible: F. Molina ... 102
8.4 Hemifacial Microsomia: Distraction Osteogenesis: F. Molina ... 103
8.5 A.S. Case# AY-46 Vertical Growth Pattern ... 106
8.6 Vertical Growth Pattern ... 106

# 9 Complete Bilateral Cleft Lip and Palate ... 107
9.1 Lip Surgery in Complete Bilateral Cleft Lip and Palate ... 108
    9.1.1 Mucosa and Muscle Joined Behind the Prolabium ... 108

|        |                                                                                                           |
|--------|-----------------------------------------------------------------------------------------------------------|
| 9.2    | Variations of Palatal Segments to Each Other, and Premaxilla Size in Bilateral Cleft Lip and Palate........109 |
| 9.3    | Protruding Premaxilla with Overexpanded Palatal Shelves........110                                        |
| 9.4    | Growth of Premaxillary Vomerine Suture (PVS)........110                                                   |
| 9.5    | Various Possible CBCLP Treatments........111                                                              |
| 9.6    | Complete Bilateral Cleft Lip and Palate Conservative Treatment........111                                 |
|        | 9.6.1 Protruding Premaxilla Anterior and Posterior Cleft Spaces........112                                |
| 9.7    | Lateral Head X-Ray Shows The Kirschner Wire........112                                                    |
| 9.8    | Premaxillary Surgical Setback........113                                                                  |
| 9.9    | Kirschner Wire Placed in Premaxilla But Missing the Vomer........113                                      |
| 9.10   | A Case Where Kirschner Wire Was Used, Hopefully to Stabilize Retropositional Premaxilla........113        |
| 9.11   | The Value of Longitudinal Facial and Dental Cast Record in Clinical Research and Treatment Analysis........114 |
|        | 9.11.1 Serial Cephaloradiographs and Casts of the Maxillary and Mandibular Dentition and Occlusion........114 |
| 9.12   | The Reasons for Success or Failure Are Multifactorial and Are Not Often Related to the Surgeon's Surgical Procedure........115 |
|        | 9.12.1 Good Jaw Relationships........115                                                                  |
| 9.13   | Variations in the Inclination of the Premaxilla at Similar Ages (Handelman)...116                         |
| 9.14   | Gradual Flattening of the Facial Profile (Hans Friede)........117                                         |
| 9.15   | Two-Stage Lip........118                                                                                  |
| 9.16   | Various Analyses to Show Facial Growth Changes........119                                                 |
| 9.17   | Bringing the Central Incisors Together to Allow for the Eruption of the Lateral Incisors........120       |
| 9.18   | Incomplete BLCLP........122                                                                               |
| 9.19   | Bilateral Cleft Lip and Palate........123                                                                 |
| 9.20   | Serial Dental BCLP Casts........127                                                                       |
| 9.21   | Excellent Facial Growth Pattern........131                                                                |
| 9.22   | Excellent Facial Growth and Occlusion........133                                                          |
| 9.23   | Incomplete Bilateral Cleft Lip and Palate: Both Lateral Incisors Are Missing—Excessive Symphysis Growth........134 |
| 9.24   | Exceptional Forward Mandibular Growth Flattening the Facial Profile........143                            |
| 9.25   | CBCLP Demonstrating Facial Profile Going from Protrusion to Retrusion....144                              |
| 9.26   | Concave Facial Profile........151                                                                         |
| 9.27   | Gradual Reduction in the Anterior and Posterior Cleft Spaces as Seen in Computerized Serial Palatal Cast (Casts Are Not Drawn to Scale Relative To Size)........158 |
| 9.28   | Excellent Facial Growth Pattern........159                                                                |
| 9.29   | Final Photographs........160                                                                              |
| 9.30   | CBCLP: Ideal Treatment Results........161                                                                 |
|        | 9.30.1 Columella Lengthened, Nasal Tip Elevated........162                                                |
|        | 9.30.2 Profile Flattened Lip/Nose Revisions........163                                                    |
|        | 9.30.3 Nasal and Lip Revisions........164                                                                 |
| 9.31   | Serial Dental Casts........167                                                                            |
| 9.32   | Superimposed Outlines of Selected Serial Palatal Casts........169                                         |
| 9.33   | Palatal Growth........171                                                                                 |
| 9.34   | Zurich Switzerland: Rudolph and Margaret Hotz Procedure........173                                        |
|        | 9.34.1 Cases by Wanda Gnoinski DDS, Orthodontist........173                                               |
| **10** | **Presurgical Orthopedics........175**                                                                    |
| 10.1   | A Historical Perspective of Cleft Palate Orofacial Growth and Dentistry......175                          |
| 10.2   | Brophy Procedure 1920........176                                                                          |
| 10.3   | Prior Use of Presurgical Appliances........176                                                            |
| 10.4   | Controlling the Protruding Premaxilla........177                                                          |

| | | |
|---|---|---|
| **11** | **Presurgical Orthopedics with Lip Adhesion and Periosteoplasty (POPLA)** | **179** |
| | 11.1 Latham–Millard Presurgical Orthopedics with Periosteoplasty | 180 |
| | 11.2 Latham–Millard Procedure | 181 |
| |     11.2.1 CUCLP | 181 |
| | 11.3 Pre-Surgical Orthopedic Periosteoplasty with Lip Adhesion (POPLA) | 182 |
| |     11.3.1 Periosteoplasty | 182 |
| | 11.4 The Latham Pinned Appliance | 183 |
| | 11.5 Complete Unilateral Cleft Lip and Palate Treated with POPLA | 184 |
| |     11.5.1 After Molding with PSOT | 185 |
| | 11.6 Facial Photographs | 186 |
| | 11.7 Facial Photographs | 187 |
| | 11.8 CBCLP: Change in premaxillary position with Latham's PSOT (POPLA) | 192 |
| | 11.9 CUCLP: Presurgical Orthopedic with Periosteoplasty and Lip Adhesion (POPLA) | 194 |
| | 11.10 Frontal and Lateral Facial Photos | 195 |
| | 11.11 Recessiveness of the Midface Slowly Develops | 196 |
| | 11.12 Loss of the Lateral Incisor Space | 198 |
| |     11.12.1 Midfacial growth retardation is now evident | 199 |
| | 11.13 POPLA Treated CUCLP and Its Effect on the Facial Profile | 201 |
| |     11.13.1 Early Midfacial Recessiveness Due To Excessive Mandibular Growth | 201 |
| | 11.14 Miami | 205 |
| | 11.15 Nijmegen | 205 |
| | 11.16 Maxillary Protraction Facial Mask | 206 |
| | 11.17 Lateral Head X-Rays Show Good VPC | 208 |
| | 11.18 Skeletal and Soft Tissue Profile Changes | 209 |
| | 11.19 Superimposed Polygons | 209 |
| | 11.20 CBCLP Case Which Required Midfacial Advancement at Adolescence | 210 |
| | 11.21 CBCLP: Ideal Treatment Results | 211 |
| | 11.22 Progressive Changes in Facial Profile Leading To a Flattened Midface | 213 |
| | 11.23 Nasal Revision | 215 |
| | 11.24 Recessed Mid-face With Concave Facial Profile After Surgery | 218 |
| | 11.25 The Result of the Early Surgical Setback of the Premaxilla | 224 |
| | 11.26 Orthodontic Treatment to Reduce the Anterior Openbite | 225 |
| |     11.26.1 Will the Premaxilla Descend or Will the Teeth Extrude? | 226 |
| **12** | **Serial Palatal Growth Studies: Outcomes Analysis** | **229** |
| | 12.1 Molding Complications | 229 |
| | 12.2 Latham Presurgical Orthopedic Procedure | 231 |
| | 12.3 Latham Presurgical Orthopedic Procedure | 232 |
| | 12.4 Northwestern: Rosenstein and Kernahan | 233 |
| | 12.5 Serial Palatal Growth Changes After Various Forms of Treatment | 234 |
| **13** | **A Multicenter Retrospective International 3D Study of Serial CUCLP and CBCLP Casts: To Determine When to Close the Palatal Cleft Space and the Need for Stages of Treatment as the Palate Grows** | **235** |
| | 13.1 Study Design | 235 |
| | 13.2 3D Palatal Cast Velocity and Surface Area Growth Changes | 235 |
| | 13.3 The Need for Three-Dimensional Measuring Techniques | 236 |

**14 Questions to Be Answered** ............................................. 237
    14.1   To Determine When to Close the Palatal Cleft Space ................ 237

**15 Making of 3D Measurements of Serial Cleft Palate Casts** .................. 239
    15.1   Palatal Landmarks ................................................ 240
    15.2   Rapid Palatal Growth the First Year ............................... 242

**16 Surgery Conclusions** .................................................. 247
    16.1   Berkowitz Best Time Ratio (BBTR) for Performing Cleft Palate Surgery .... 247

**The Facial Growth Pattern and the Amount of Palatal Bone Deficiency**
**Relative to Cleft Size Should Be Considered in Treatment Planning** ............. 249
    References ....................................................... 262

# The Normal Face

1

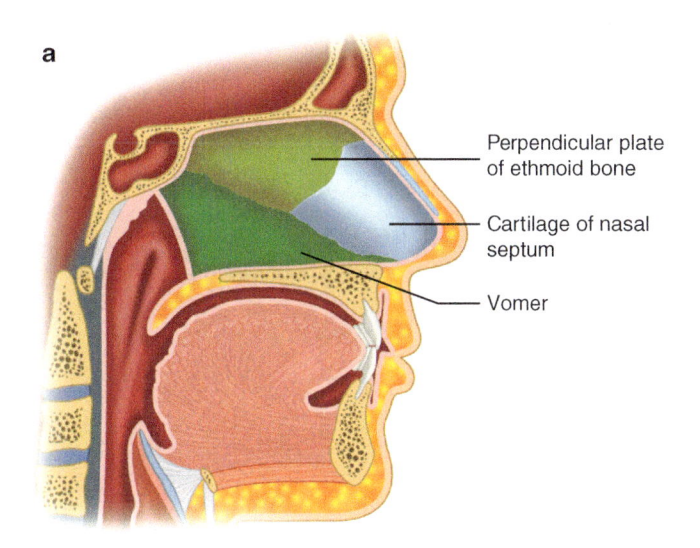

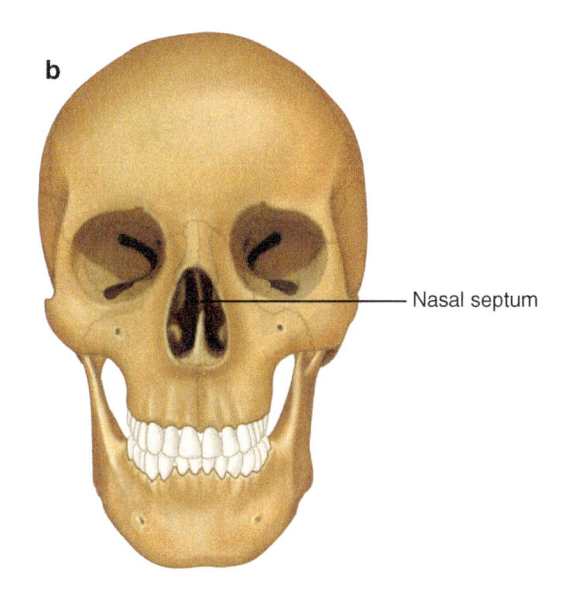

## 1.1 Balanced Muscle Forces

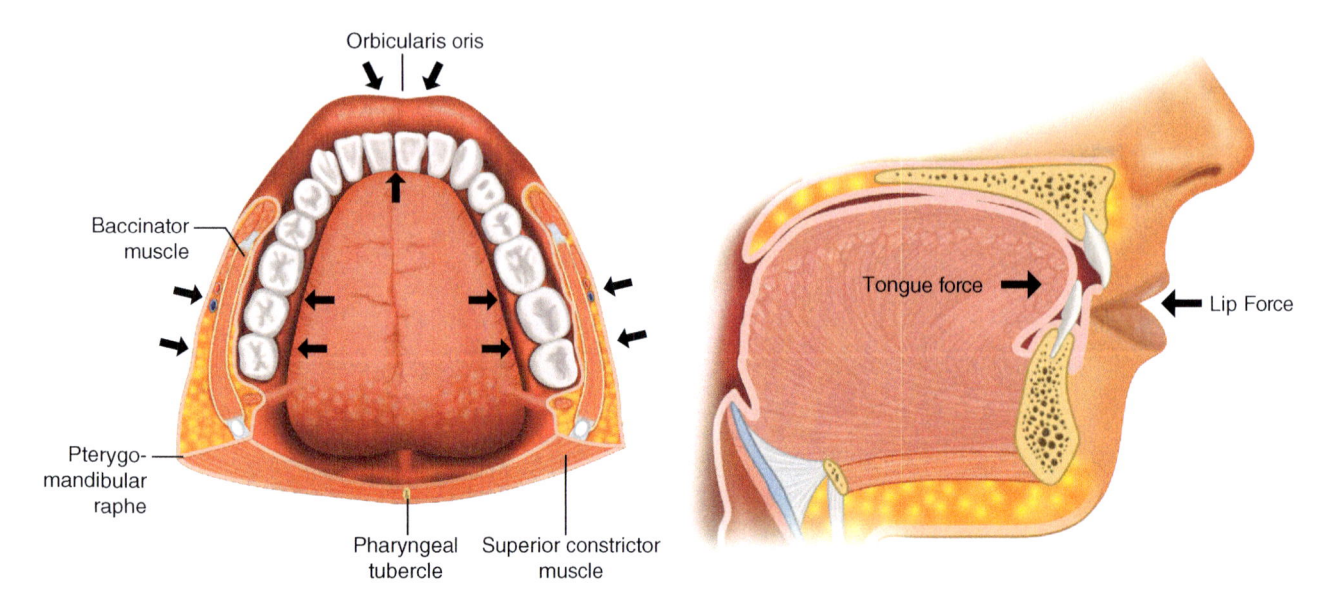

## 1.2 Normal Facial Musculature

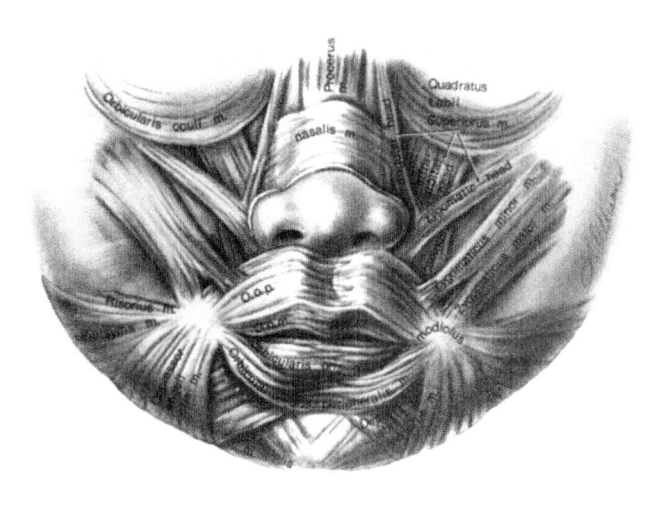

## 1.3 BCLP

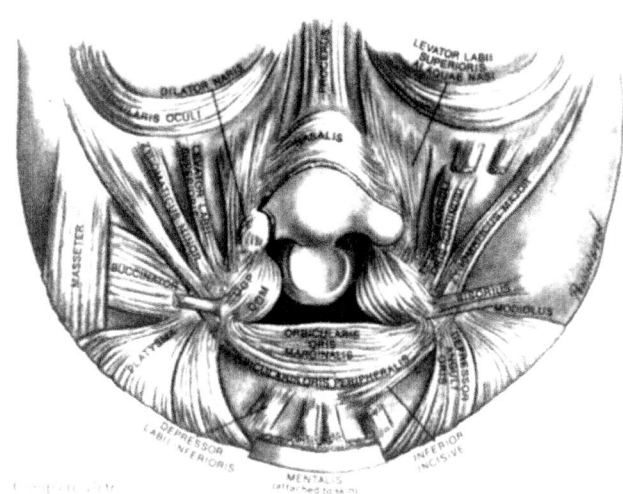

## 1.4 UCLP

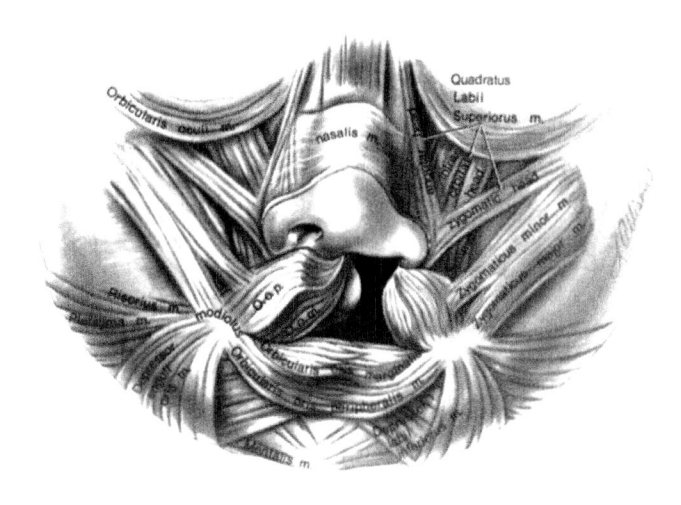

# Causes of Clefts of the Secondary Palate

*1. Tongue Resistance:* The tongue arched up between the shelves, delays palatal movement.

*2. Decreased shelf forces:* Teratogen has invoked this mechanism—no known genes.

*3. Failure to fuse:* Associated with delayed shelf reorientation.

*4. Narrow shelves:* Shelves can be elevated but are too narrow to reach each other—deficiency in facial mesenchyme to the palatal segments.

*Slavkin*—Development Craniofacial Biology. 1979.

## 2.1 Migration of Undifferentiated Mesenchymal Cells to Various Parts of the Face

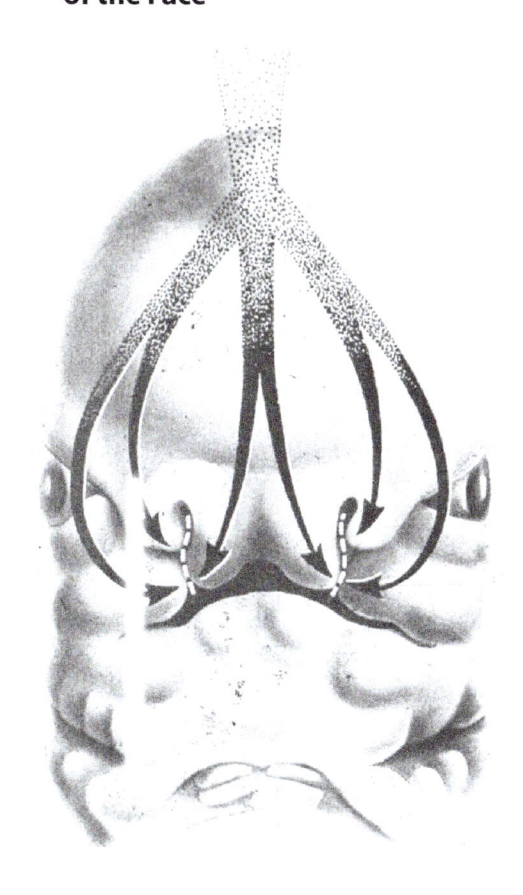

## 2.2 Various Problems that Can Arise

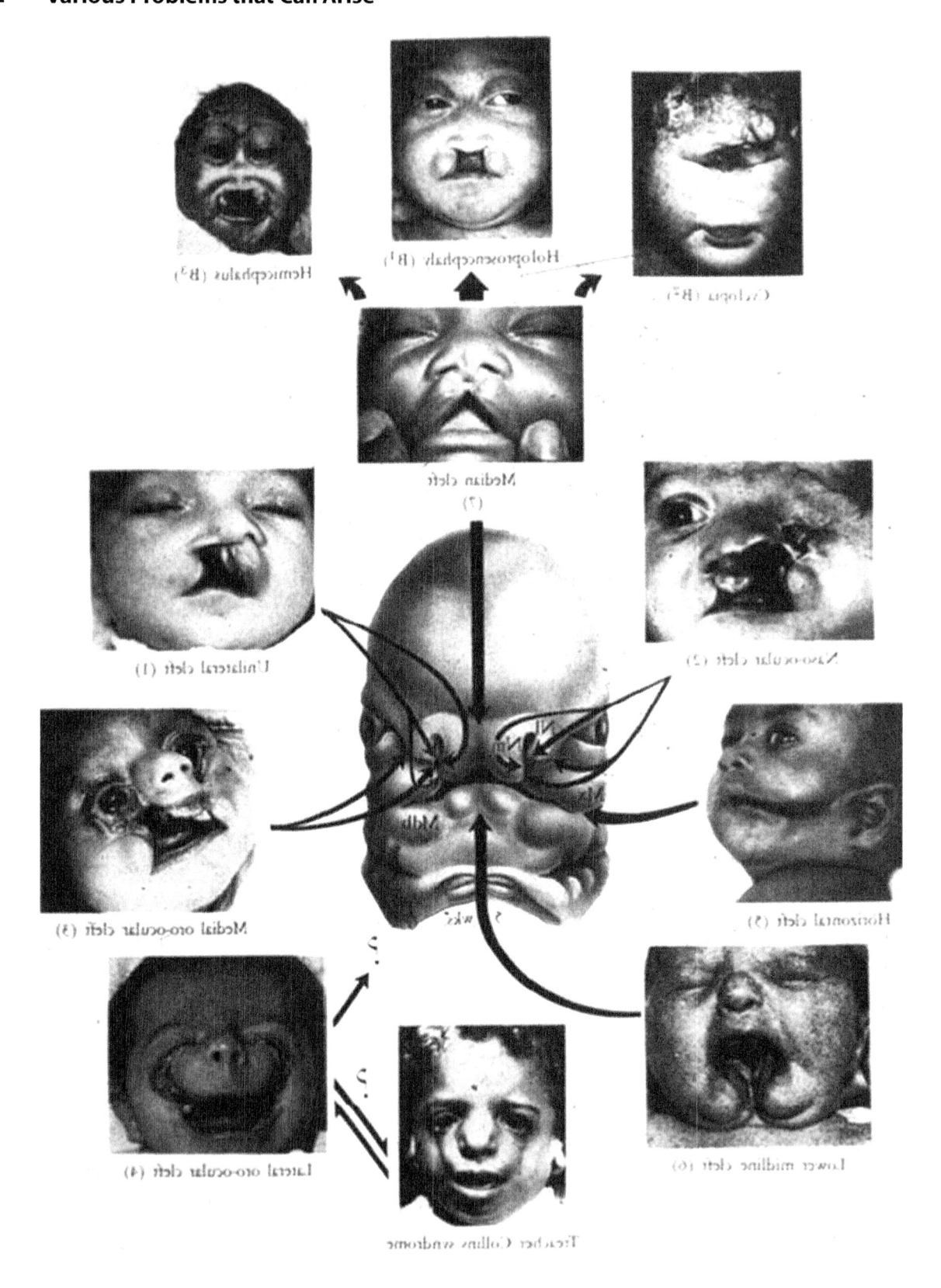

Courtesy Millard, D.R., Jr. *Cleft Craft III: Alveolar and Palatal Deformities*

## 2.3 Neural Crest

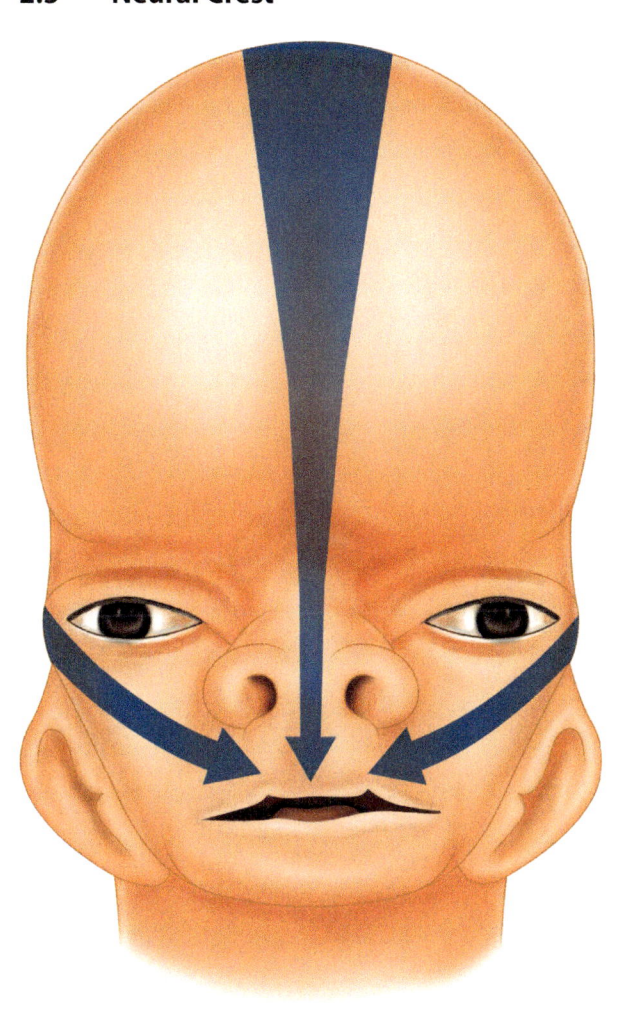

Migration of undifferentiated mesenchymal cells

## 2.4 Lip Areas of Cell Penetration

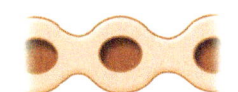

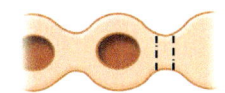

Normal

Unilateral HL

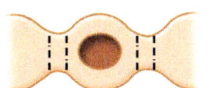

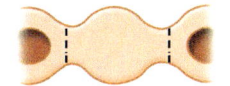

Bilateral HL

Median c left

Family History of Clefting

| Number of affected parents | Number of affected siblings | Cleft lip with or without cleft palate (%) | Isolated cleft palate (%) |
|---|---|---|---|
| – | – | 0.12 | 0.05 |
| – | 1 | 4–5 | 2–3 |
| 1 | – | 2 | 1.7 |
| 1 | 1 | 13–14 | 14–17 |
| 2 | – | 13–14 | 14–17 |
| – | 2 | 13–14 | 14–17 |
| 2 | 1 | 20–25 | 25–50 |
| 2 | 2 | 15–50 | 50 |

Studies indicate that about a third of children born with oral-facial clefts have a family history of clefting. In the United States and Western Europe, there is a family history of clefting in approximately 40% of cases, leaving approximately 60% of cases without any known familial occurrence. There is a greater chance of having a child with a cleft if the mother or father, or other siblings (i.e., first-degree relatives) have had a cleft. There is less risk of clefting if only the grandparents, aunts, uncles, nieces, or nephews (i.e., second-degree relatives) have had a cleft, and even less risk if only first cousins (i.e., third-degree relatives) have had a cleft.

# Embryoparthenogenesis 3

## 3.1 Facial Development Between 5½ Weeks and 8 Weeks

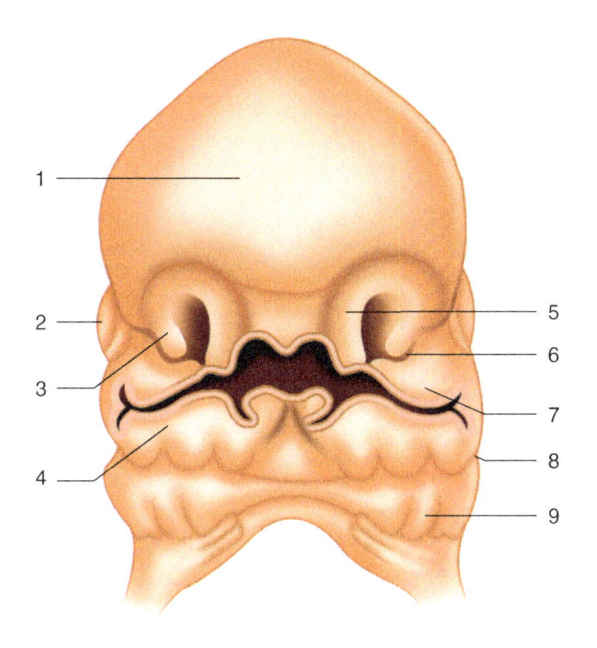

Facial region at about 5½ weeks. 1, Forebrain. 2, Optic vesicle. 3, Lateral nasal swelling. 4, Mandibular process. 5, Medial nasal swelling. 6, Nasolacrimal groove. 7, Maxillary process. 8, Hyomandibular cleft. 9, Hyoid arch. (Modified from Patten, B. M.: Human Embryology, 3rd ed. New York, McGraw-Hill, 1968)

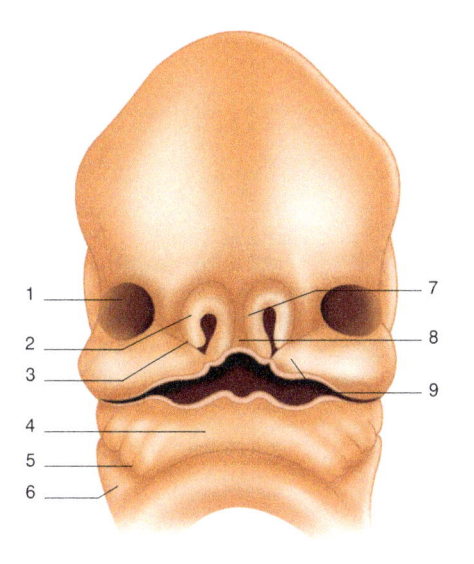

The face between 6 and 7 weeks. 1, Eye. 2, Lateral nasal swelling. 3, Nasolacrimal groove. 4, Mandibular swelling. 5, Hyomandibular cleft. 6, Hyoid arch. 7, Medial nasal swelling. 8, Midline nasal region where nasal septum is forming. 9, Maxillary swelling

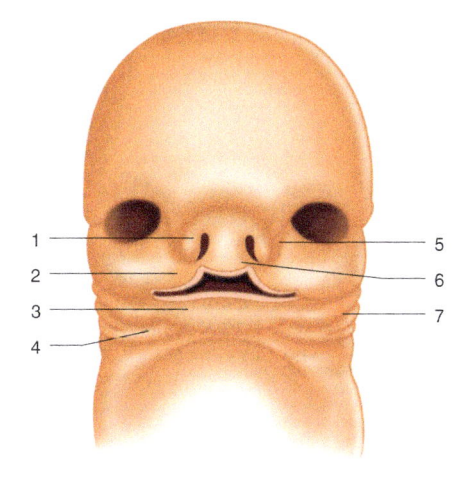

The face between 7 and 8 weeks. 1, Nasolateral process. 2, Maxillary process. 3, Mandible. 4, Hyoid arch (note formation of external ear lobes). 5, Merger line of nasolacrimal groove. 6, Philtrum. 7, Hyomandibular cleft

© Springer Nature Switzerland AG 2022
S. Berkowitz, *Orthodontic-Surgical Partnership in Cleft Lip and Palate Treatment*,
https://doi.org/10.1007/978-3-030-54300-6_3

## 3.2 7½ Week Embryo

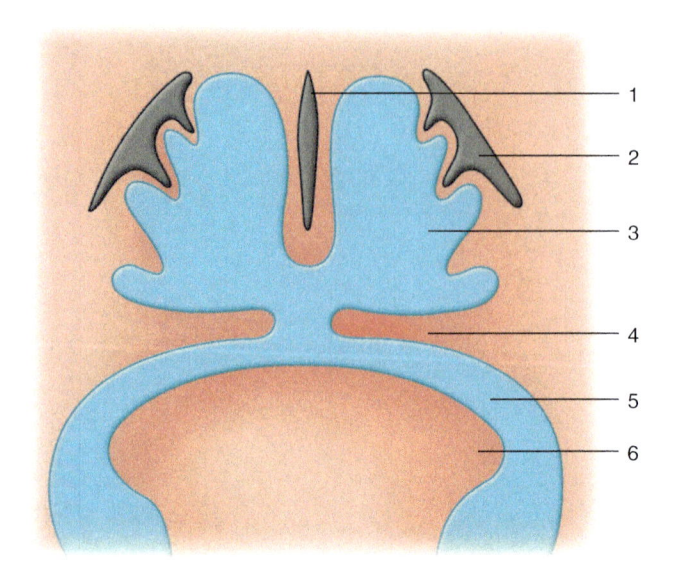

Frontal section through the oronasal region of a 7½-week embryo. 1. Cartilage of the nasal septum. 2. Cartilage of the nasal conchae. 3. Nasal chamber. 4. Palatal shelf. 5. Oral cavity. 6. Tongue. (Adapted from Langman, J.: Medical Embryology. Copyright 1969, The Williams & Wilkins Company, Baltimore)

## 3.3 10 Week Embryo

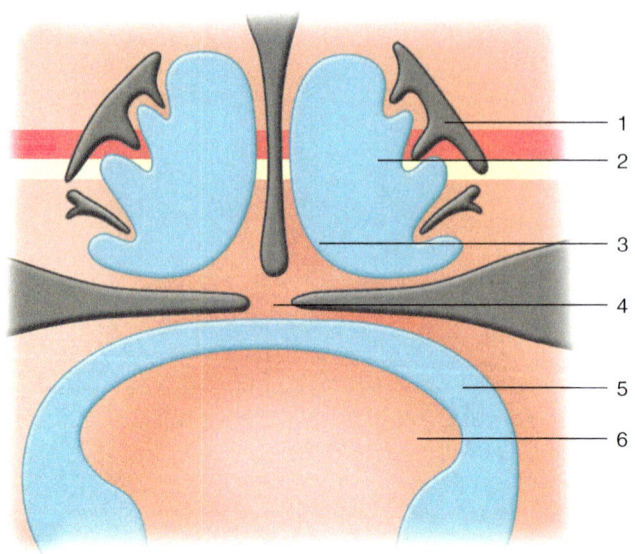

Frontal section through the oronasal region of a 10-week embryo. 1. Nasal conchae. 2. Nasal chamber. 3. Nasal septum. 4. Palatal shelves, fused at midline and fused with nasal septum. The intramembranous bone of the palatal shelves (from the maxilla) is beginning to form. 5. Oral cavity. 6. Tongue. (Adapted from Langman, J.: Medical Embryology. Copyright 1969, The Williams & Wilkins Company, Baltimore)

## 3.4 Pattern of Palatal Fusion

### 3.4.1 7½ Week Embryo

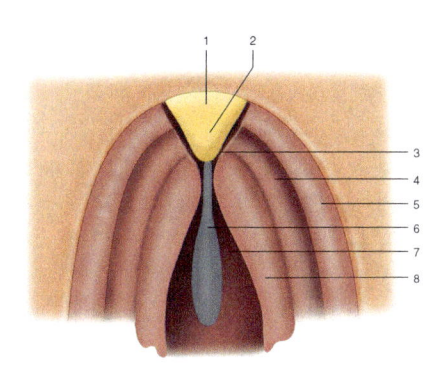

Oral view of the palatal shelves in a 7½-week embryo. 1. Philtrum of upper lip. 2. "Premaxillary" segment from medial nasal processes. 3. Primary palate. 4. Upper arch (part derived from maxillary swellings). 5. Cheek. 6. Nasal septum. 7. Open oral and nasal cavities. 8. Palatal shelves. In this stage, the philtrum and premaxillary segment have already merged with the maxillary swellings

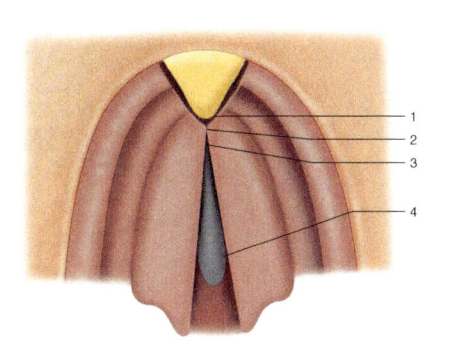

Oral view of palate showing beginning of fusion. 1. Merger of midline primary palate with bilateral secondary palatal shelves. 2. Incisive foramen. 3. Palatal raphe (midline fusion). 4. Open nasal and oral chambers

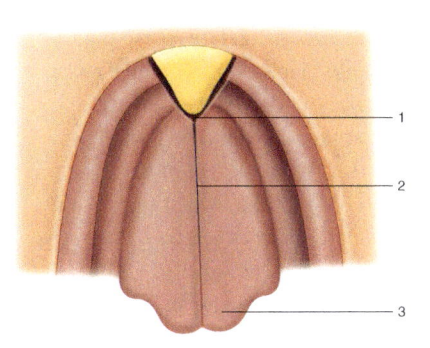

Full length palatal fusion. 1. Incisive foramen. 2. Palatal raphe. 3. Uvula

## 3.5 Causes of Clefting

1. **Failure of the palate to fuse.**
   The palatal processes are positioned vertically on either side of the tongue. As the mandible descends away from the cranial base, it frees the palatal processes to become horizontal and then fuse from an interior to posterior direction. However, in some instances such as in the Pierre Robin syndrome where a micrognathic mandible exists the tongue is positioned within the nasal chamber preventing the change in position of the palatal processes. Thus, the failure of the palatal processes to fuse results in an isolated cleft palate of various dimensions.

2. **Delayed fusion.**
   With increase in head width, the palatal processes fail to come together and fuse.

3. **Osteogenic Deficiency.**
   This is believed to be the most prevalent cause of clefting in both the anterior and posterior palates. The migration of mesenchymal cells to the midface can vary in time and degree resulting in various sizes of the cleft defect.

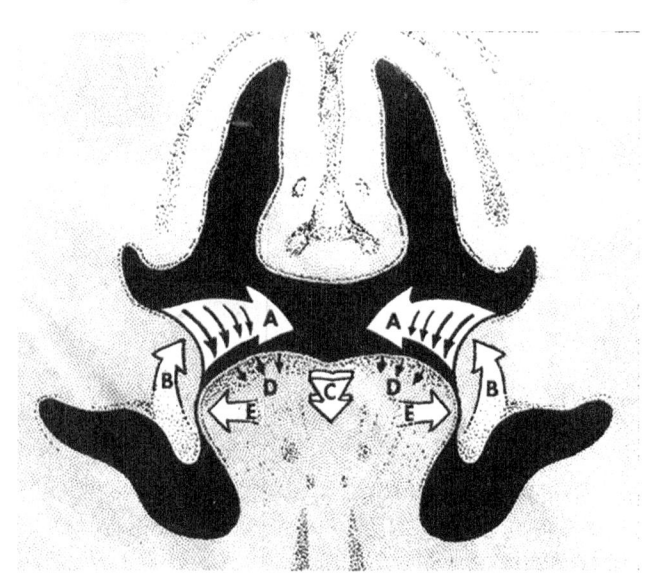

## 3.6 Palatal Osteodeficiency is Usually Found in ALL Cleft Types

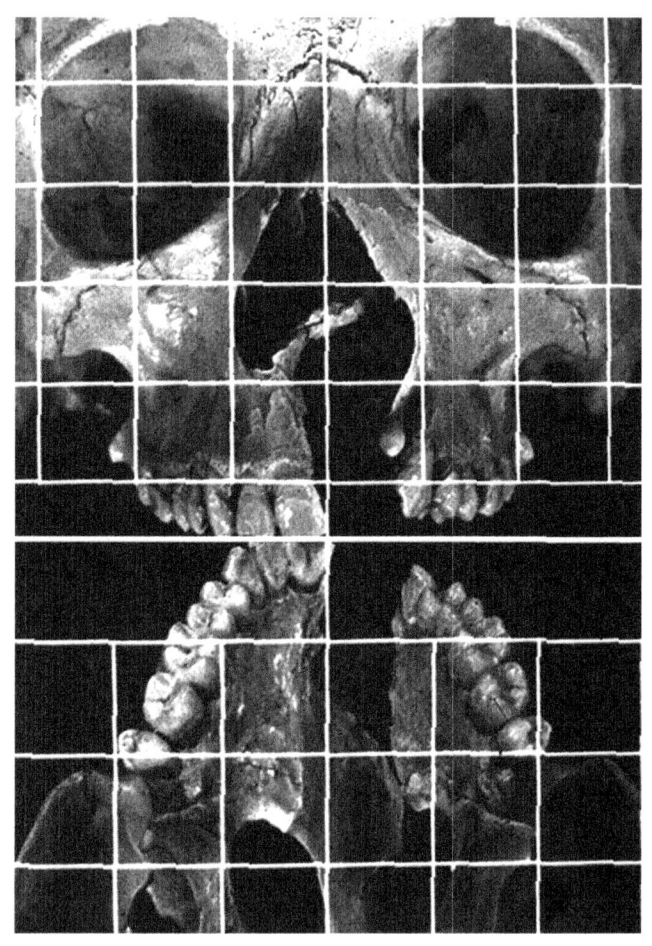

## 3.7 Example of Severe Osteogenic Palatal Deficiency

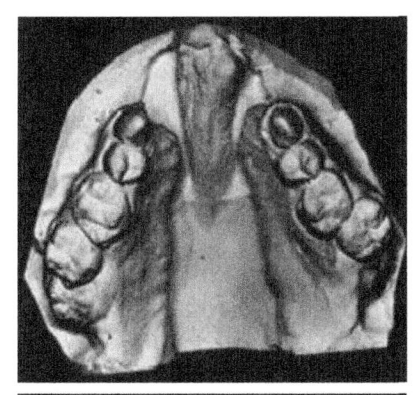

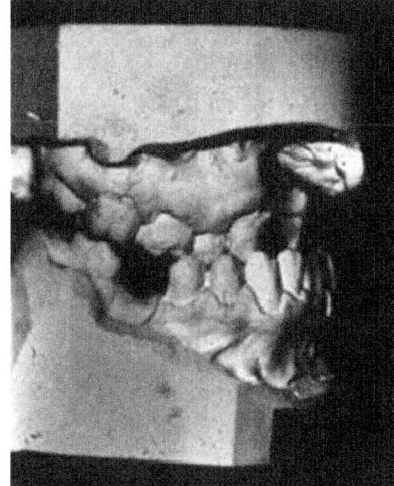

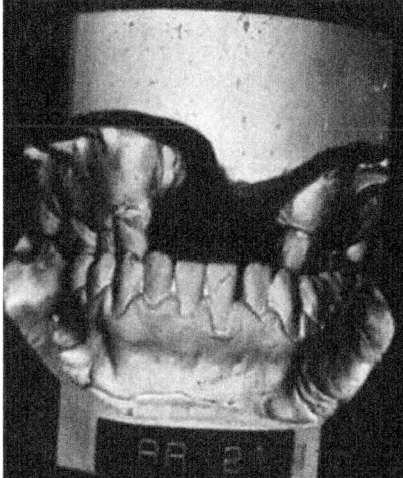

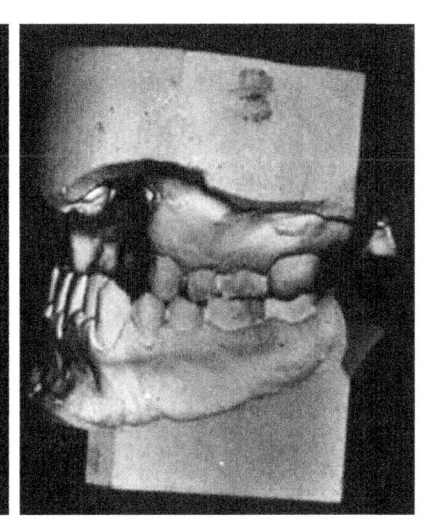

## 3.8 Variations in Submucous Cleft Palate

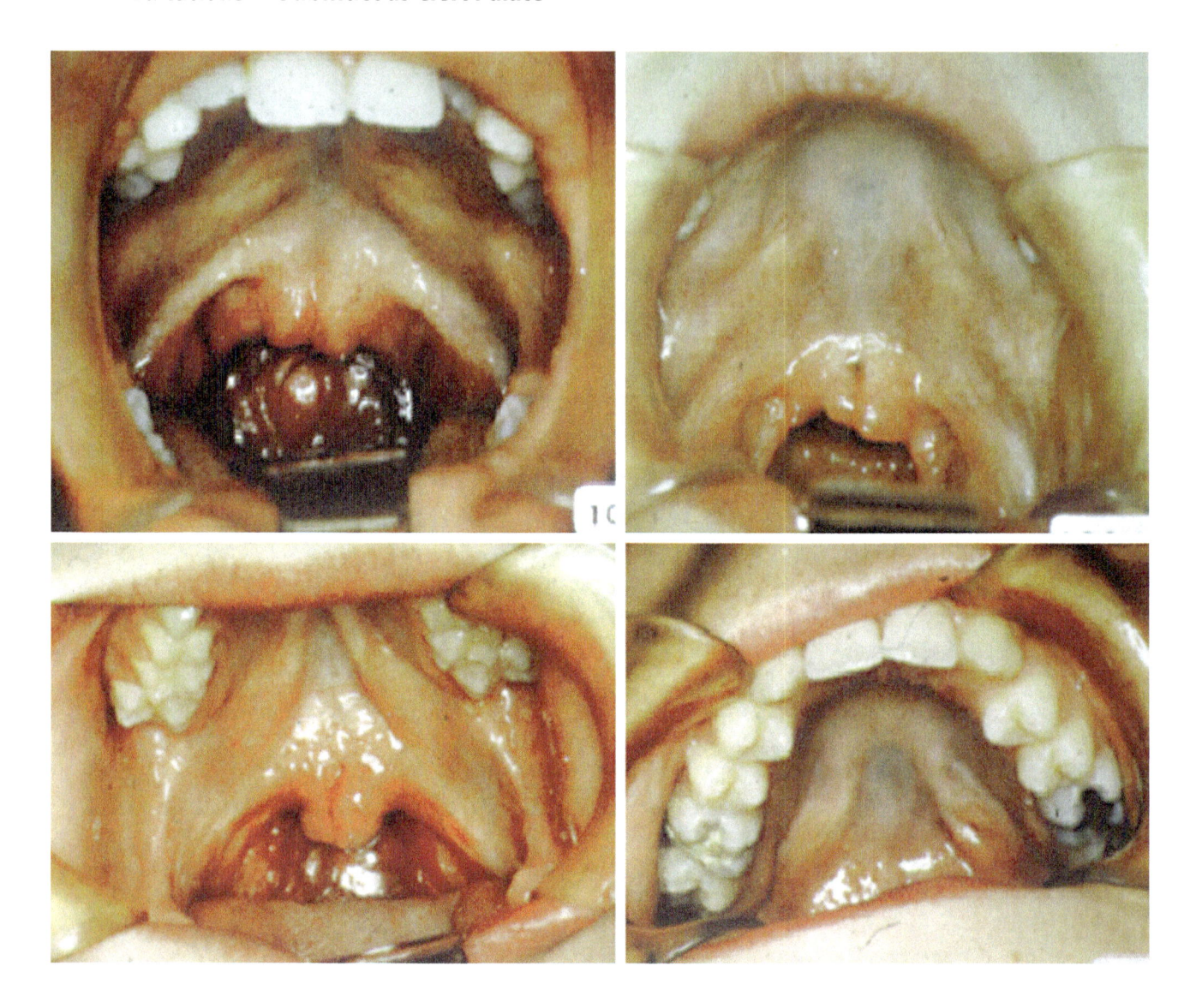

This cleft is characterized by a bifid uvula, lack of muscle continuity across the soft palate, and a pink zone of mucosa (zona pellucida) across the cleft in the hard palate. A palpable notch in the posterior border of the hard palate is always indicative of the presence of a cleft. Not all patients with submucous cleft have VPI.

## 3.8 Variations in Submucous Cleft Palate

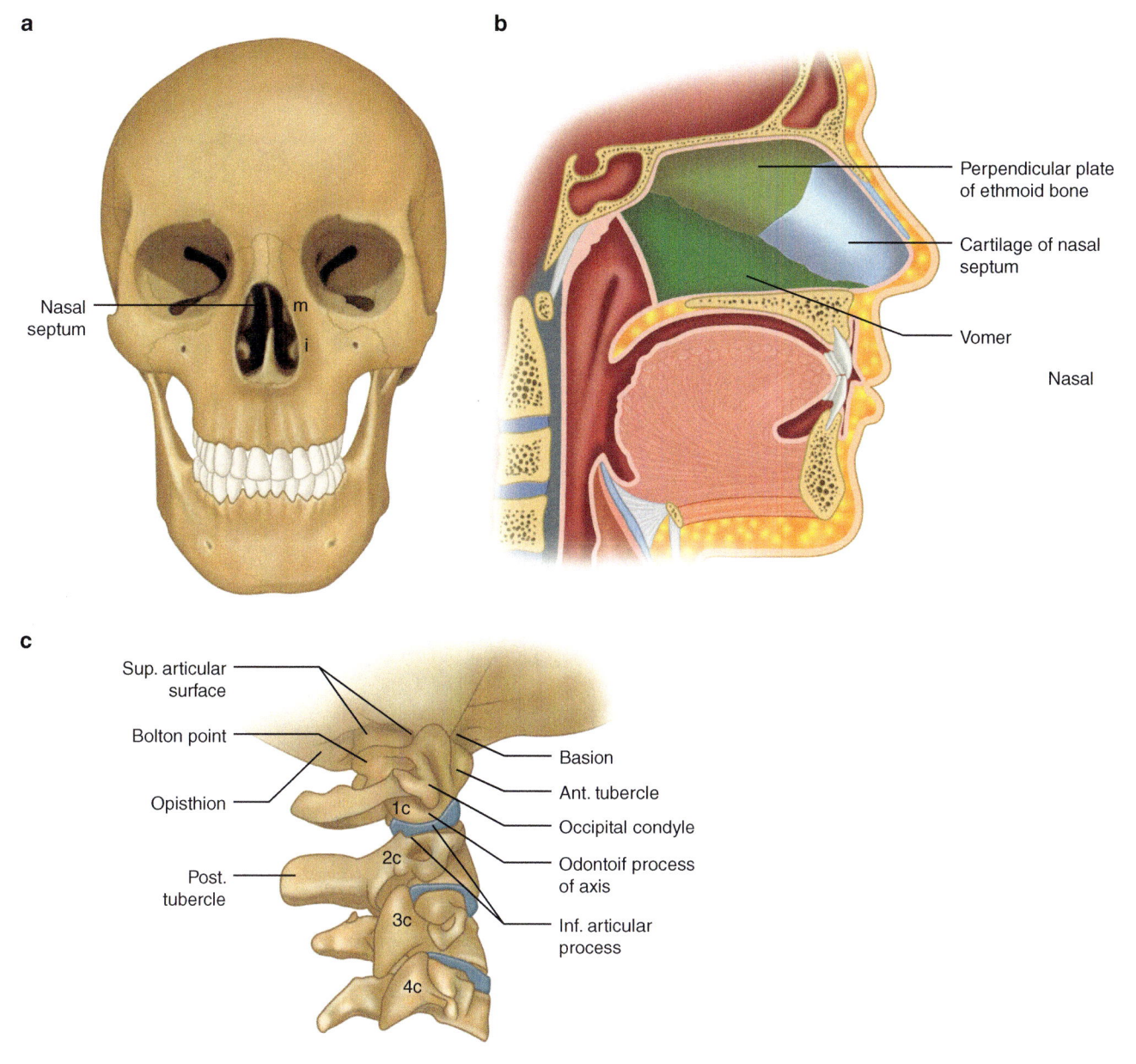

(**a**) The normal nasal septum: the inferior (i), middle (m), and superior turbinates are attached to lateral nasal walls. (**b**) The nasal septum is composed of the perpendicular plate of the ethmoid, the cartilage of the nasal septum and the vomer. In complete clefts of the lip and palate at birth, the nasal septum is displaced to the non-cleft side in varying degrees. The configuration of the nasal septum and the turbinates on the cleft side limits the medial movement of the cleft palatal segment after lip and palate repair. (**c**) Cervical spine: The condition and the relationship of the various vertebrae to each other can influence the depth and configuration of the pharyngeal space. For example, the anterior tubercle of the Atlas (1C = first cervical vertebrae) supports the posterior pharyngeal wall. If it is absent or dislocated, the functional pharyngeal depth may increase to a nonfunctional state

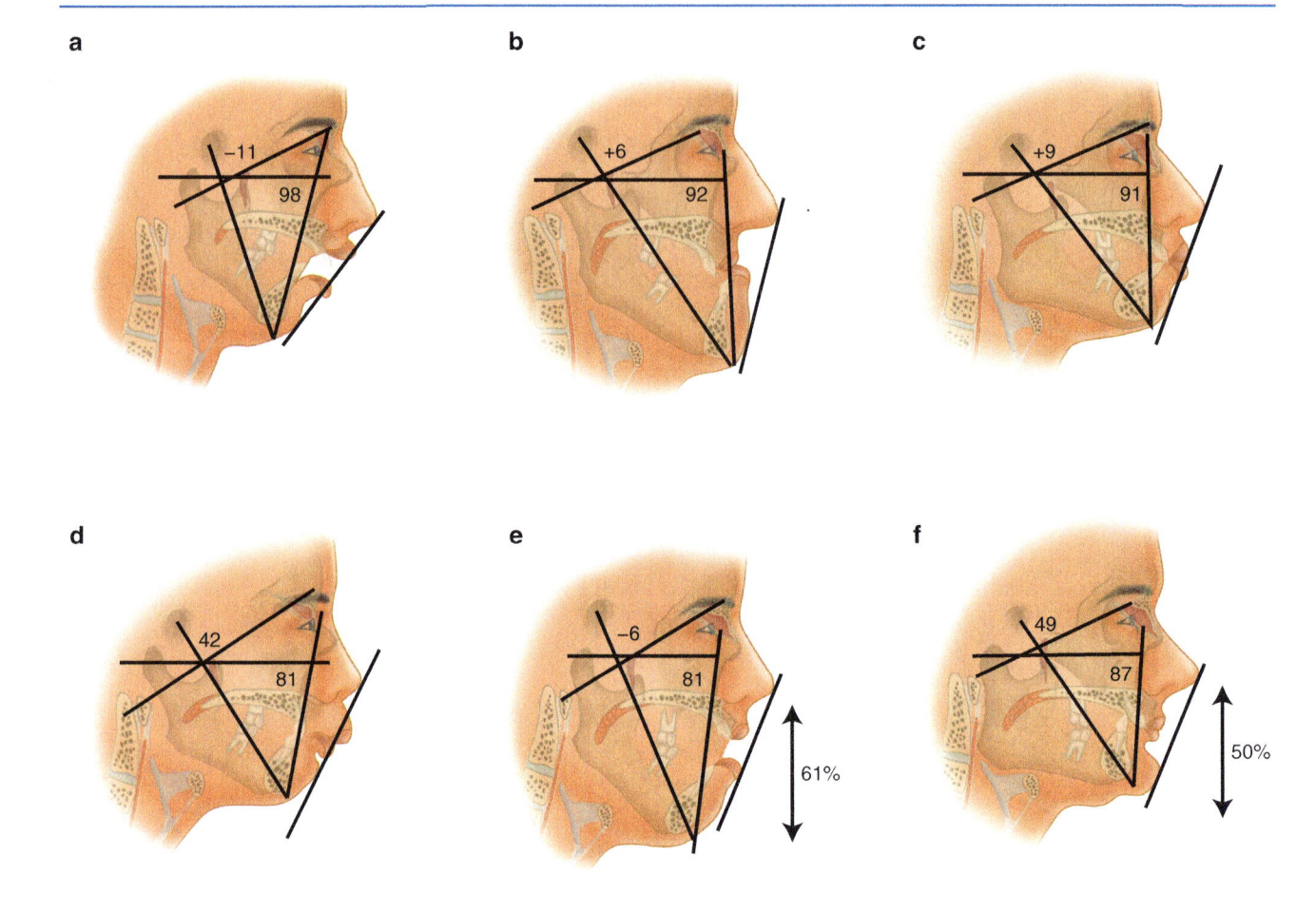

A child with a cleft may have any of these faces, therefore, no one procedure performed at birth can be satisfactory for all different facial types. Treatment planning must be individualized according to the patient's growth pattern, and must be staged.

## 3.9 Obtuse CB

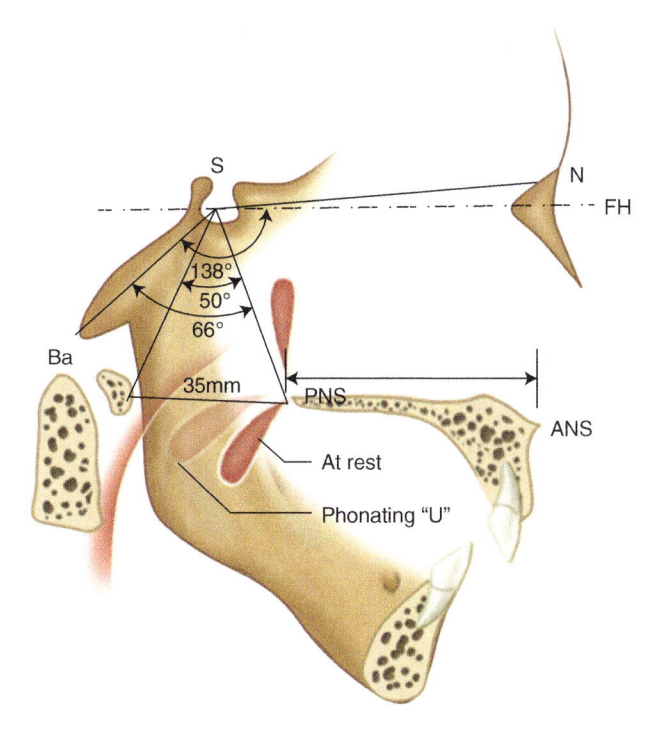

## 3.10 Acute CB

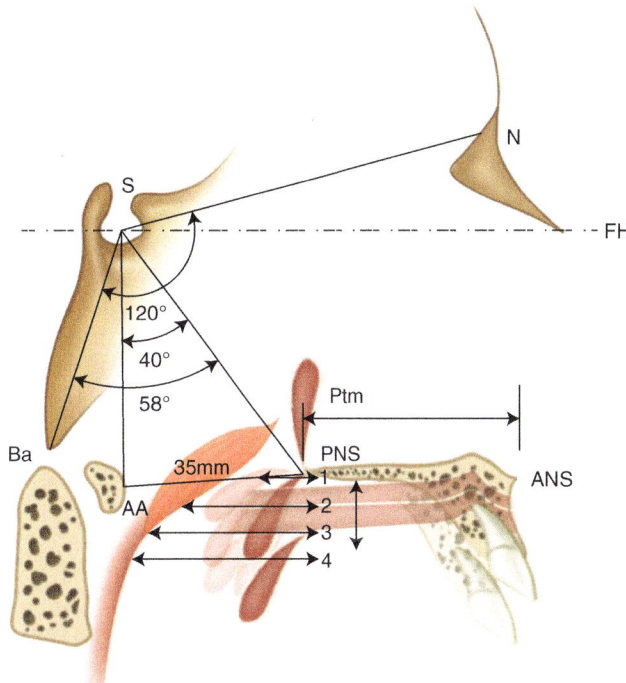

**The influence of the skeletal architecture on the pharyngeal form and size.** The pharyngeal space is bounded superiorly by the cranial base and laterally by the cervical spine on one side and the tongue/hard palate complex on the opposite side. The odontoid process (axis) of the cervical spine points to the posterior extent (Basion—Ba) of the basilar portion of the occipital bone. It is the median point of the anterior margin of the foramen magnum. The hard palate of the maxillary complex is anatomically associated with the anterior cranial base and can vary in its anteroposterior dimension.

*Left:* obtuse cranial base angle. In cases with a severe obtuse cranial base angle, the pharyngeal space is usually deeper than normal even in the presence of a long hard palate. An obtuse cranial base positions the cervical spine more posteriorly since it must be associated with the basilar portion of the occipital bone. This condition is usually seen when hypernasality exists in the absence of an overt palatal cleft and is called congenital palatal insufficiency (CPI).

*Right:* With an acute cranial base angle, the cervical spine is positioned close to the hard palate creating a shallow pharyngeal depth.

## 3.11 Nasopharyngeal Space

**At rest**

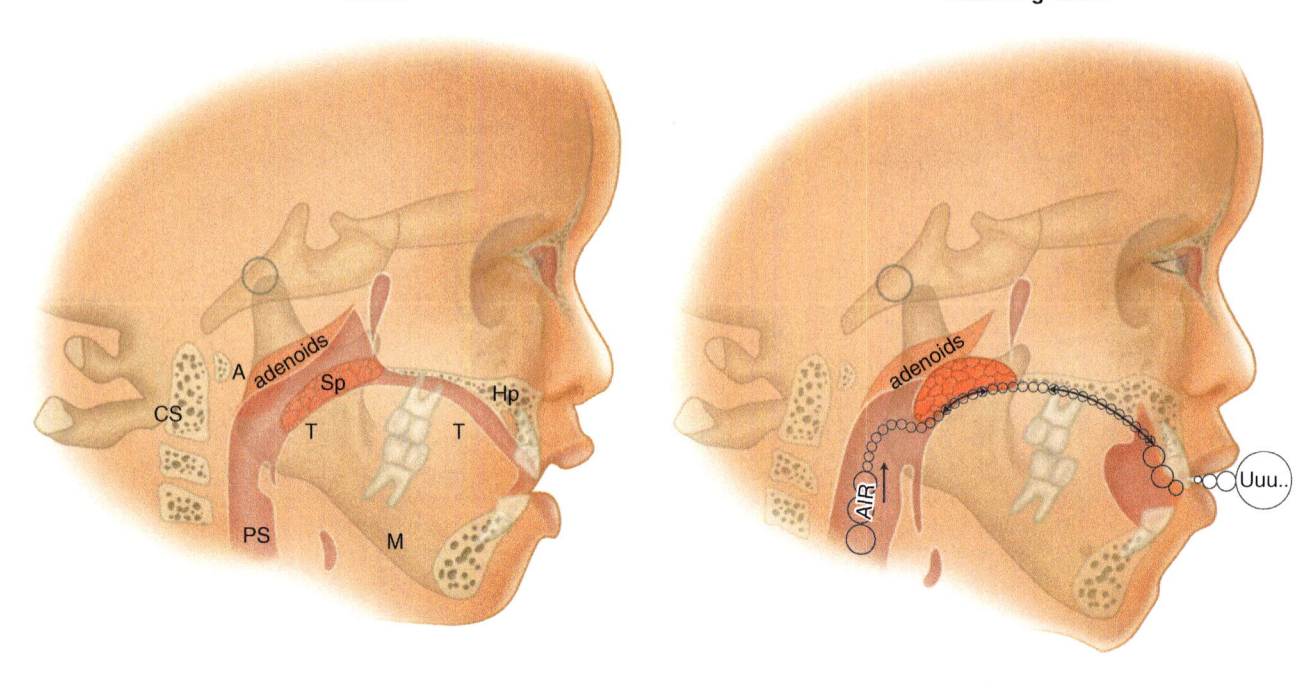

**Vocalizing Uuu...**

**Lateral cephaloradiograph shows the skeletal structures surrounding the pharyngeal space and allows evaluation of the pharyngeal depth, shape of cervical spine, soft palate size and length, and extent of soft palate elevation.** Because it is a two-dimensional representation of the velopharyngeal area and does not show lateral pharyngeal wall motion, this record cannot be used to diagnostically determine velopharyngeal functions. **a.** Left: Structures involved in controlling airflow as seen in a lateral cephalograph at 5 years of age (A = Anterior tubercle of the atlas, CS = Cervical spine, S = Odontoid process, W = Posterior pharyngeal wall, PS = Pharyngeal space, SP = Soft palate (velum), HP = Hard palate).

## 3.12 Variations in Facial Growth Patterns

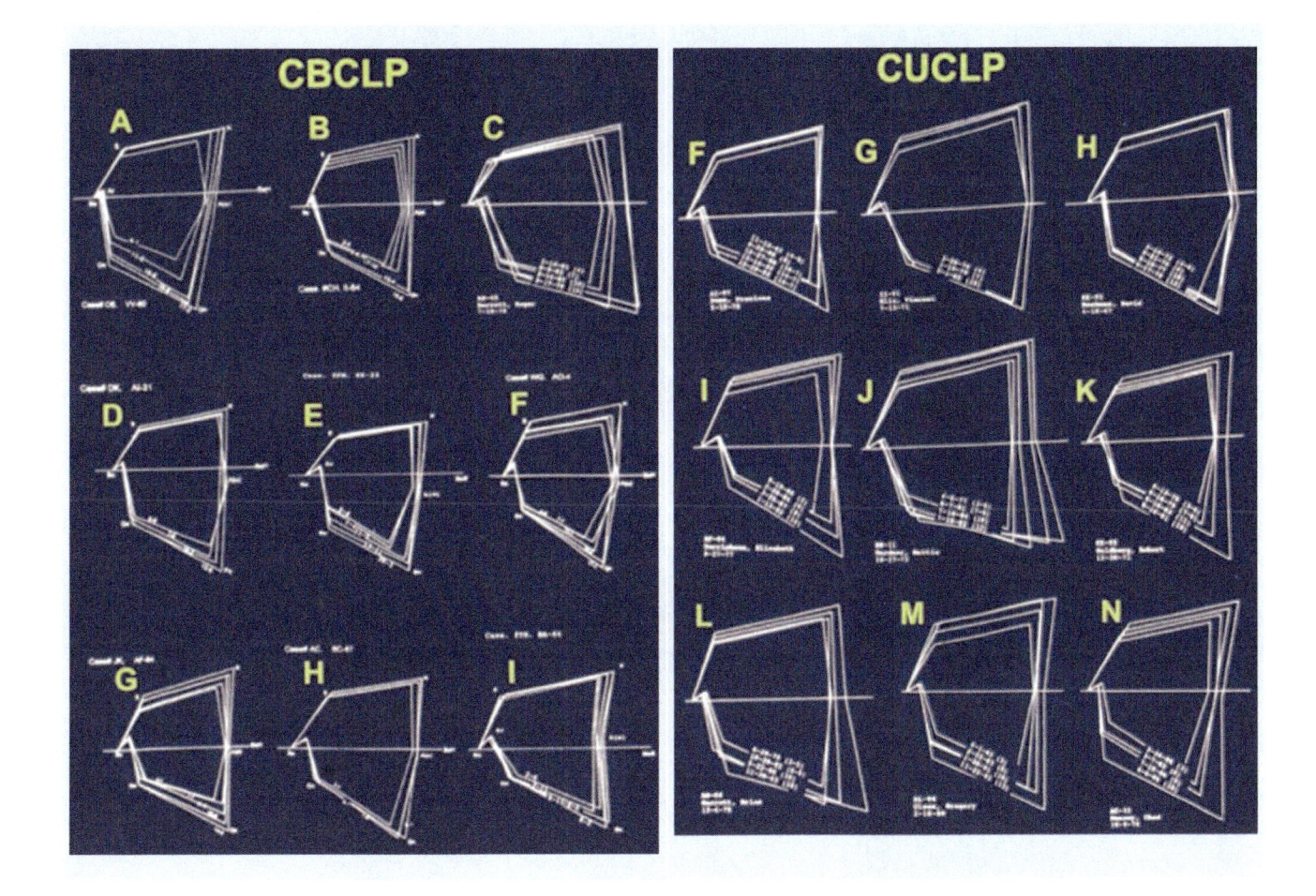

## 3.13 In Both CBCLP and CUCLP the Facial Growth Pattern Determines the Final Facial Profile

**All Goals Are Attainable When:**
- Reduced Palatal Scarring
- Normal Palatal Vault Space
- Normal Maxillary Anterior Teeth Alignment
- No Primary Bone Grafts
- No Gingivoperiosteoplasty
- No Palatal "Pushback" Surgery
- Palatal Closure Between 18 and 24 Months In Most Cases Sometimes Earlier Or Even Later
- Palatal Surgical Closure When Cleft Space is 10% of Palatal Size
- Consider Variations In Nasopharyngeal Architecture And Muscle Function
- The Need For Differential Diagnosis Based On Facial Growth Changes

## 3.14 Velopharyngeal Closure Patterns

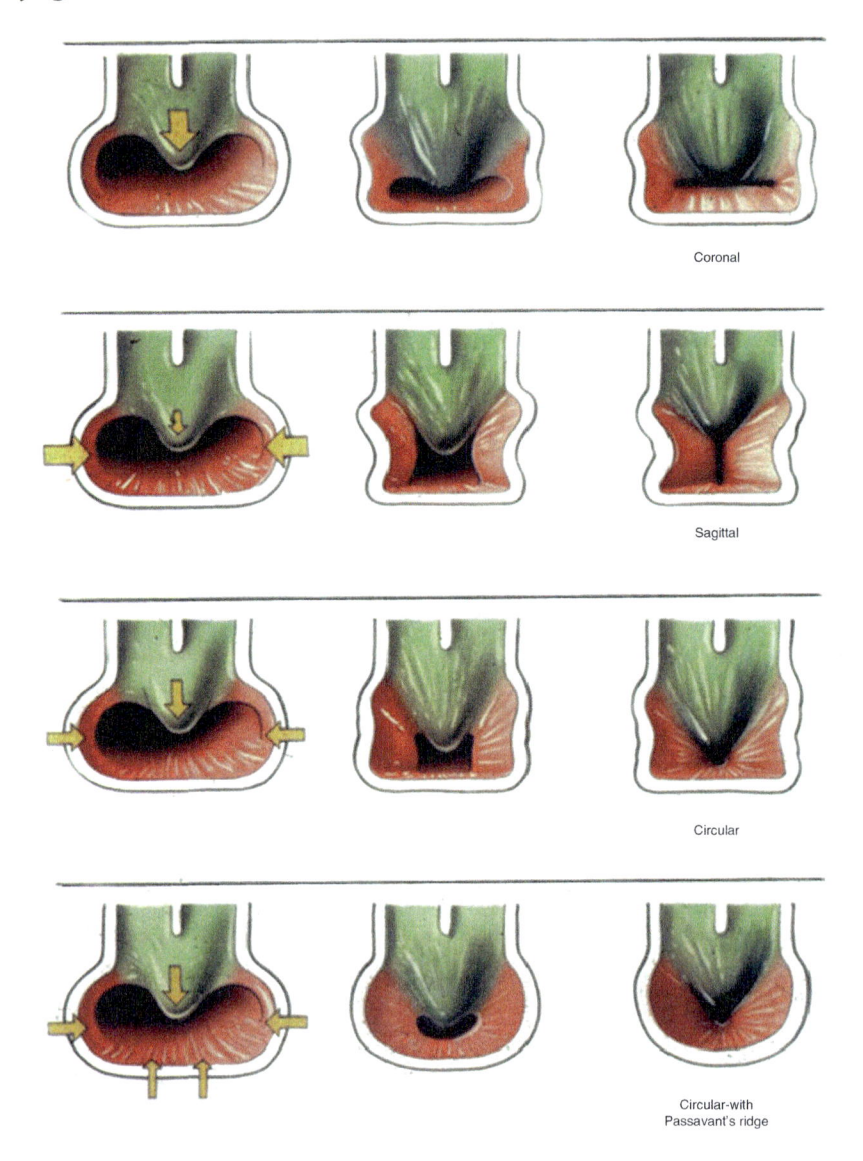

Coronal

Sagittal

Circular

Circular-with Passavant's ridge

Four basic velopharyngeal closure patterns. The size and shape of velopharyngeal valving patterns is very variable (see Skolnick, Vol. 2). Although the closure patterns are not actually discrete, for convenience sake, Skolnick et al. (1973) categorized velopharyngeal valving into four patterns. These patterns are:

**Coronal pattern:** The majority of valving is palatal with the full width of the velum contacting the posterior pharyngeal wall. The lateral walls move medially to the lateral edges of the velum. There is no motion in the posterior wall.

**Sagittal pattern:** The majority of valving is pharyngeal. The lateral walls move to the midline and approximate each other. The soft palate does not contact the posterior pharyngeal wall, but instead abuts up against the approximated lateral pharyngeal walls, thus completing the closure pattern.

**Circular pattern:** There is essentially equal contribution from the velum and lateral pharyngeal walls with the bulk of the musculus uvulae acting as the focal point. The dorsum of the musculus uvulae contacts the posterior wall (which does not move). The lateral walls squeeze around the bulk of the musculus uvulae.

**Passavant's ridge pattern:** As in the circular pattern, there is essentially equal contribution from the velum and lateral pharyngeal walls, but in addition, the posterior pharynx moves forward. The musculus uvulae also serves as the focal point for closure in this pattern. (Reproduced with permission from Siegel-Sadewitz VL, Shprintzen, RJ. Nasopharyngoscopy of the normal velopharyngeal sphincter: an experiment of biofeedback. Cleft Palate J. 1982; 19:196.)

## 3.14 Velopharyngeal Closure Patterns

**At rest**  **Vocalizing Uuu...**

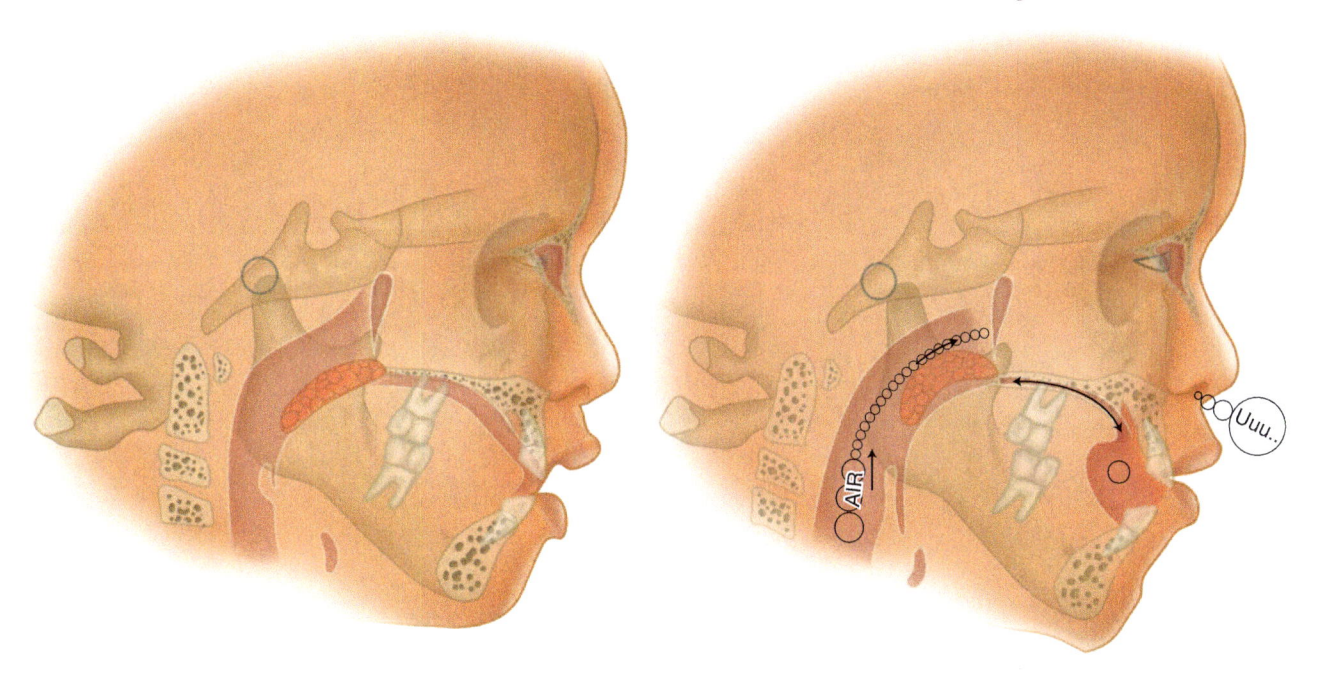

T = tongue, M = mandible. Right: Airflow when vocalizing "Uuu" during normal speech. The soft palate elevates and makes contact with the adenoids (if present) or the posterior pharyngeal wall during normal speech and swallowing. (**a**) When the lateral pharyngeal muscles operate in coordination with a competent (adequate length, width, and timing of action) soft palate in a normal skeletal environment, most of the air is channeled through the mouth while some enters the nose. This is designated as velopharyngeal competency (VPC). (**b**) Velopharyngeal incompetency (VPI). There are usually many reasons for inadequate airflow control. Some are: (1) A relatively deep pharynx when related to velar length; (2) Inadequate velar elevation and/or pharyngeal wall motion (neuromuscular function); and (3) Poor timing of speech with pharyngeal and velar muscle (sensory-motor) function

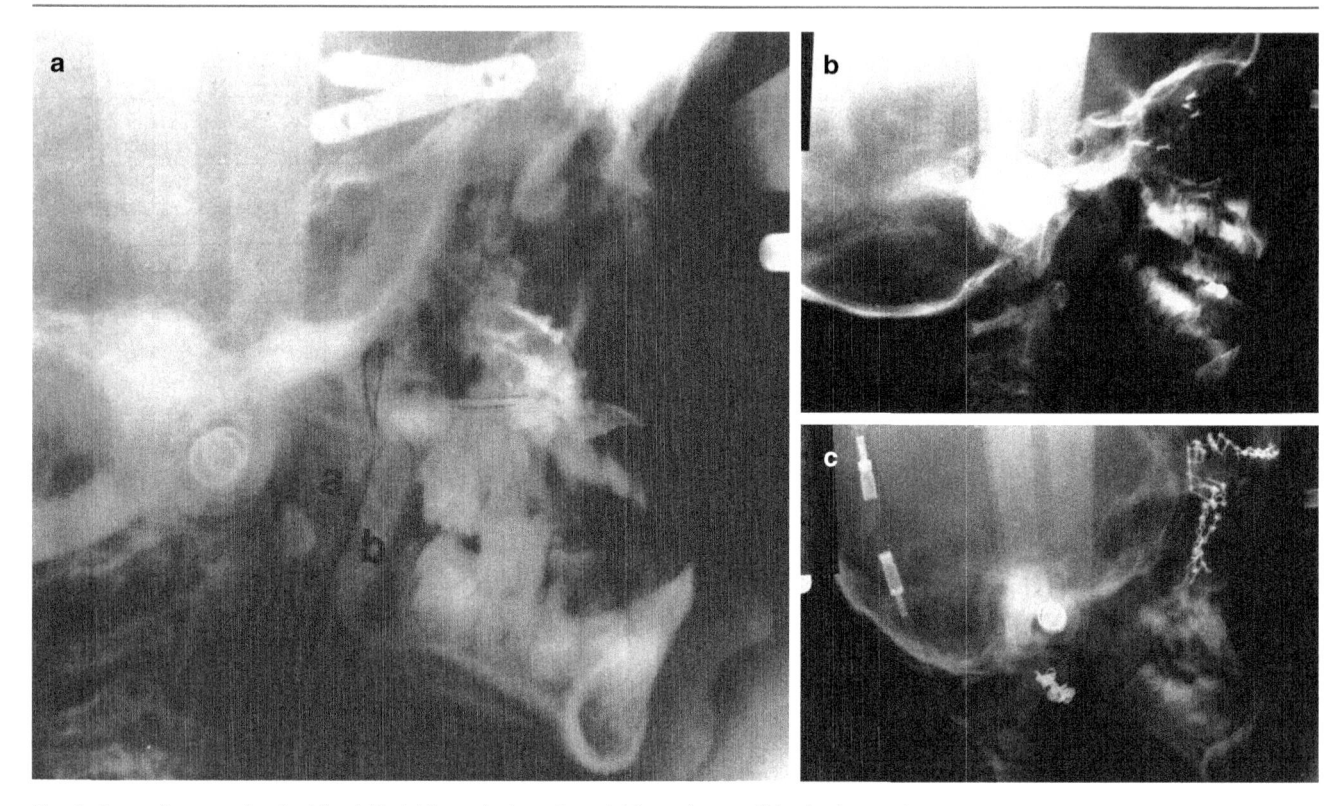

Nasal obstruction associated with midfacial hypoplasia and cranial base abnormalities in three different craniofacial syndromes: (**a**) Aperts (a = adenoid, b = soft palate), (**b**) Mandibulo-facial-dysostosis, and (**c**) Crouzon Syndrome

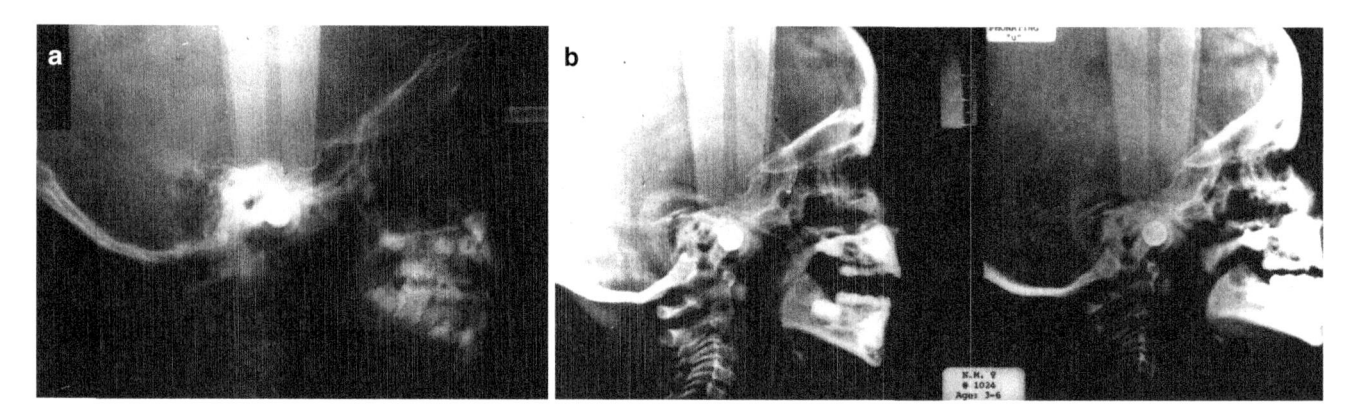

Cervical spine anomalies and their effects on the pharyngeal space configuration. (**a**) The absence and (**b**) malformation or dislocation of the anterior tubercle of the atlas result in the lack of support to the posterior pharyngeal wall, thus increasing the depth of the pharyngeal space. These anomalies coupled with a small velum will compound the problem. Left: Velum at rest. Right: Velum in function. No contact with the posterior pharyngeal wall

## 3.14 Velopharyngeal Closure Patterns

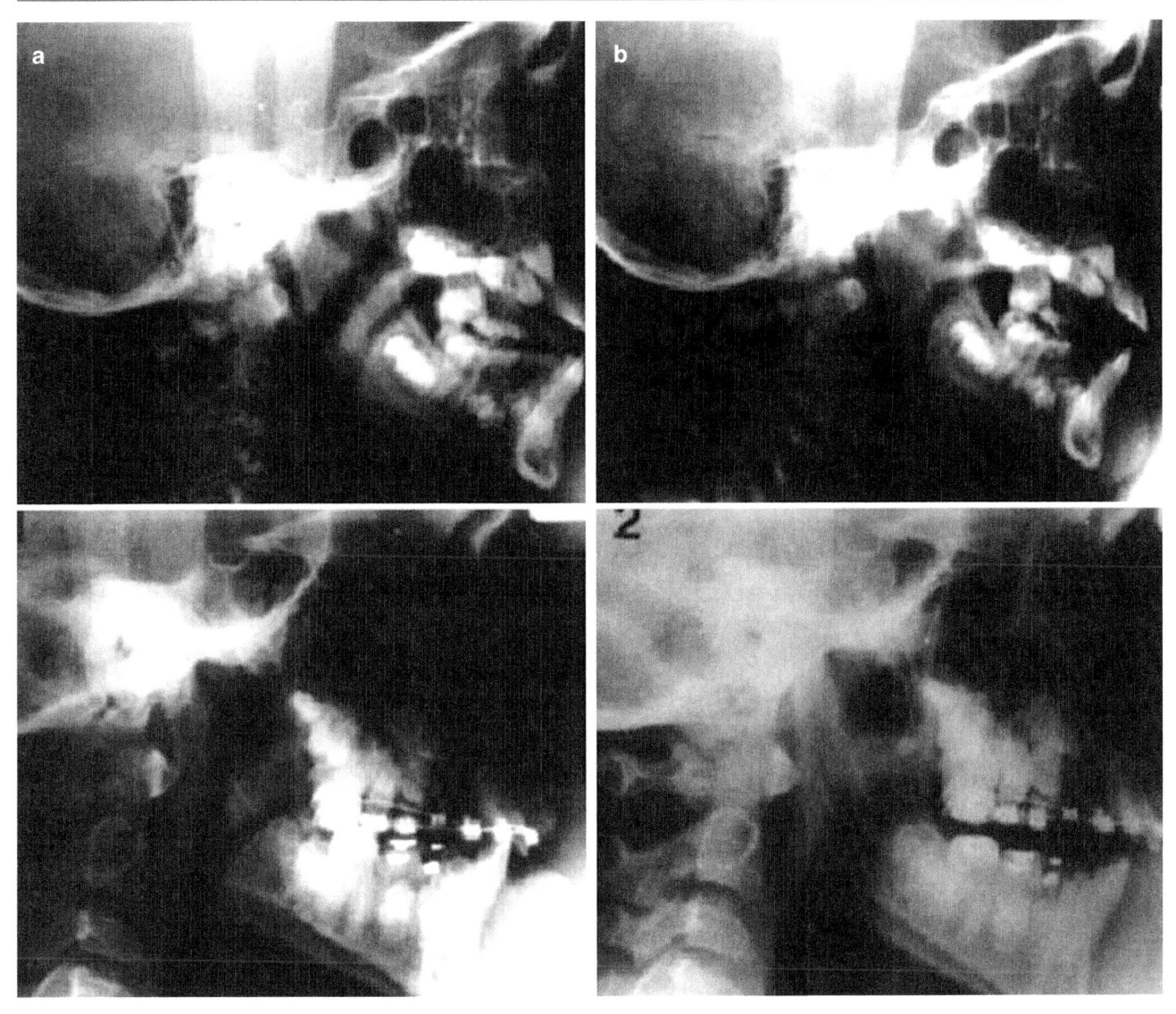

Variations in the pharyngeal space, velar elevation, and adenoid size. (**a**) *Left:* normal pharyngeal architecture at rest, 10 years of age. *Right:* while vocalizing "Uuuu." Note to the velum of good length making contact against a small adenoid—the hard palate is positioned above the anterior tubercle. (**b**) Short, stubby velum in a relatively small pharyngeal space making good contact with the posterior pharyngeal wall at the level of the anterior tubercle, 12 years of age, no adenoids. 1. At rest, 2. Vocalizing "Uuuu…"

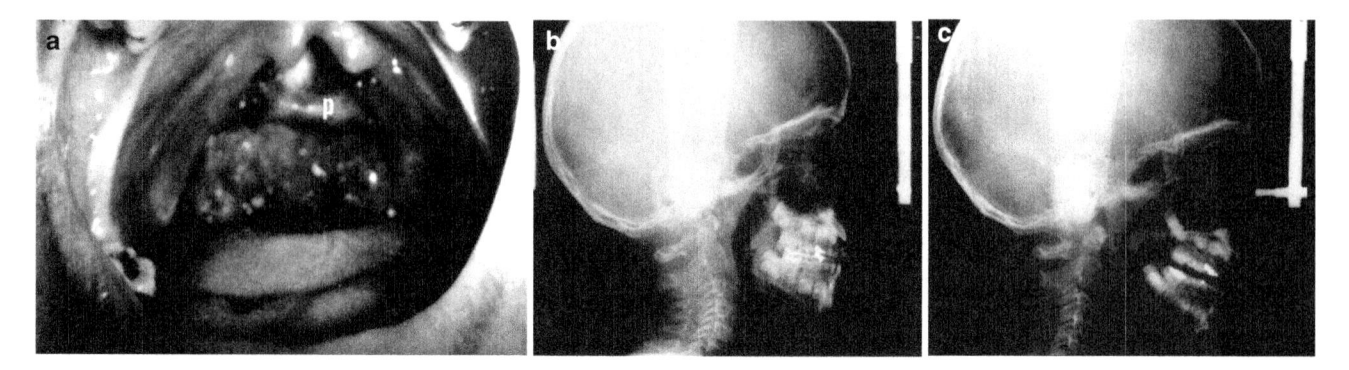

**Passavant's Pad.** The superior border of the superior constrictor pharyngeous muscle on contraction forms a ridge or pad on the posterior wall. It is observed in both non-cleft and cleft patients. There is no consistent relationship of the pad to the velum and it is usually seen during swallowing as well as during speech, whistling, and blowing. Some state that it functions adequately for compensatory purposes and does not appear to contribute to velopharyngeal closure in all patients. (**a**) An intraoral view of Passavant's pads (p). (**b**) Lateral cephaloradiograph—at rest. (**c**) While phonating "Uuu," showing Passavant's pad (p) at the level of the anterior tubercle of the atlas making contact with the uvula.

## 3.15 Lateral Cephs Before and After Surgery To Lengthen the Soft Palate

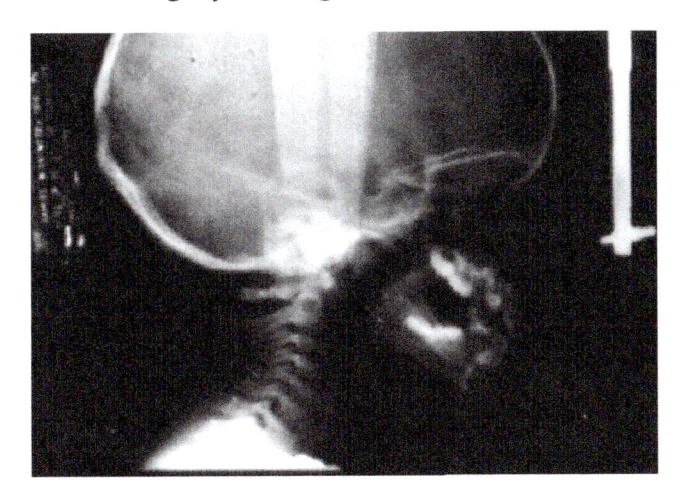

Velum at rest

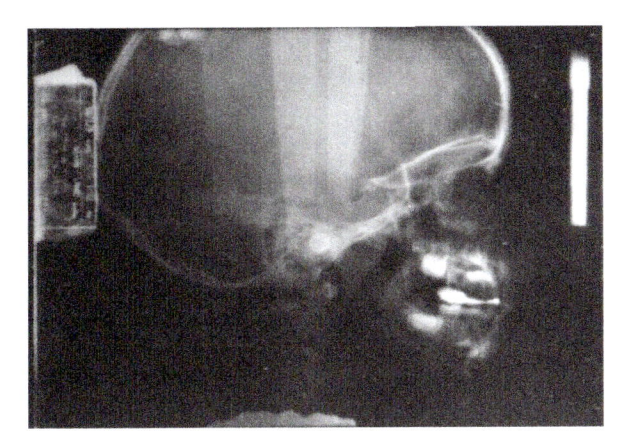

Vocalizing uuu… poor elevation of soft palate

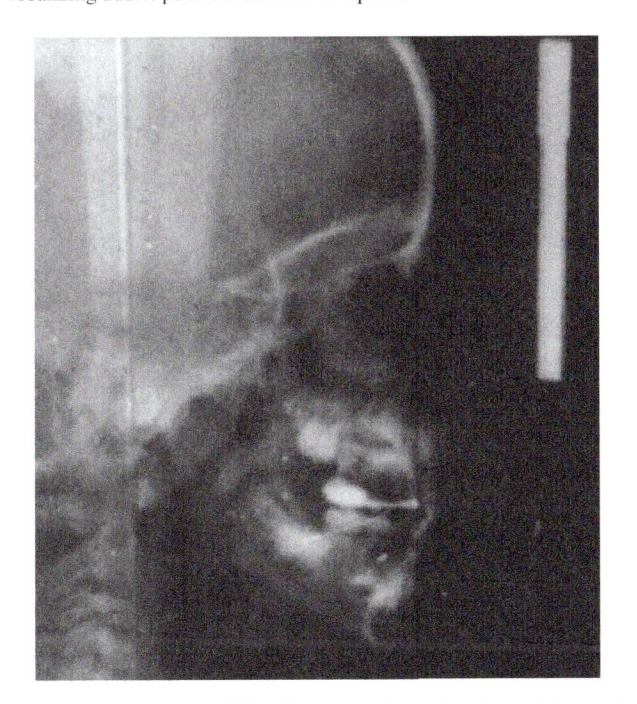

After velar lengthening VPI still present. Poor elevation while vocalizing uuu…

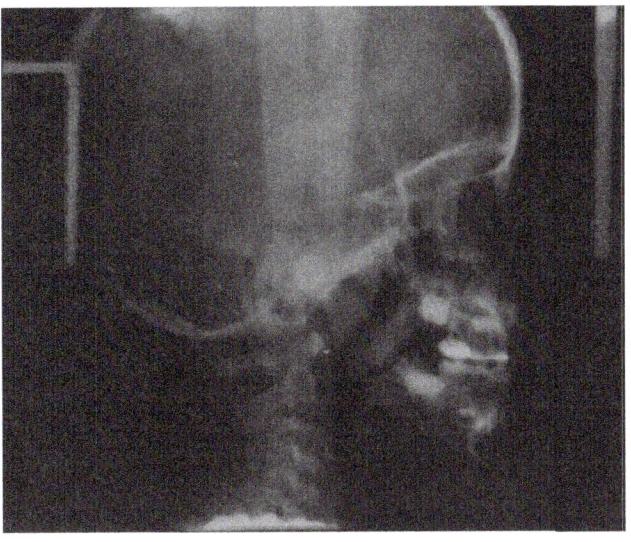

VPI—Vocalizing Sss… poor velar motion

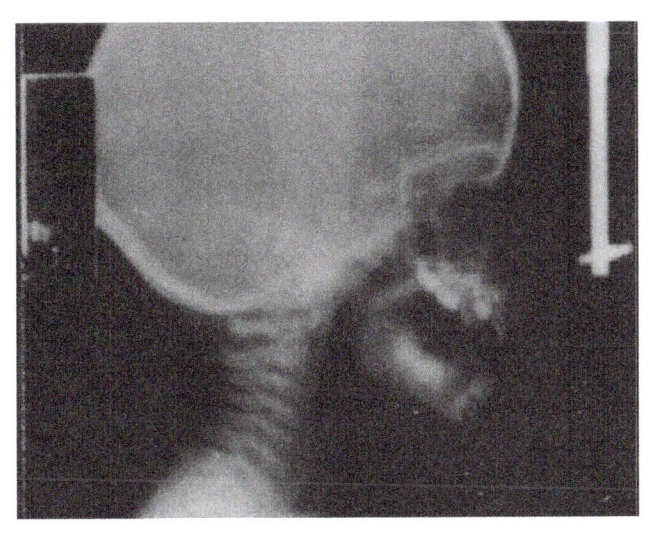

Velum at rest

**Final Treatment: Pharyngeal Flap**
**Comment:** The velum has good length but does not elevate sufficiently. Need to know neuromuscular activity potential before performing corrective velar surgery.

# Variation in Cleft Types

## 4.1 Isolated Cleft Palate

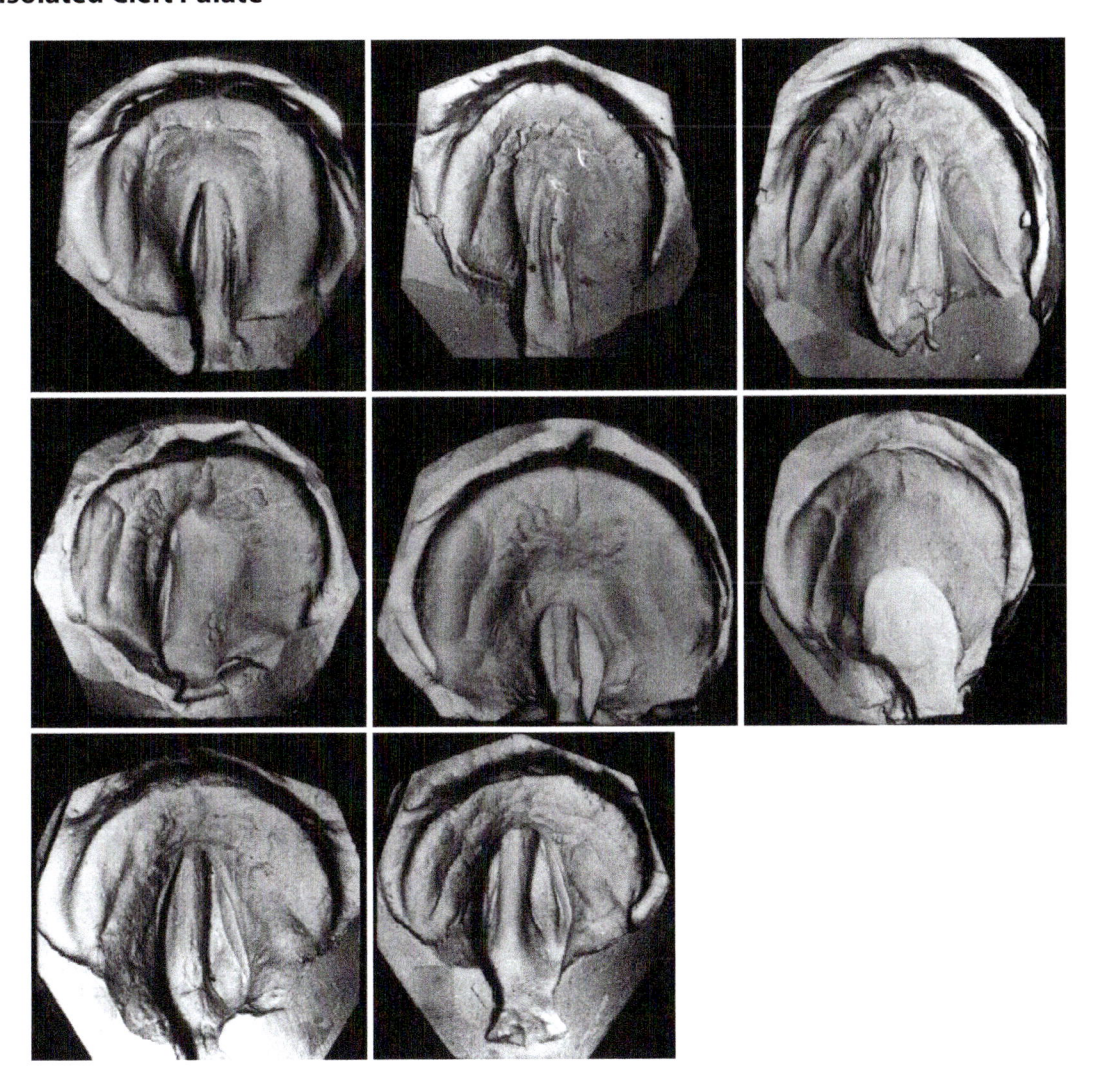

Variations in isolated cleft palate. The length and width of the cleft space is highly variable. The cleft extends anteriorly to various distances but not beyond the incisal canal.

Note the relative size of the cleft palate space which reflects differences in the degree of osteogenic deficiency.

In some instances, the cleft space diminishes with time; however, there are occasions when the cleft's relative size remains the same.

© Springer Nature Switzerland AG 2022
S. Berkowitz, *Orthodontic-Surgical Partnership in Cleft Lip and Palate Treatment*,
https://doi.org/10.1007/978-3-030-54300-6_4

## 4.2 Variations in Anterior-Posterior Length of the Two Segments in Unilateral Cleft Lip and Palate

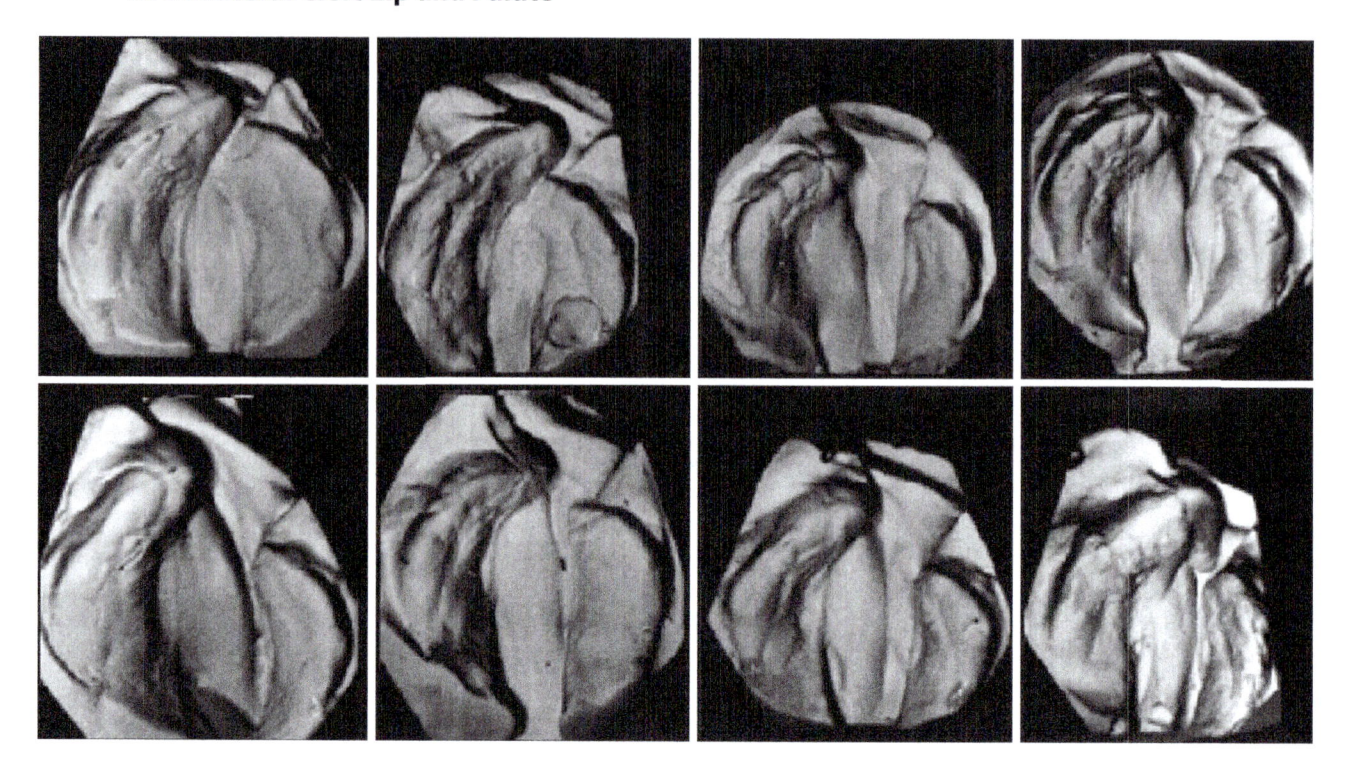

## 4.3 Effect of Lip and Palatal Clefting on Maxillary Segments

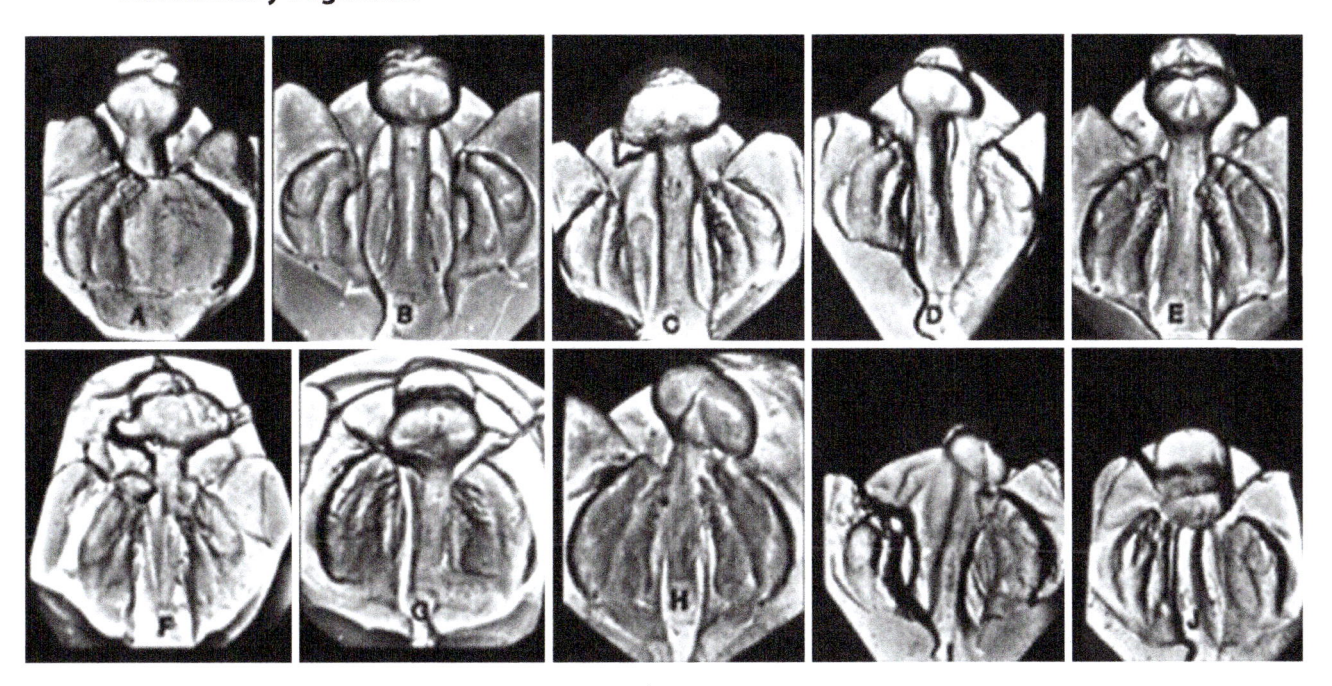

## 4.4 Variations in Bilateral Cleft Lip and Palate Types

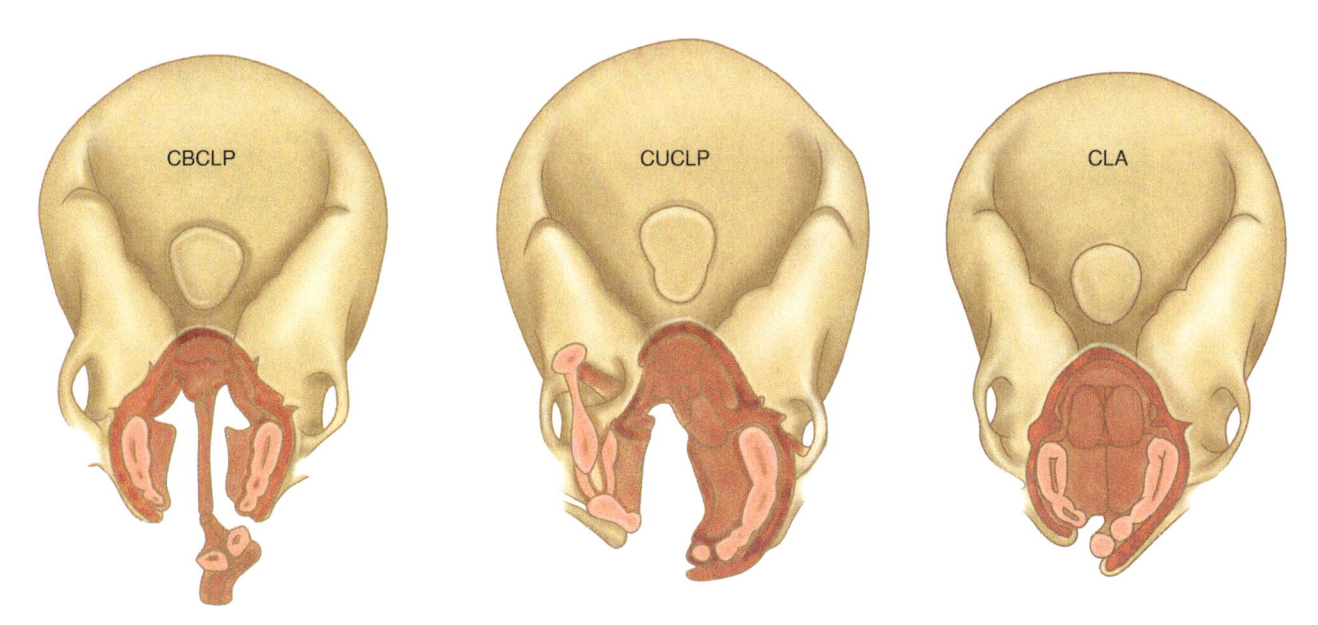

The anatomic classification system on the location, completeness, and extent of the cleft deformity. Because the lip, alveolus, and hard palate develop from different embryonic sources, any combination of clefting can exist.

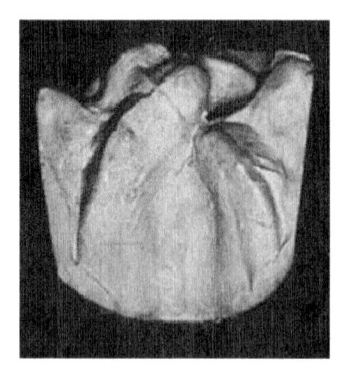

**A.** Cleft of the lip and alveolus. Normal palate

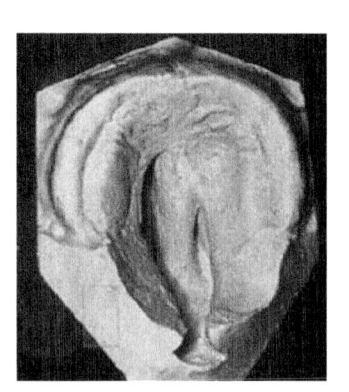

**B.** Isolated cleft of the hard and soft palate. Normal lip and alveolus

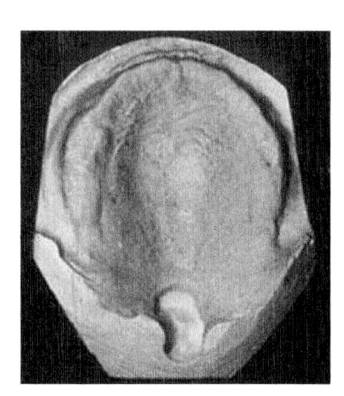

**C.** Cleft of the soft palate and uvulae

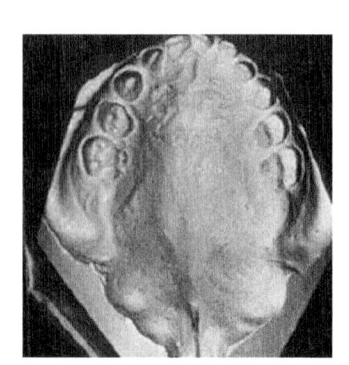

**D.** Cleft of the uvulae

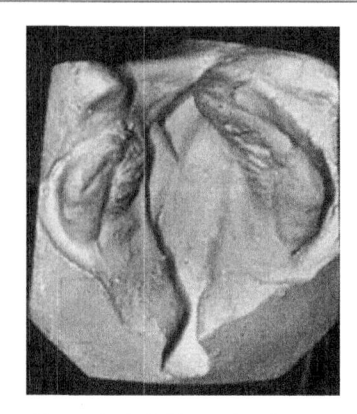

**E.** Complete unilateral cleft lip and palate

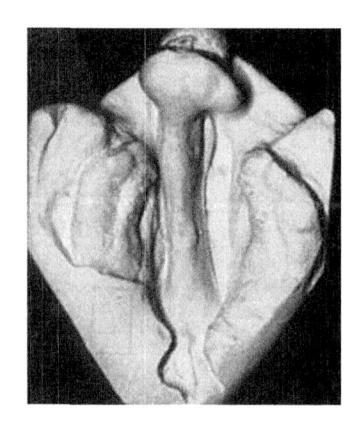

**F.** Complete bilateral cleft lip and palate

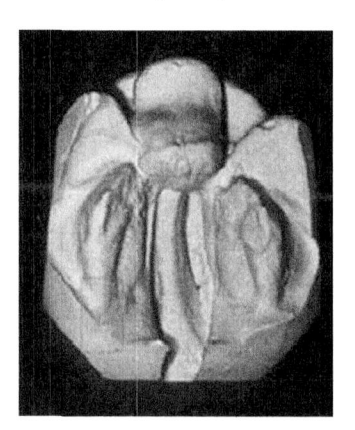

**G.** Incomplete bilateral cleft of the lip and palate

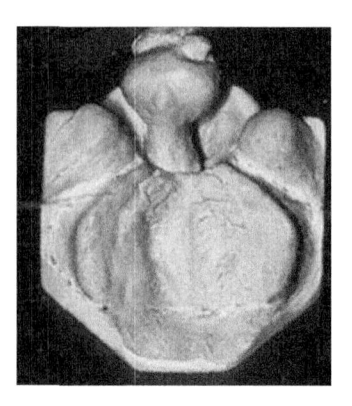

**H.** Complete bilateral cleft of the lip and alveolus

## 4.5 Review of the Literature

### 4.5.1 Surgical Procedure (Type and Timing)

There is currently a great deal of controversy over which surgical procedure should be used to close the palatal cleft, when such procedure should occur, and whether neonatal maxillary orthopedics has any long-term utility and stimulates palatal growth.

The history of cleft palate surgery reveals that poorly conceived, badly executed and ill-timed operations, performed at birth, have resulted in poor surgical results in many individual cases (Graber (1), (8)). After a series of such findings were reported in the 1950s, there was a movement to delay surgical treatment in the cleft child until school age, in order to avoid deleterious effects from surgery on palatal and facial growth (Schweckendiek (3), Hotz (4), Hotz et al. (5)). Proponents of this newer view recommended the interim use of prosthetic obturators in the young patient while waiting for a significant proportion of maxillary growth to occur.

The proponents apparently assumed that all surgical procedures on the palate posed a definite impediment to the natural maxillary growth process and the use of the obturator (designed a certain way) would stimulate palatal growth almost eliminating the need to use releasing incisions and mucoperiosteal undermining.

Opponents of this school of thought advocated surgical repair of the cleft palate before one year of age in order to avoid perverted patterns of speech that would require prolonged and difficult correction at a later age (Holdsworth (6), Jolleys (7), Robertson and Jolleys (8), Dorr and Curtin (9)). This latter group gave priority to speech over palatal and facial development. Still others (Slaughter and Pruzansky (10), Slaughter et al. (11), Blocksma et al. (12), Dingman et al (13) (14), Berkowitz (15), (16)) took a middle of the road position, suggesting that palatal surgery be performed between 12 and 24 months of age.

No matter what type of treatment any of them favored, surgeons could not explain why their particular surgical methods, performed on similar clefts at the same age, often yielded different results. Why some cases showed "catch-up-growth" with good facial and palatal growth and functional dental occlusion while others showed poor facial and palatal development. Catch-up-growth has been defined by Hughes (17) as growth with a velocity above the statistical limits of normality for age during a defined period of time. Such an increase in the rate of growth, before and after palatal surgery, with or without neonatal maxillary orthopedics, may allow it to attain its normal adult size, or despite the increase in velocity the palate may still fail to do so. In the latter case, it is called incomplete "catch-up-growth." Wilson and Osbourn (18) showed that the duration and severity of the insult (the surgical procedure used to close the cleft space in the hard palate) may positively or negatively affect the ability of the palate to recover and undergo "catch-up-growth."

The morphometric analysis of the changing form and size of the palate will permit some insight into the appropriate surgical procedure (age and type) to prevent growth retardation caused by the reduction in blood supply to the specific palatal area with the creation of growth inhibiting scar tissue. Comparing inter-institutional differences of total palatal surface area (osseous and soft tissue, between the crests of the alveolar ridges) will reflect on the physiological attributes of the various surgical or orthopedic procedures.

Among specific unanswered questions:

Were the different outcomes due to different levels of skill on the part of the operators?

Were there significant differences within each cleft type that should have been differentially diagnosed?

*Feinstein (19) has written:*

In the biostatistical architecture of clinical research, the first operational principle is to specify the components and choose the logic of the objective of the research. The components consist of a sequence of initial state, maneuver and subsequent state. The logic consists of suitable scientific judgement in the decisions made to demarcate the diagnostic and prognostic conditions of the initial state of the population; to identify differentiate and prognostically correlate the diverse targets of the subsequent state; and to choose maneuvers that are satisfactory in potency, comparison, multiplicity and concurrency.

In speaking of the initial and the subsequent states, emphasis will be placed on studies of casts starting at birth and extending through adolescence.

**Initial State:**

Analysis of the initial (newborn) state suggests that under certain conditions surgical repair of the palate is feasible quite early while, in other instances, optimal conditions for repair will not become evident until a later age. In our experience, a selected number of cases with very small cleft spaces underwent palatal repair at or before one year of age without detriment to midface and palatal growth. On the other hand, there are cases where the cleft space is too large when compared to the amount of available soft tissue and surgery needs to be postponed to avoid creating growth inhibiting scare tissue. This is an example of individualized differential diagnosis and treatment planning.

**Maneuver:**

If we assume that qualified surgeons within a given institution or region, practicing a specific series of techniques, over a given period of time, represent a constant, the differences in success or failure should reside in the initial state (the geometric and size relationship of the palatal segments to the size and shape of the cleft space). Also to other factors, such as surgery that governs the subsequent state. Of course, the sample must separate cases subjected or not subjected to presurgical maxillary orthopedics: cases subjected to vomer flaps should be considered separately since these variable can influence the subsequent state. Of the three components, the maneuver presented the greatest number of confounding variables. Differences between surgeons, variance in the performance by the same surgeon from day to day and over the course of several years, and difference in techniques which are difficult to identify and compare, complicate the analysis but our biostatistician and anthropologist still believe the research objectives could be reached.

**As Feinstein stated:**

We believe that within certain defined limits, the success or failure of the surgical procedure depended more on the initial state than on the variables inherent with the maneuver. To put it another way, variables within the patient were more prognostic of the subsequent state than differences between surgeons.

Serial studies starting at the newborn period have shown that too many factors were operating in relation to the patients under study to permit the formulation of simple, all-inclusive rules, such as any suggestion regarding the age at which clefts of the palate should be repaired. Berkowitz, therefore, hypothesized that the ratio of the useful mucoperiosteal tissue available for surgery present at the time of closure of the cleft space to the size of the cleft space determined the area of denuded bone left at the surgical site. This area heals by epithelial ligation which in turn becomes scar tissue. The amount and degree of scarring could spell the difference between therapeutic success and failure since it influences the palate's ultimate size (osseous plus soft tissue) and form.

This hypothesis needs to be tested using quantitative measurements for only in this way will surgeons change their focus to include the size and form of the palate, the extent of the cleft defect as well as the surgical procedure. Pruzansky (20) frequently stated that his most important contribution to the cleft palate literature was the conclusion that "cleft lip and palate does not represent a single fixed entity subject to generalizations of description and classification and least of all to rigid therapeutic formulas." Although his anecdotal reports support this conclusion, he did not have a sufficient number of cases and proper measuring equipment to test his conclusion using biostatistical analyses. The question of tissue adequacy or inadequacy could not be explored until a 3-dimensional measuring tool and proper CadCam software became available.

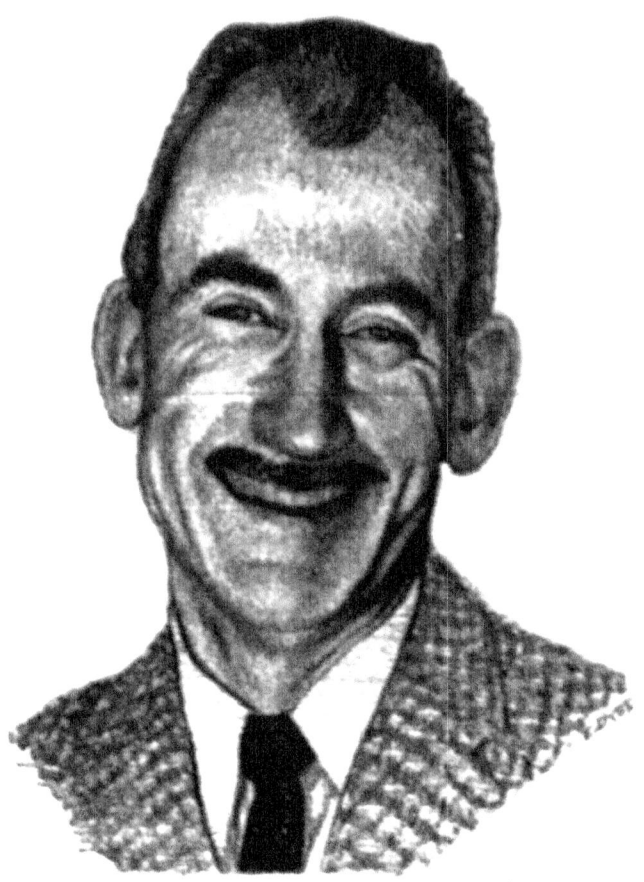

*Paul Tessier*

Paul-Tessier of Paris differentiated between two types of medial oro-ocular clefts, *vertical* and *oblique*. He noted differential features. In the eyelids, localization of the cleft seems to be outside the punctum lacrimale in vertical clefts and inside the oblique cleft. The medial canthal ligament is almost normal in direction and insertion in vertical clefts but atrophic, obliquely directed and associated with ectopia in oblique clefts.

Paul Tessier's classification of craniofacial clefts is based on his lifetime collection of cases. Craniofacial and orbital maxillary clefts are rare malformations, compared to cleft lip and cleft palate, and extend through constant lines or axes through the eyelids or eyebrows, nostrils, lips, and maxillae. Bone and soft tissue are seldom involved to the same extent. Soft tissue defects are more common from the midline to the infraorbital foramen while boney defects are more severe lateral to the infraorbital foramen.

Courtesy Millard, D.R., Jr. *Cleft Craft III:*
*Alveolar and Palatal Deformities*

It is Tessier's theory that facial clefts have their origin on the cranial base and thus can be traced from the cranium through the orbit to the face regardless of main blood vessels or growth centers.

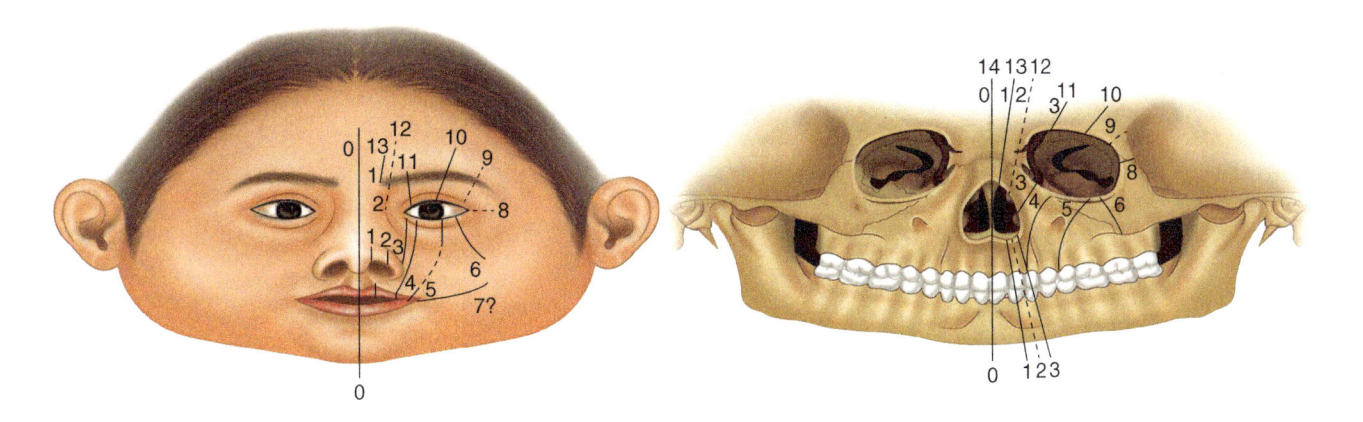

## 4.5 Review of the Literature

Courtesy Millard, D.R., Jr. *Cleft Craft III: Alveolar and Palatal Deformities*

Here is an example of a bilateral medial oro-ocular cleft patient. In cleft patient with turning of the edges for lining and rotation of a cheek flap for cover while aligning the lateral and medial vermilion of the lip.

Fogh-Andersen in 1965 reported three oblique facial clefts out of 3,988 clefts. One was a severe oblique cleft combined with bilateral cleft lip and palate, nasal defect, and preauricular appendages. He also published an account of a less severe incomplete oblique cleft of the lip involving the medial portion of the lower eyelid. His surgery corrected the lip and cheek with a Z-plasty.

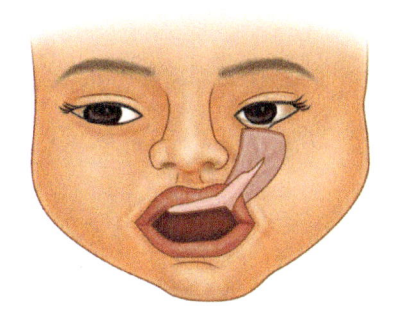

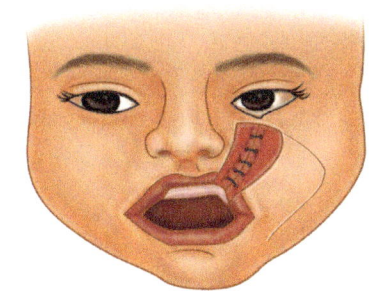

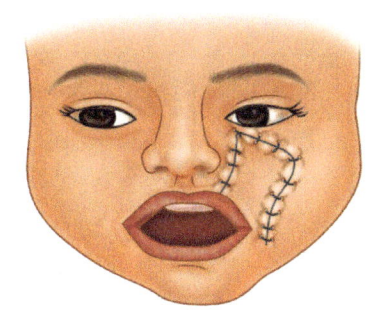

Courtesy Millard, D.R., Jr. *Cleft Craft III: Alveolar and Palatal Deformities*

# Surgery 5

## 5.1 The Vomer Flap: Good or Bad?

The longitudinal data of the Oslo group is critical of those who condemn the vomer flap. Friede and Pruzansky observed more favorable growth in patients treated without a vomer flap; however, this is not a uniform finding in the comparative studies. Some clinical centers not using a vomer flap have shown results similar to those where a vomer flap has been utilized.

The effects of a vomer flap on facial growth have been considered. Some reported the flap to be clinically significant. Illustrations by Dr. Millard Jr. *Cleft Craft* 1980

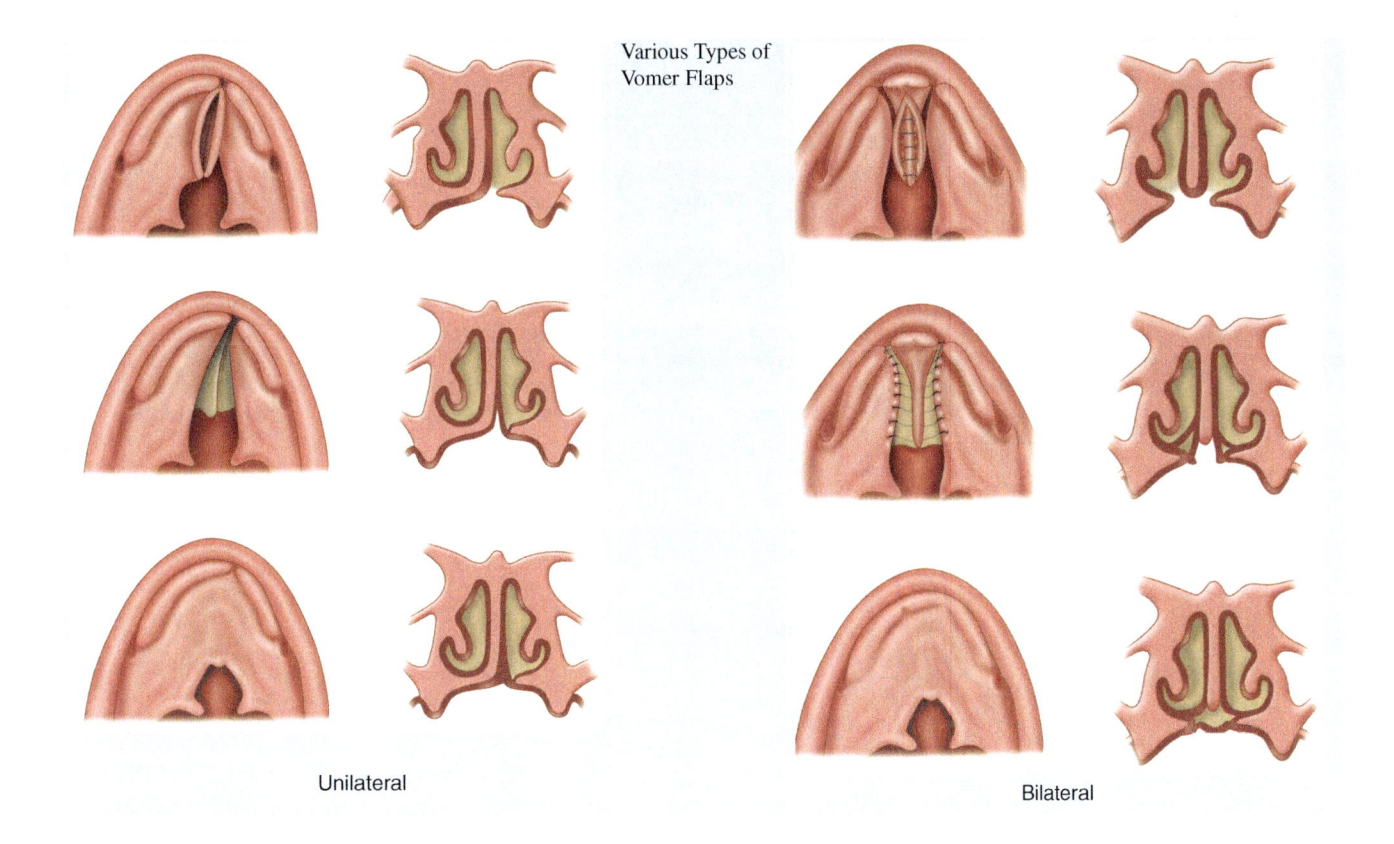

Various Types of Vomer Flaps

Unilateral | Bilateral

© Springer Nature Switzerland AG 2022
S. Berkowitz, *Orthodontic-Surgical Partnership in Cleft Lip and Palate Treatment*,
https://doi.org/10.1007/978-3-030-54300-6_5

## 5.2 Von Langenbeck (Simple Closure)

### 5.2.1 Palatoplasty

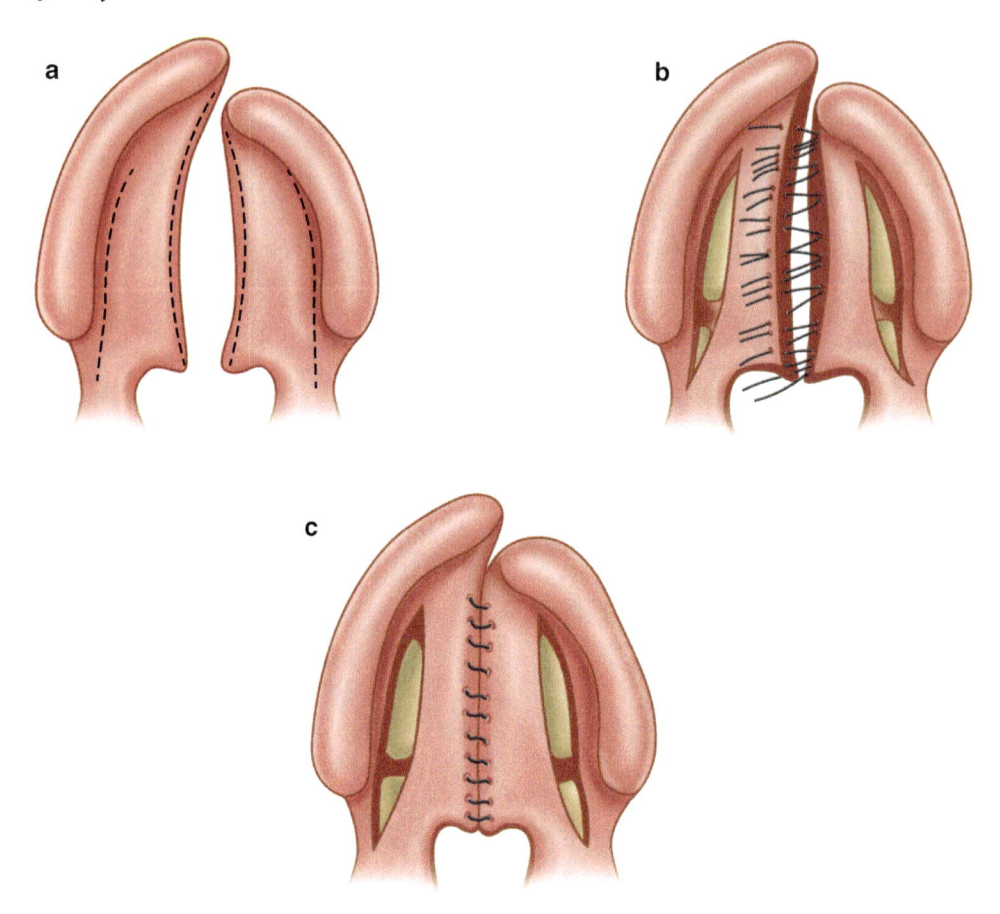

(**a**) The incision lines. (**b**) Mucoperiosteal flaps have been elevated, although this is not well shown in this diagram. The nasal mucosa is closed. In this anomaly, the nasal mucosa on the non-cleft or medial side is continuous with the septum and vomer. More is available to manipulate. Vomer flap can be used on nasal sides as well. (**c**) Oral mucosa closure. Note that it is impossible to obtain a two-layer closure of the alveolar portion of the cleft with this operation. Lateral raw areas are relatively smaller because the mucoperiosteum is not detached anteriorly. The anterior cleft space is closed simultaneously with a secondary alveolar bone graft.

## 5.3 V-Y Lengthening Veau-Wardill-Kilner Procedure

This procedure creates large anterior denuded bone space which becomes highly scarred leading to growth disturbance.

(a) Flap design

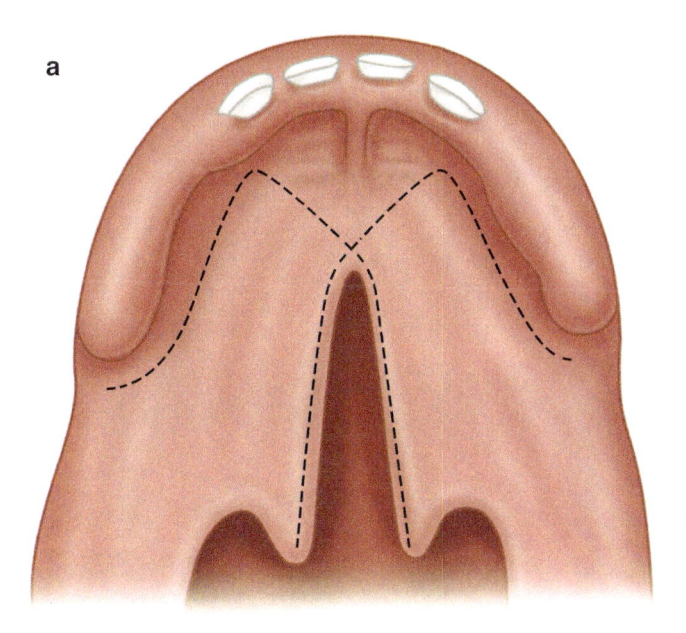

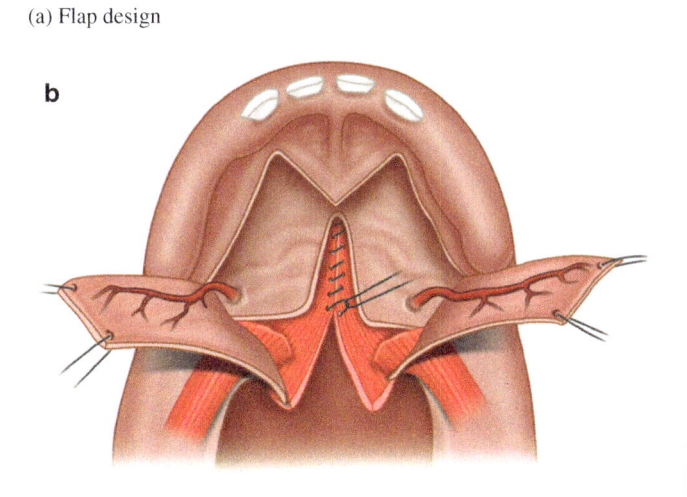

(b) Bilateral pedicle flap elevation, muscle disinsertion, and nasal lining closure

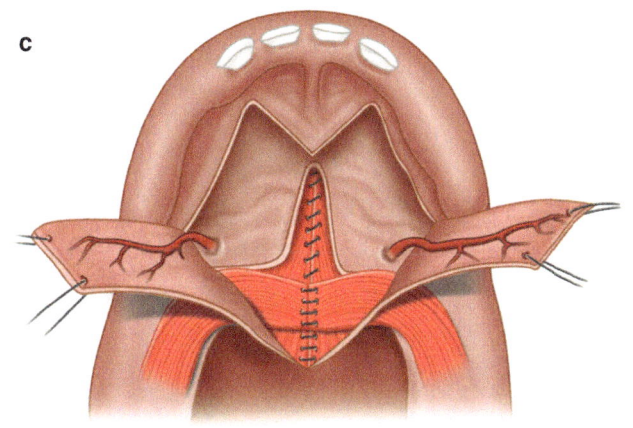

(c) Levator sling creation (intravelar veloplasty)

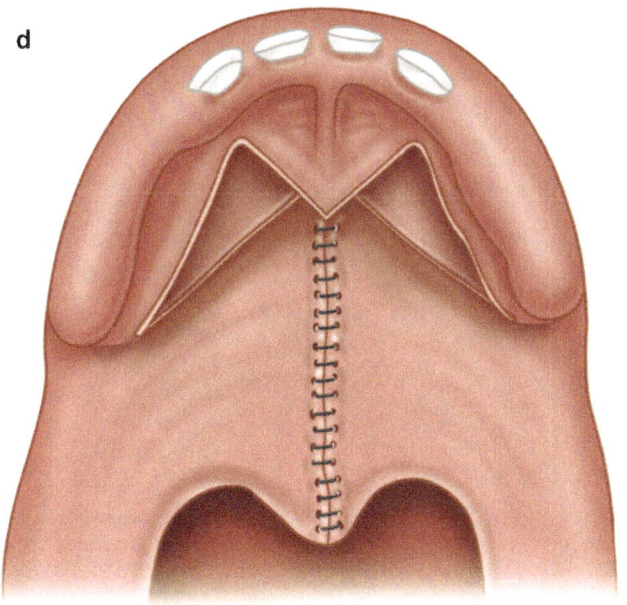

(d) Oral flap closure with palatal lengthening

## 5.4  Double-Reversing Z-Plasty (Furlow Procedure)

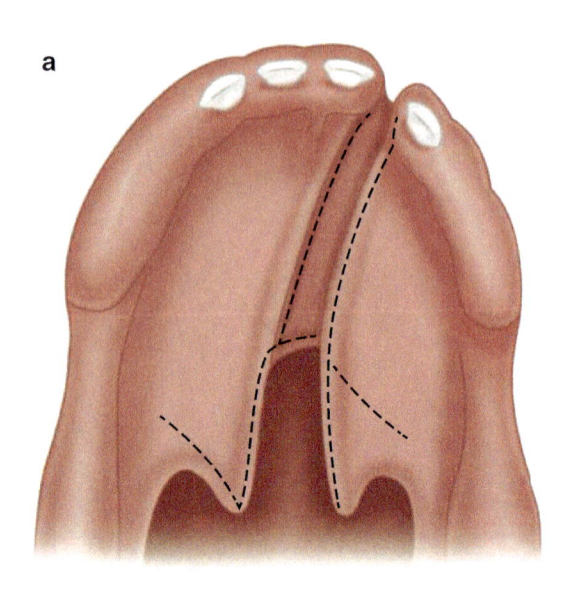

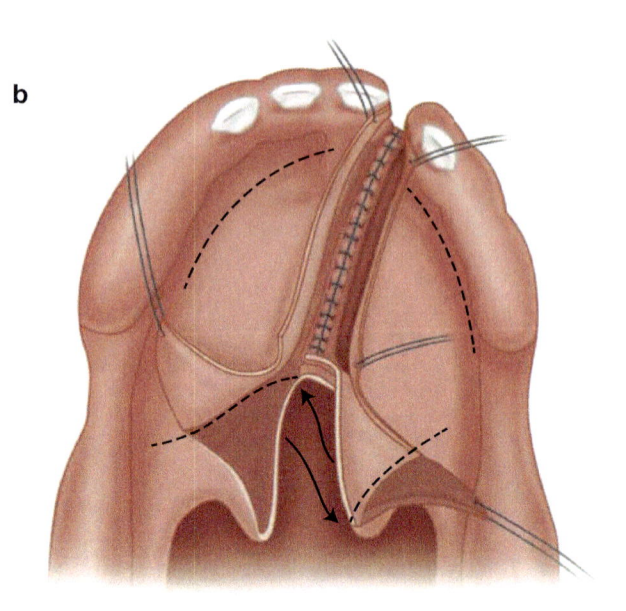

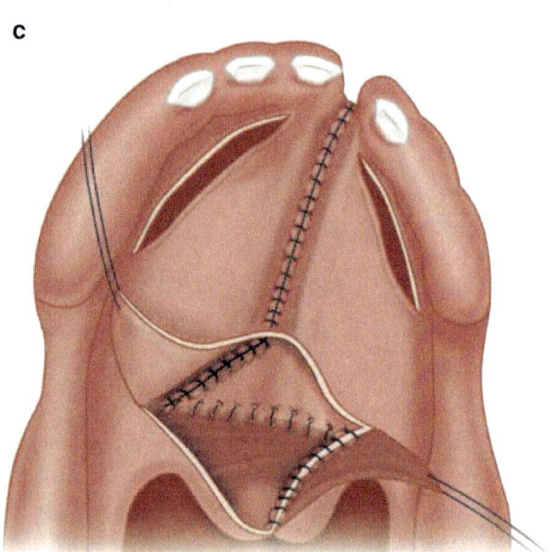

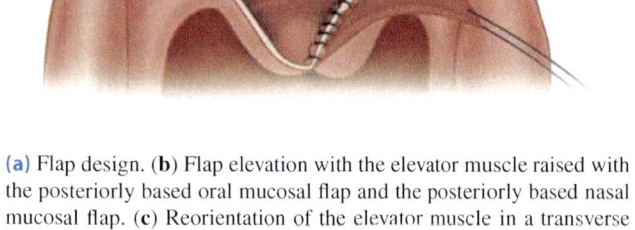

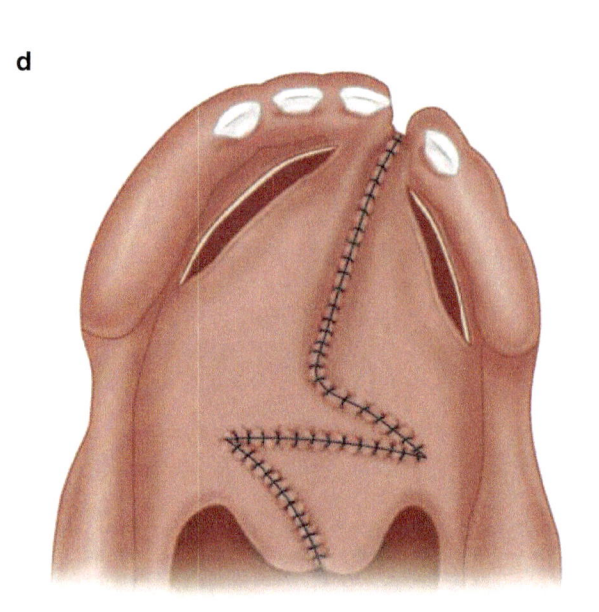

(a) Flap design. (b) Flap elevation with the elevator muscle raised with the posteriorly based oral mucosal flap and the posteriorly based nasal mucosal flap. (c) Reorientation of the elevator muscle in a transverse end-end or overlapping fashion. (d) The oral mucosal flaps interdigitate in a Z orientation opposite that of the nasal mucosal flaps. (May extend soft palate 5 mm but no more)

## 5.5 Palatal Surgery

### 5.5.1 Procedure

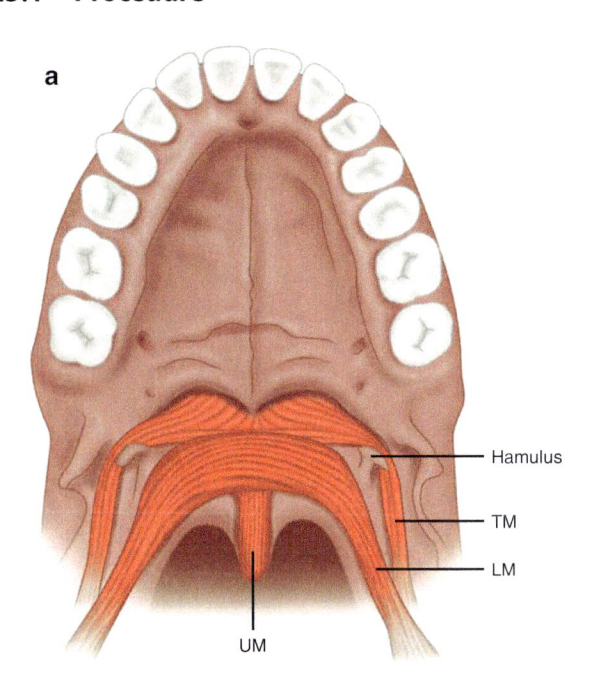

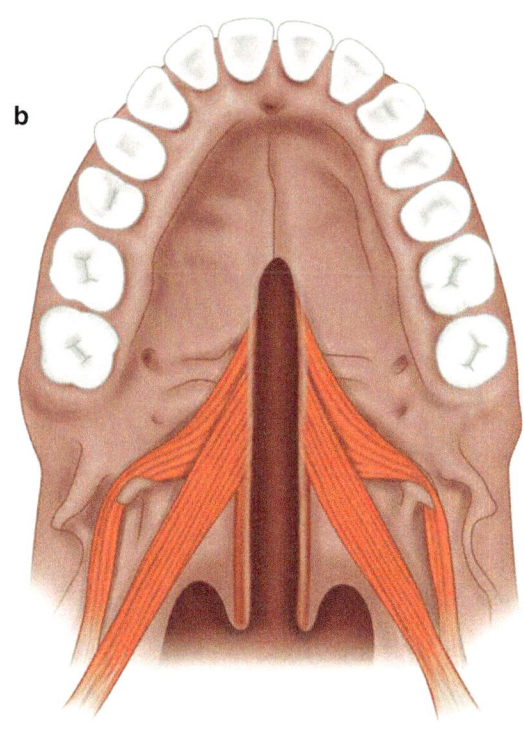

### 5.5.2 What Should Not Be Done

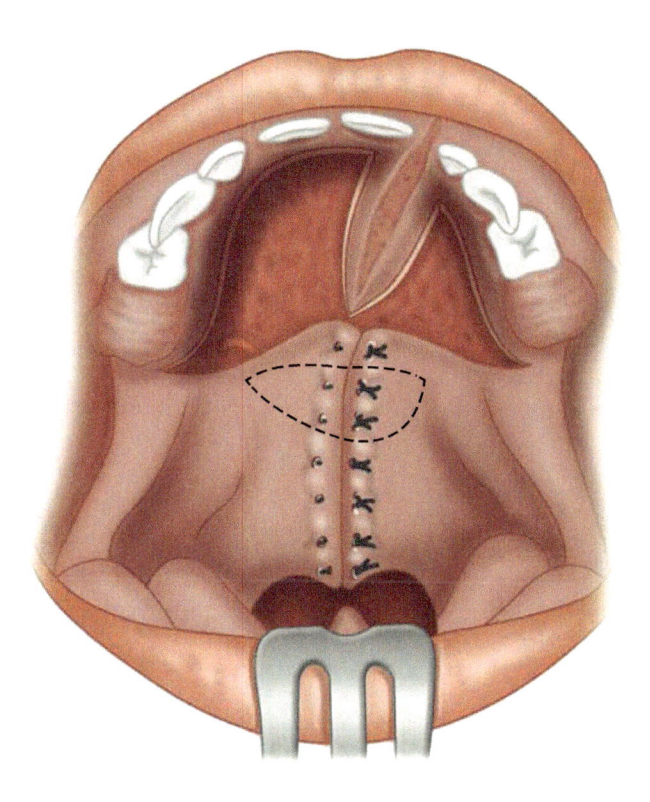

Island flap pushback procedure used to lengthen the soft palate at 16 months of age. This surgery involved leaving extensive areas of denuded bone anteriorly and laterally.

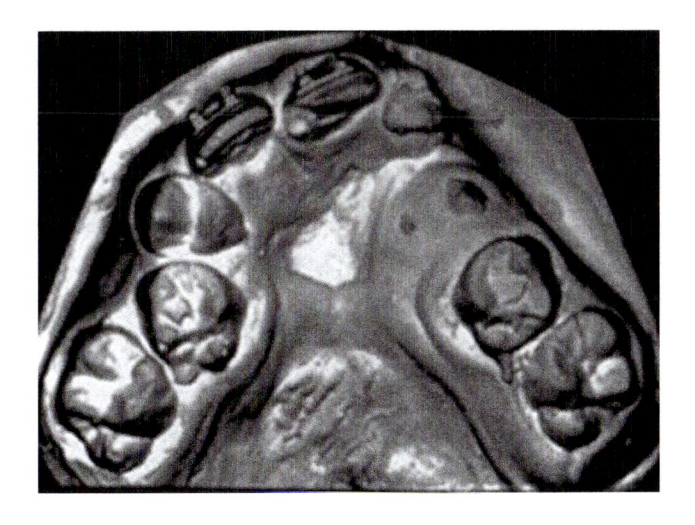

9 years of age. The severe scarring caused palatal deformation and retardation of growth as seen by the lack of arch length.

(a) Normal velar musculature. The levator palatini muscles produce a transverse sling in the middle third of the soft palate which is primarily responsible for posterior-superior movements during contraction. LM = levator palatini muscle. TM = tensor palatini muscle. UM = uvulus muscle. (b) Cleft velar musculature. In cleft deformities, the sling is disrupted with a longitudinal rather than a transverse orientation. The elevator and tensor muscles are inserted into the posterior and medial bony margins of the hard palate.

## 5.6 Osteotomies: To Close the Cleft Space—Not Acceptable

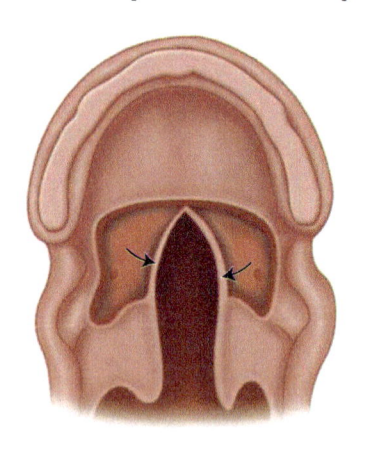

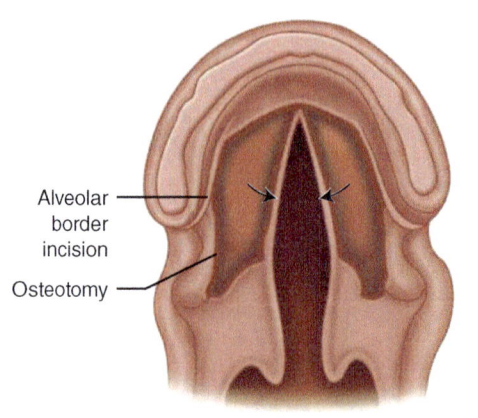

Alveolar border incision
Osteotomy

Incomplete cleft palate
Small bone defect
Osteotomy into notch

Incomplete V-shaped cleft palate
Osteotomy to anterior notch

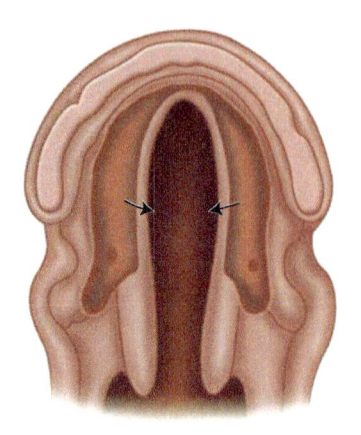

Incomplete horseshoe cleft palate
Osteotomy to tip of notch

Illustrations by Dr. Millard Jr. *Cleft Craft* 1980

## 5.6 Osteotomies: To Close the Cleft Space—Not Acceptable

### After Maxillary Surgery Advancement with Lefort I

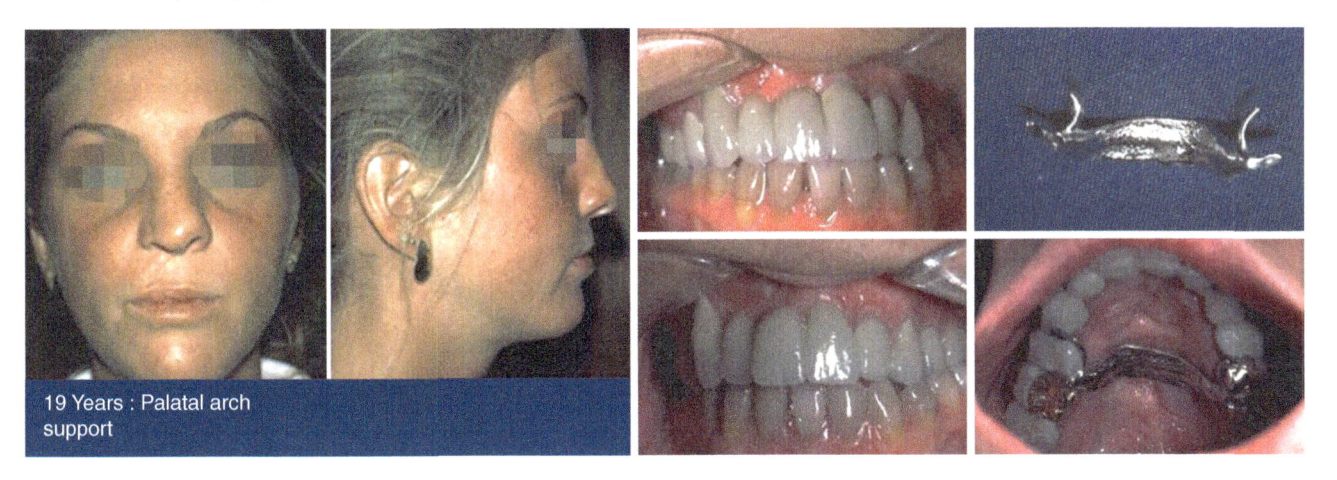

19 Years : Palatal arch support

Palatal bar to hold expansion

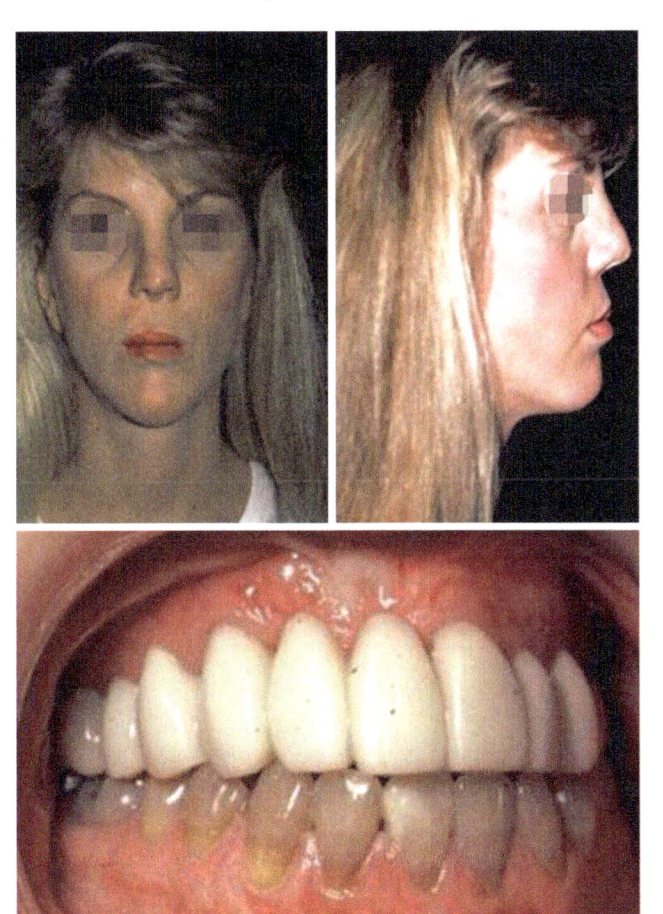

24 years: An extensive upper anterior fixed bridge

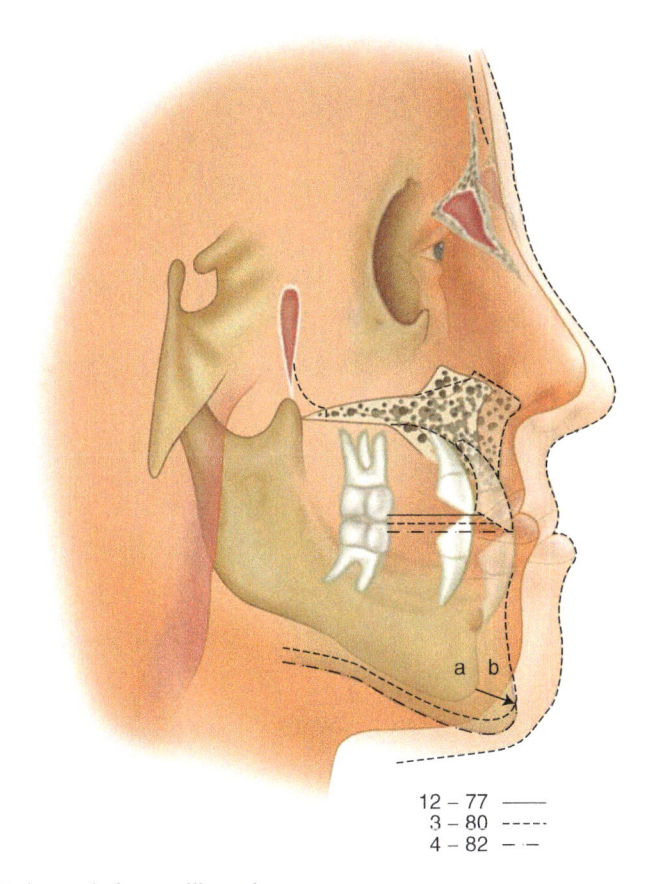

Before and after maxillary advancement

12 – 77 ———
3 – 80 - - - - -
4 – 82 – –

**Present-day treatment planning is an educated art**

Yet, clinical reports of various treatment protocols are usually anecdotal and supportive of the clinic's own treatment concepts.

**There is a failure studying palatal deformity due to:**

- Dearth of serial cleft palate casts.
- Lack of lateral cephalometric records.
- Lack of accurate palatal cast measuring devices to quantify growth changes and permit computer analysis.

# Orthodontics

Orthodontists are involved with the study and guidance of the growth and development of the face and dentition of the child with a cleft or craniofacial anomaly, from birth to maturity.

As a result of special training to become a developmental anatomist, their role includes recording the changing facial morphology and jaw function as a result of surgery and growth.

They provide orthodontic/orthopedic treatment, if necessary, and general expertise for consultation with all of the other members of the cleft and craniofacial team. Orthodontists are involved in one way or another with virtually all of the treatment procedures provided by all of the team's specialists.

Since palatal clefts vary in the extent of osteogenic and muscular deficiencies, surgeons should recognize that all clefts, although similarly classified, are not the same.

Therefore, each case requires differential diagnosis and treatment planning. What may be the treatment of choice for one patient may be totally different for another, even with the same cleft type at birth.

To assess changes during the course of general growth and treatment, head radiographs of the same individual taken at separate times are traced. The tracings are then superimposed to ascertain the changes that have occurred. A common method is to register the two tracings at the point sella with the sella-nasion lines superimposed.

This method provides a gross overview of changes in the dentofacial complex and in soft tissue but is useful only in evaluating what has already occurred. In this material, we also use the Coben superimposition procedure (basion horizontal) because it more accurately reflects actual craniofacial growth direction.

The use of "landmark" or baseline images associated to the basicranium is to show the composite results of facial growth. This can provide meaningful information because it is the enlargement of the face relative to the cranial base that is being evaluated. In the child, further growth changes in the anterior part of the cranial base slow considerably at about 5–6 years of age, whereas facial growth continues actively through adolescence or beyond. Comparing the relative growth between these two regions, rather than simply focusing on a single fixed point, provides clinically useful information when cephalometrically evaluated.

All orthodontic records of cephaloradiographs, panorex, facial and intraoral photographs, and dental casts of both jaws should be taken at least once in each of the subsequent age periods and even more frequently if orthognathic surgery has been performed to monitor the treatment protocol and outcome.

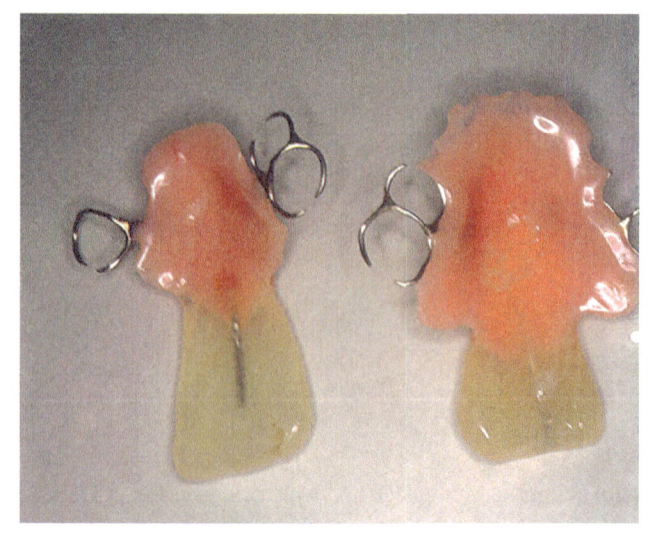

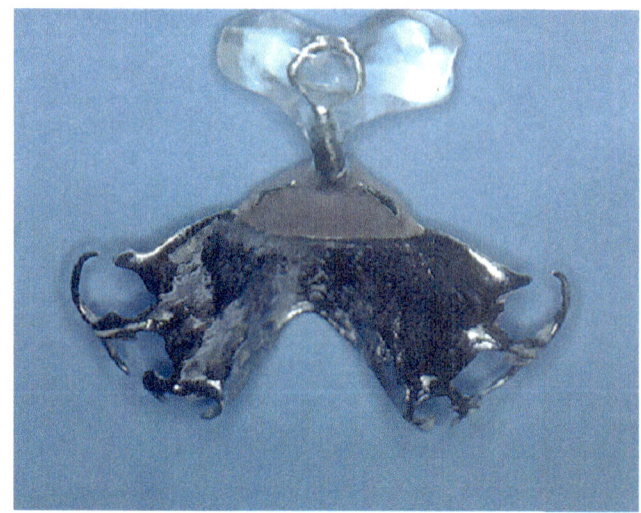

A temporary acrylic resin speech appliance with wire clasps and full palatal coverage designed for a 4-year-old child.

A permanent cast-gold speech appliance with partial palatal coverage for an adult with no missing teeth.

## 6.1 Speech Aid Appliances

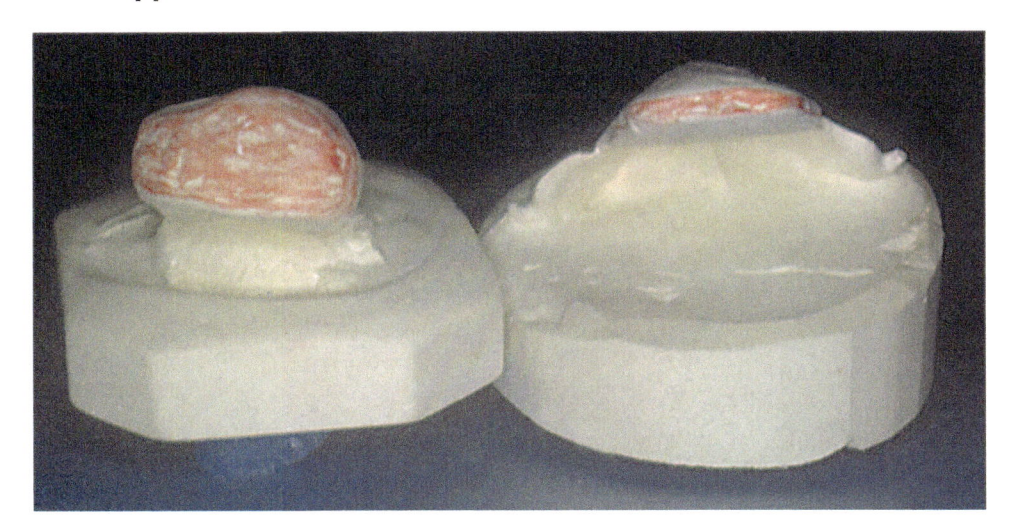

As a result of our studies, we have concluded that the inferior-superior dimensions of the speech bulb do not have a significant effect on speech quality as long as the bulb is properly placed to facilitate good velopharyngeal closure. This dimension was reduced to one quarter of its original size, as shown in cast made during fitting for one patient, without apparent effect on nasal resonance.

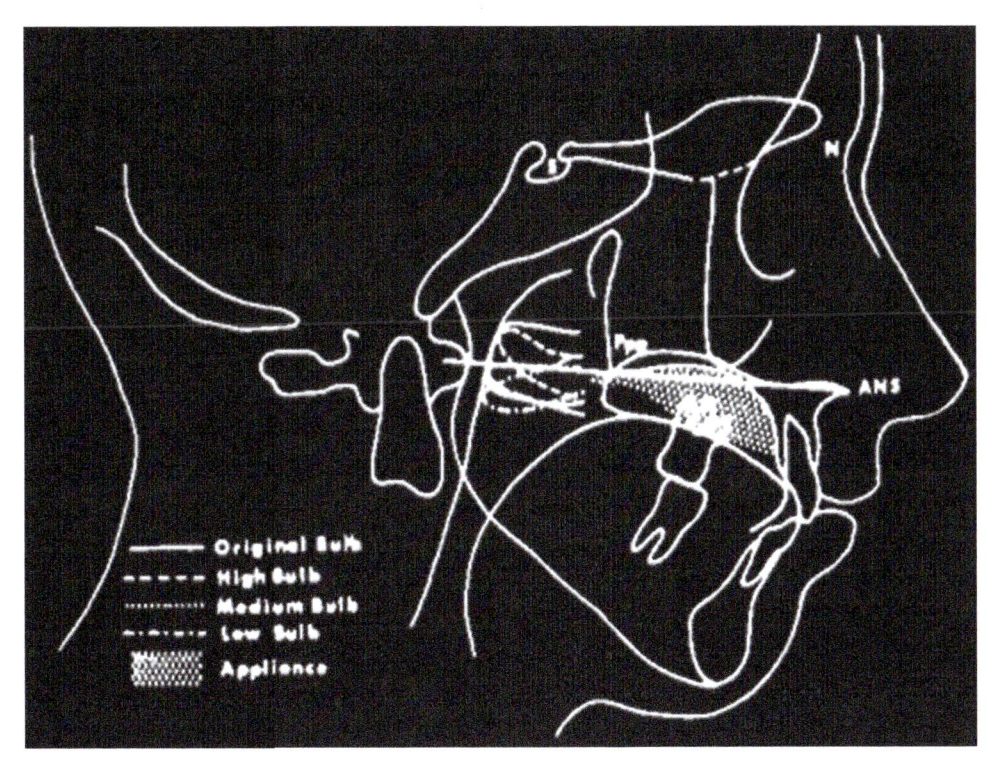

Superimposed tracing of the original speech bulb and various experimental speech bulbs. The palatal plane was used as a plane of reference along with posterior pharyngeal wall activity, muscle bulge, or Passavant's pad. The posterior nasal spine (PNS), absent in cleft palate subjects, is called *posterior palatal point* (Ppp) and represents the most posterior point of the remnants of the palatal shelves as shown in the lateral cephalometric film. Median position was judged best.

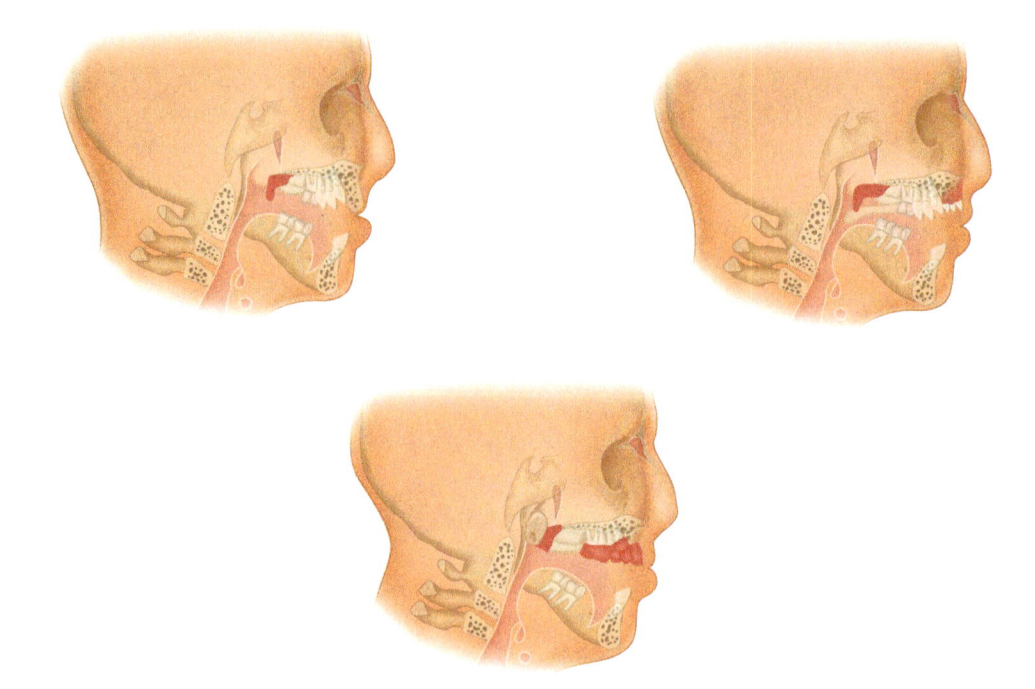

The pharyngeal bulb in a speech appliance is viewed in cross section in place in the nasopharynx. (**a**) Incompetent velopharyngeal closure. (**b**) Inadequate nasopharyngeal bulb. (**c**) Pharyngeal bulb (pharyngeal extension) is well positioned within the nasal chamber (Courtesy *J.D. Subtelny*)

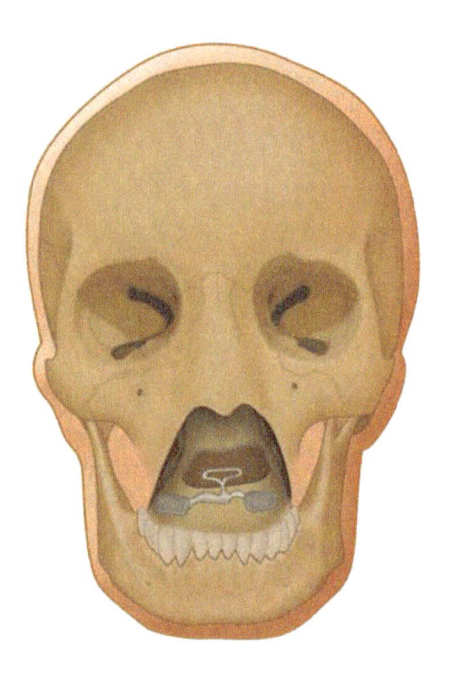

REST

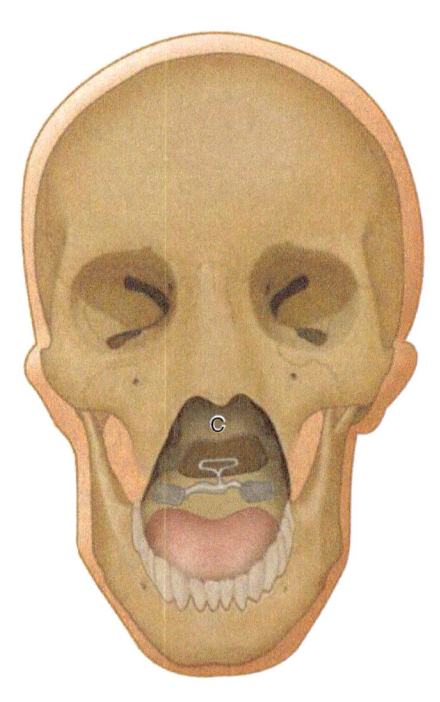

Phonation of [a]

**The pharyngeal bulb on a speech aid appliance is viewed in the nasopharynx**. At rest (left), a lateral space on either side of the bulb allows for normal nasal drippings to enter the mouth. When phonating /a/, the lateral pharyngeal walls make contact with the speech bulb, reducing nasal airflow. (Courtesy of *J.D. Subtelny*)

## 6.1 Speech Aid Appliances

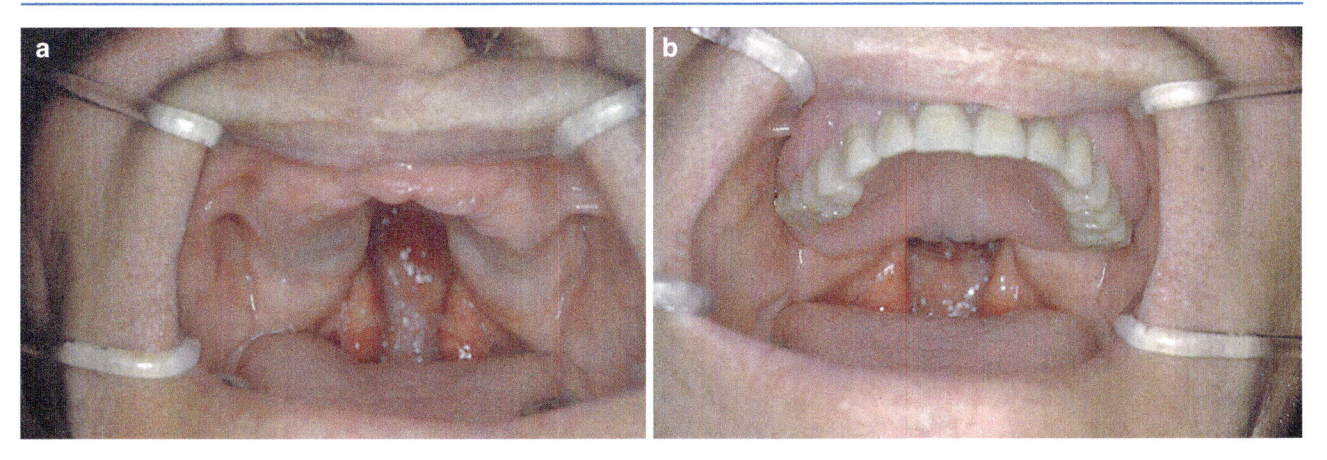

(a) An edentulous patient with an unoperated cleft of the soft and hard palate that affects the retention and support of the prosthesis. At no time should a patient with a cleft, especially an unoperated cleft, be rendered edentulous. (b) The completed prosthetic speech appliance in position

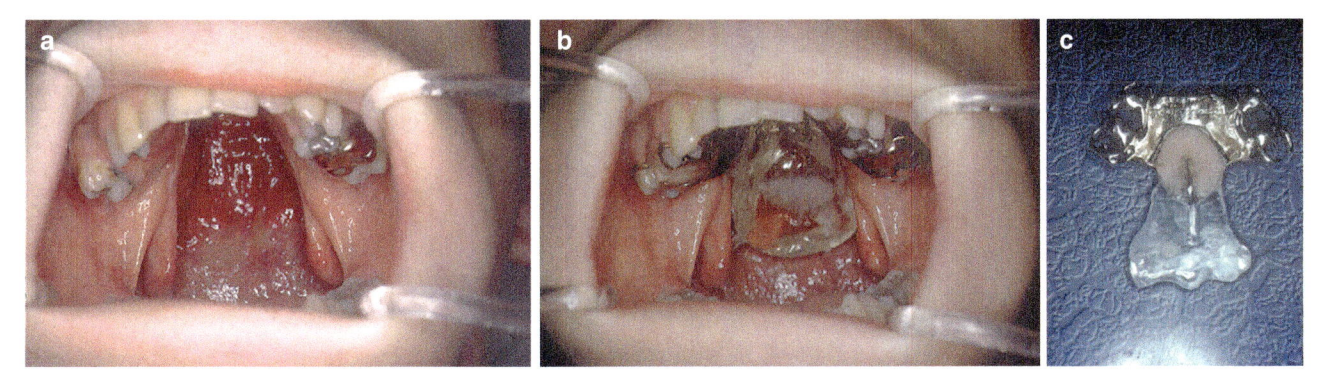

(a) Patient at the age of 16 years with a very wide cleft of the soft and hard palate. (b) Prosthetic speech aid in position. Note that the pharyngeal section of the speech aid is placed directly over the posterior and lateral pharyngeal wall muscle activities. (c) Oral view of prosthetic speech aid. The utilization of second bicuspids and first and second molars for retention and support will prevent this prosthesis from dislodging into the nasal cavity during swallowing and speaking

| Surgery | |
|---|---|
| 3 months | Lip adhesion (and soft palate) united |
| 6 months | Rotation advancement |
| 18–24 months | Hard and soft palate closure using a Von Langenbeck + modified vomer flap |
| 8 years | Secondary alveolar bone graft |

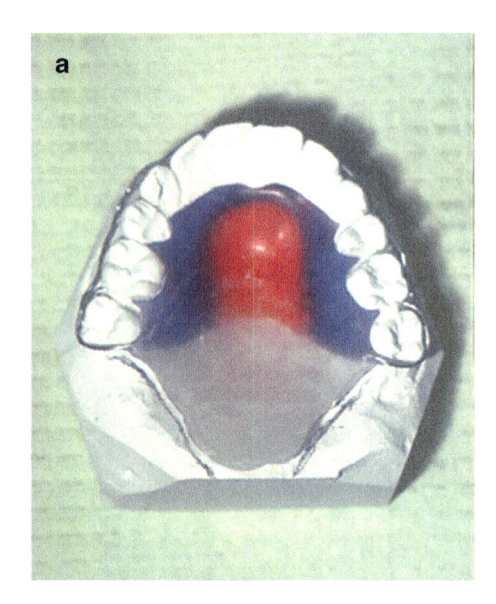

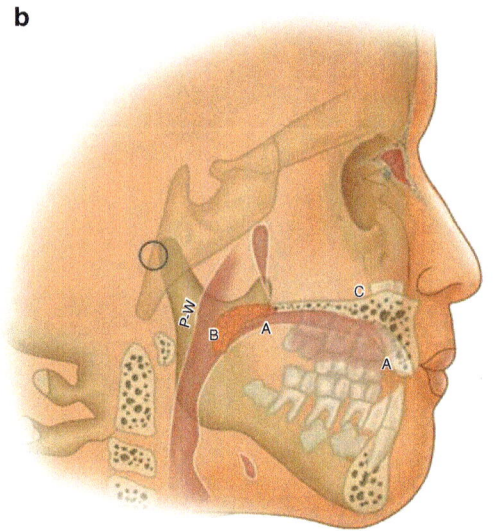

A palatal lift appliance. It is used to improve velopharyngeal function by improving velar muscle action. (**a**) The appliance on a dental model. The velar extension extends posteriorly to the uvula. (**b**) Lateral cephalometric tracing showing the appliance (A-A′) velar section making contact up to the uvula (B). The appliance can be well stabilized by using orthodontic bands with soldered buccal shelves to establish undercuts for the clasps

| Orthodontics | |
|---|---|
| 4–5 years | Buccal crossbite correction with fixed appliance |
| 7–8 years | Anterior teeth correction with secondary alveolar bone grafts |
| 11+ years | Standard orthodontics retention |

## 6.1 Speech Aid Appliances

Palatal closure at 1–5 Mos. Using Von Langenbeck procedure resulting in good occlusion

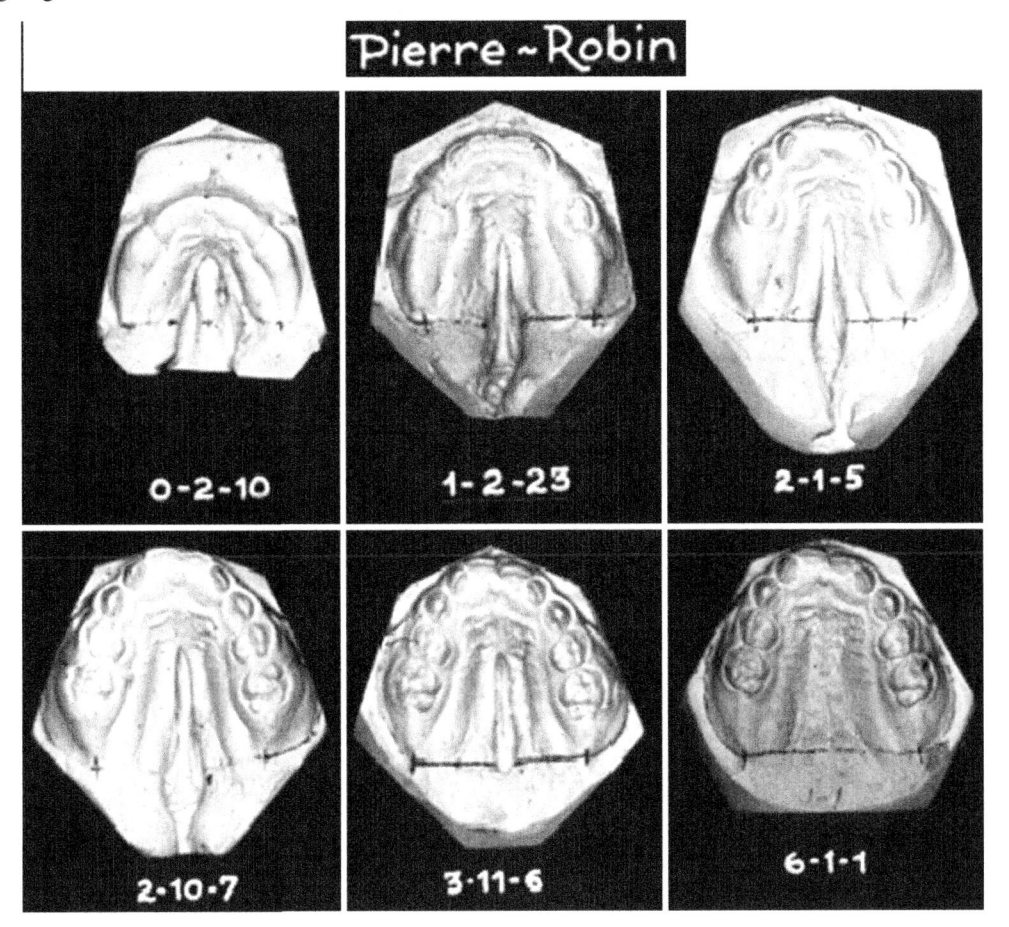

Gradual reduction in cleft space due to growth of the palatal segments joining the cleft. The degree of scarring is not growth inhibiting or distort the palatal stage.

Case: JDeG AN-92

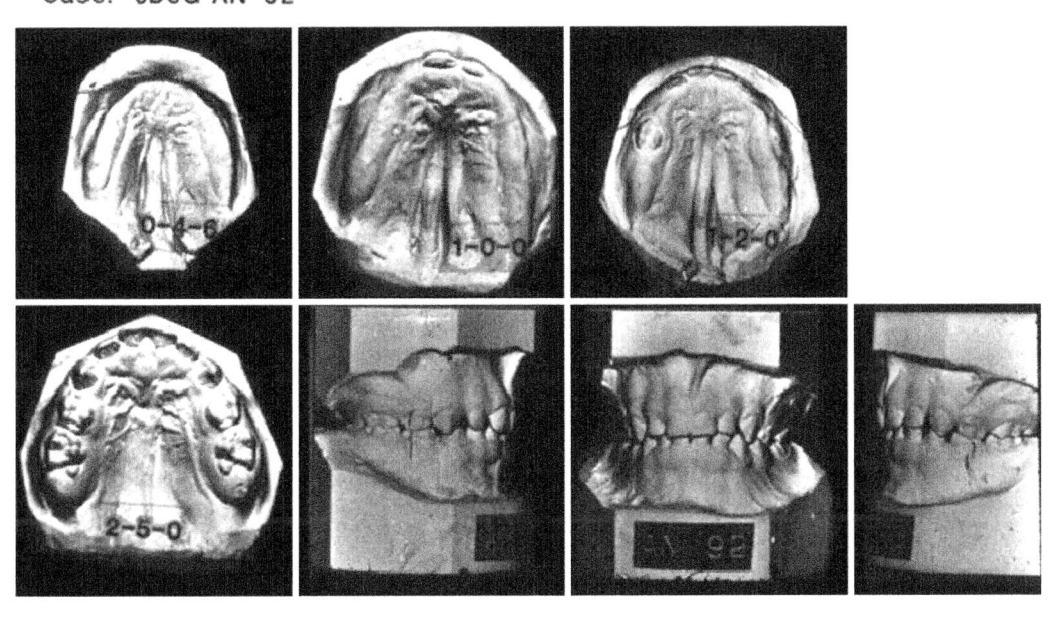

# Complete Unilateral Cleft Lip and Palate Conservative Treatment (Non-presurgical Orthopedics)

Information relating to the complexities of embryonic facial development is fundamental to an understanding of the growth potential of the primary and secondary palate. Studies (Slavkin (21), Ross and Johnston (22)) have shown that the facial mesenchyme, which give rise to the skeletal and connective tissues and ordinate form neural crest cells which undergo extensive migration and interaction.

Coalescence of the facial processes results in the formation of the primary palate, which constitutes the initial separation between the oral and nasal cavities and eventually gives rise to portions of the upper lip and anterior maxilla. The exact mechanism of primary palate formation is not clear; however, most clefts of the primary palate appear to result from variable degrees of mesenchymal deficiency in the facial processes.

The suspected causes of clefts of the secondary palate are also varied. Slavkin reports several possible mechanisms: (a) Tongue Resistance: The tongue, arched up between the shelves, delays palatal shelf movement. (b) Decreased Shelf Forces: Although there are no examples of mutant genes that can cause this, there are many teratogens for which this mechanism has been invoked. (c) Failure to Fuse: This possible cause may be associated with delayed shelf reorientation. (d) Narrow Shelves: This theory suggests that the palatal shelves can move normally enough to reach the horizontal, yet still be too narrow to reach each other. This condition could be explained by a more generalized deficiency of facial mesenchyme reaching the palatal area, making the hard palatal shelves and soft palate inherently smaller.

The causative factor has important clinical implications, since it suggests that in some unilateral clefts of the lip and palate, the size of the cleft space may be disproportionately very large and variable in shape, more so than found in other clefts of the secondary palate. Also, the velum in this cleft type may be deficient in muscular tissue and predispose the child to velopharyngeal incompetency. Thus, it would be helpful to be able to identify infants with skeleto-muscular deficiencies at an early age (within the first two years of age),

in order to customize the cleft closure procedure to enhance proper speech production as well as normal palatal growth and development. Obviously, a cleft child with palatal tissue deficiency will have a different set of problems than the cleft palate patient with palatal tissue adequacy and a cleft caused by failure of proper shelf force or failure to fuse.

## 7.1 The Neonatal Palatal Form in Complete Clefts of the Lip and Palate: The Effect of Muscle Forces

The normal palatal arch form is determined by the result of the compressive forces of the orbicularis oris-buccinator–superior constrictor pharyngeal muscle ring counteracted by the protrusive and expansive forces of the tongue. However, in the presence of clefts of the lip and palate, aberrant muscle forces cause the lip and palatal segments to be distorted in space. The lateral pull of the cleft lip musculature, coupled with the pushing forces of the tongue fitting within the cleft space, are unrestrained space, are unrestrained (Subtelny).

## 7.2 The Influence of Surgery on Palatal Form and Growth

When the cleft lip and/or soft palate are united, the cleft muscular forces are reversed, causing the laterally displaced skeletal structures to move medially into a more normal form. The increased tension of the facial musculature may vary in degree among patients and with the type of lip surgery employed. No attempt is made to measure these forces for the same reasons it is not measured in standard orthodontic treatment planning. It is impractical! The role of lip tension on palatal arch, however, does deserve further investigation.

Our observations over the last 25 years have shown that after the lip is united, the displaced palatal segments will assume various relationships to each other (some may overlap, others may butt-join, or not touch due to premature contact of the inferior turbinate on the cleft side with the nasal septum). Here seems to be a correlation of arch form, seen in the deciduous dentition, with the size and geometric relationship of the palatal segments at birth. For example, in complete unilateral clefts of the lip and palate, after the lip is united, those cases with a very long non-cleft palatal segment, and a short cleft segment coupled with a small anterior cleft space, are more likely to have their segments overlap. Other variables such as steepness of the palatal slopes and the adequacy of tissue need to be considered as well. Only through a more extensive three-dimensional analysis of the newborn's geometric palatal form, will the clinician gain the necessary insight into the possible effects of surgery on the palate's subsequent form, the occlusion in the absence of orthodontics.

Slaughter et al. (23) first recognized the many anatomic variations within similarly classified clefts and suggested that there are great differences in the amount and quality of palatal tissue among the several cleft types and even within any one type. The amount of palatal tissue relative to the cleft size increases with growth, but the timing of this growth might vary from one child to another. In some patients, the greatest proportional changes occur earlier than in other patients so that cleft space closure may have to be delayed to avoid growth inhibiting scar tissue; such finds were verified by Pruzansky (24) (25), Pruzansky and Lis (26), Pruzansky and Aduss (27), Pruzansky et al. (28), Lis et al. (29), and Berkowitz (15). Krogman et al. (30) observed post-operative "catch-up-growth" in almost every case and concluded that by the age of six years, the maxillary complex is usually acceptably normal. Berkowitz et al. (31) and Mapes et al. (32) further reported that after palate surgery there may be a growth lag from 14 to 20 months, but subsequently the processes of orderly development may take over, and the rate of growth may even accelerate.

## 7.3 Complete Unilateral Cleft Lip and Palate

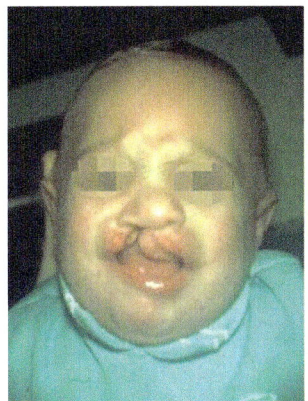

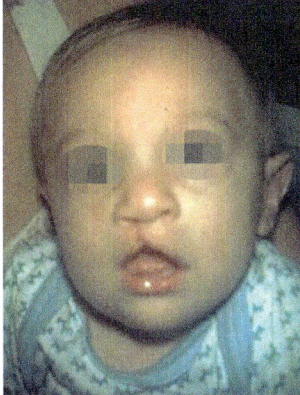

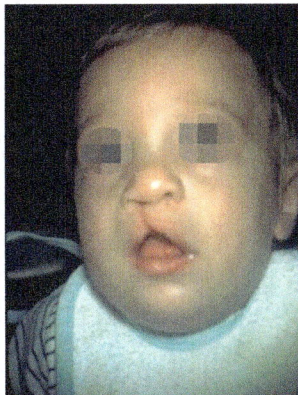

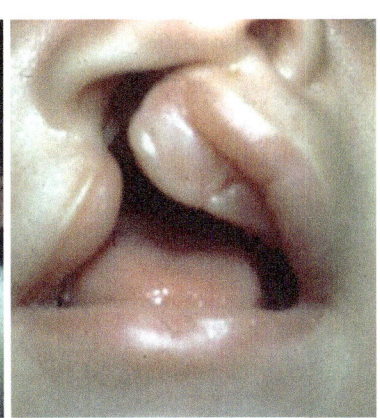

After lip adhesion

Alveolar molding led to premaxillary retrusion and closure of the cleft lateral incisor space. Orthodontics opens this space and advancing the incisors creates an ideal overbite and overjet. The cuspid was positioned into the missing lateral incisor space. No lateral incisor was present in the cleft.

## 7.4 Complete Unilateral Cleft Lip and Palate

Excessive scaring diminished maxillary development. Palate was closed with Island flap. Lefort I advancement was necessary which led to the exfoliation of the labial bony plate as the result of the loss of lateral and posterior alveolar area blood supply.

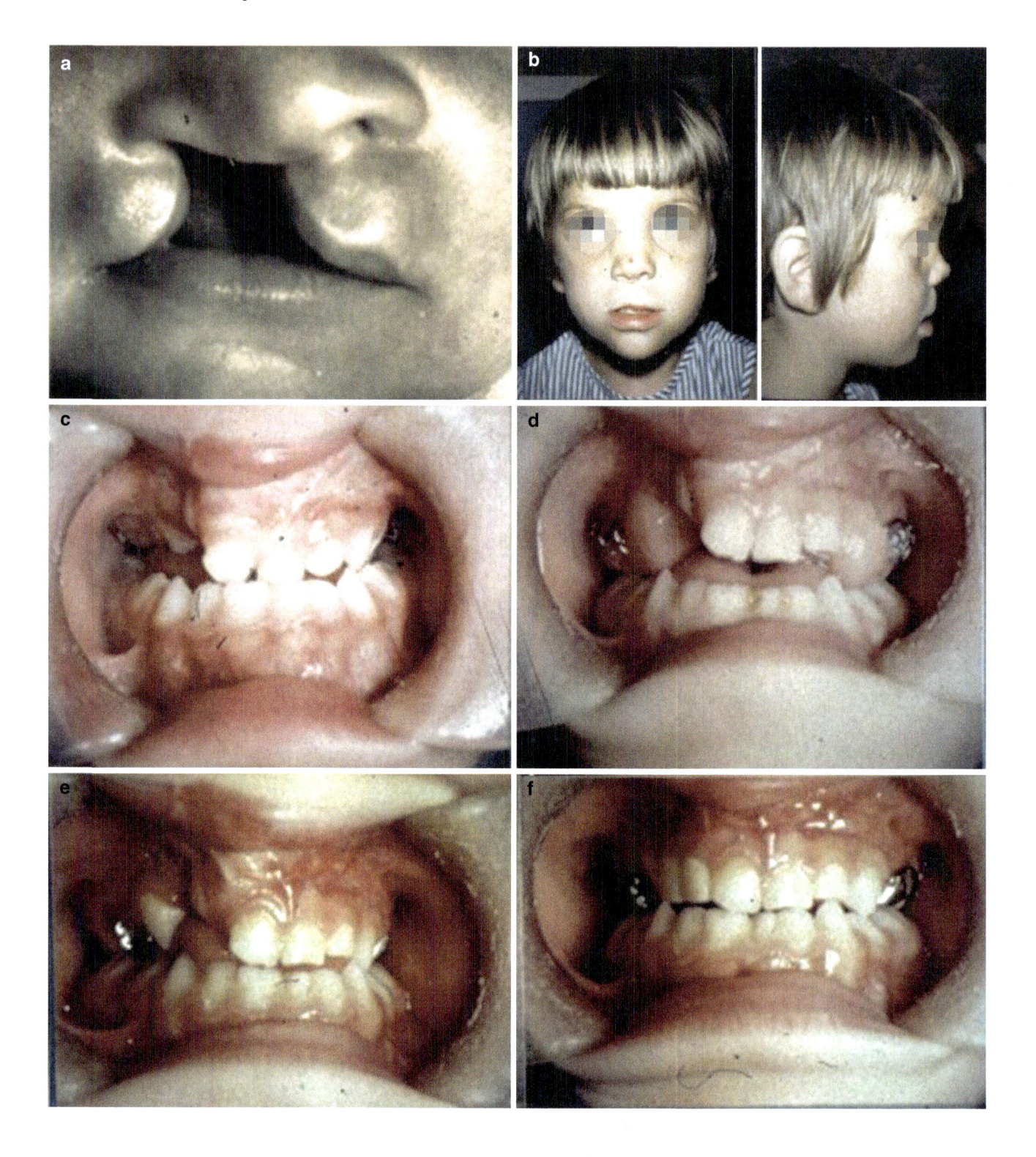

## 7.5 Two Cases Which Show Severe Overlap of Palatal Segments with Closure of the Cleft Space

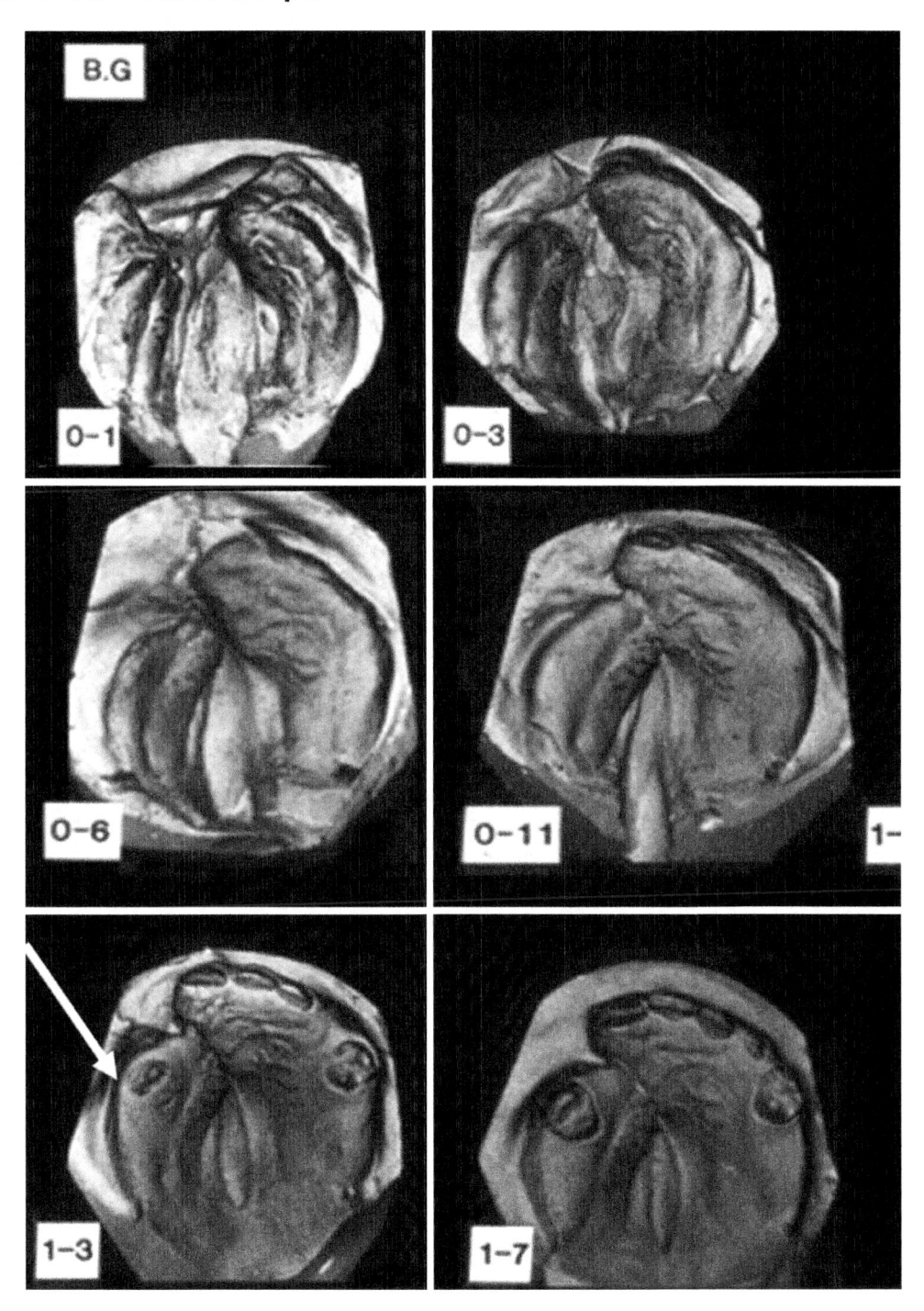

Lip Adhesion with Velar Repair

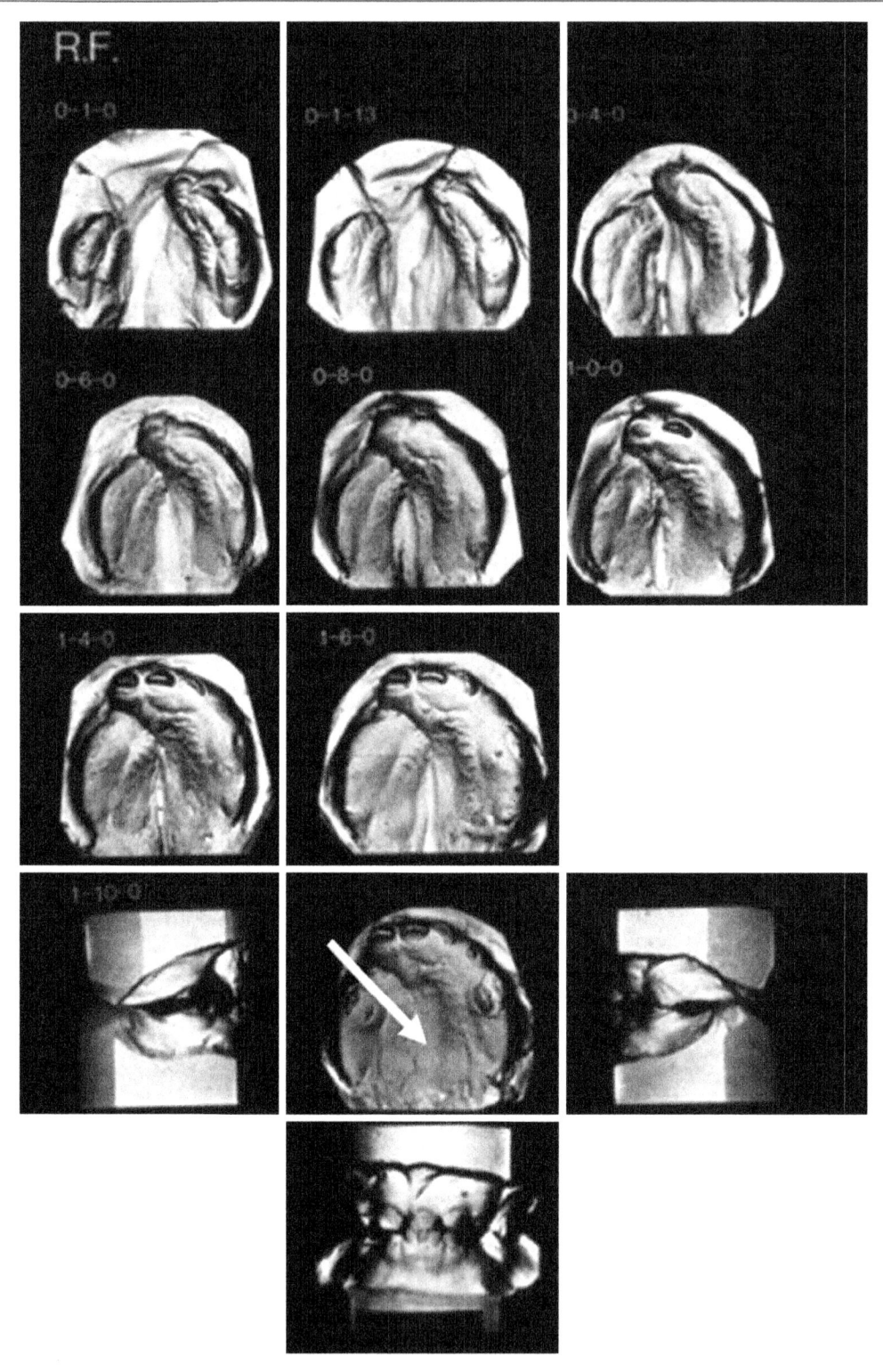

Lip Adhesion Only.

## 7.6 CASE SM XX-53

### 7.6.1 Serial Cases Show Changes in Palatal Relationships

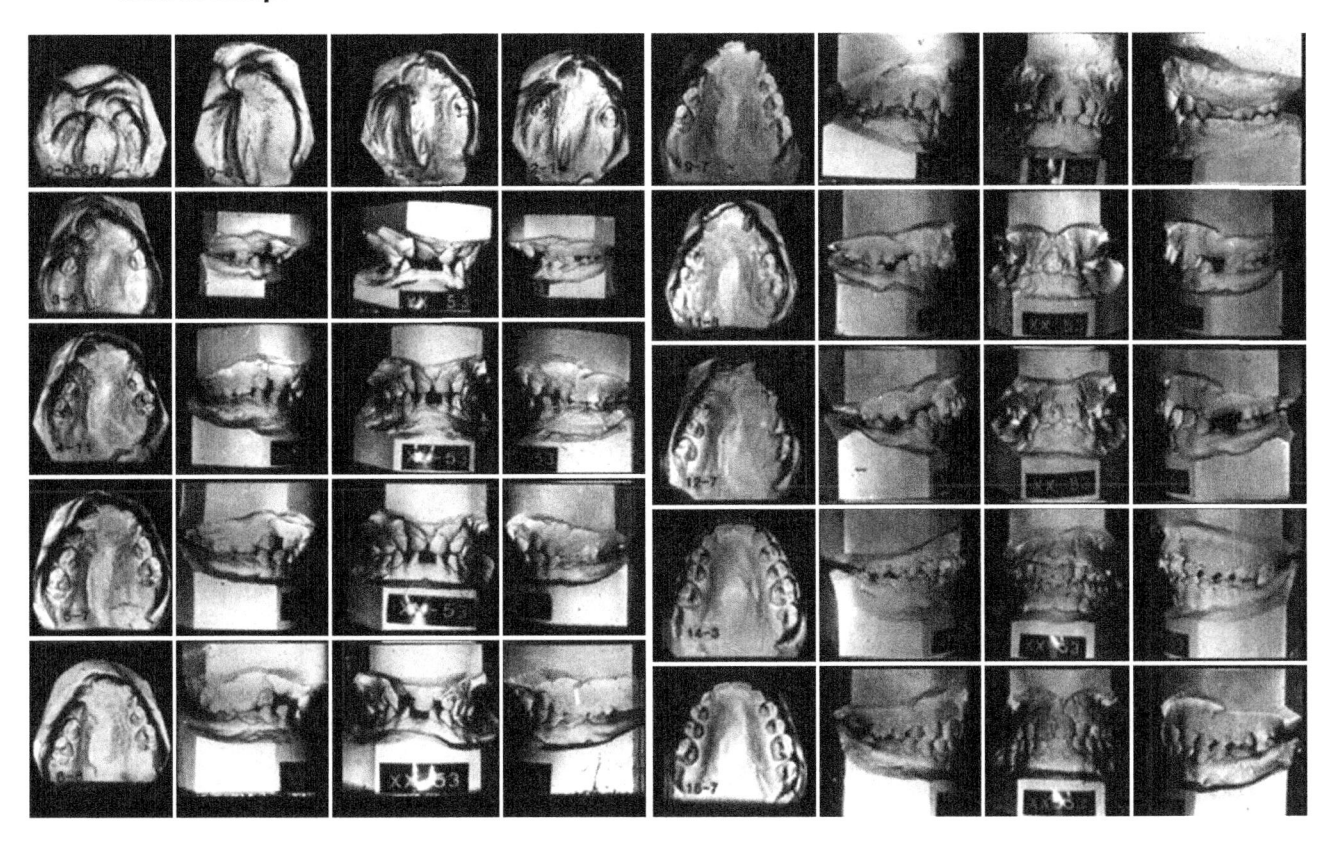

### 7.6.1.1 Patient with Isolated Cleft Palate

Notice that the relative size of the cleft space diminishes as the palate grows and increases in size.

The palate was closed with the Von Langenbeck at 18 months. The excellent occlusion reflects diminished palatal scarring. The patient had excellent speech.

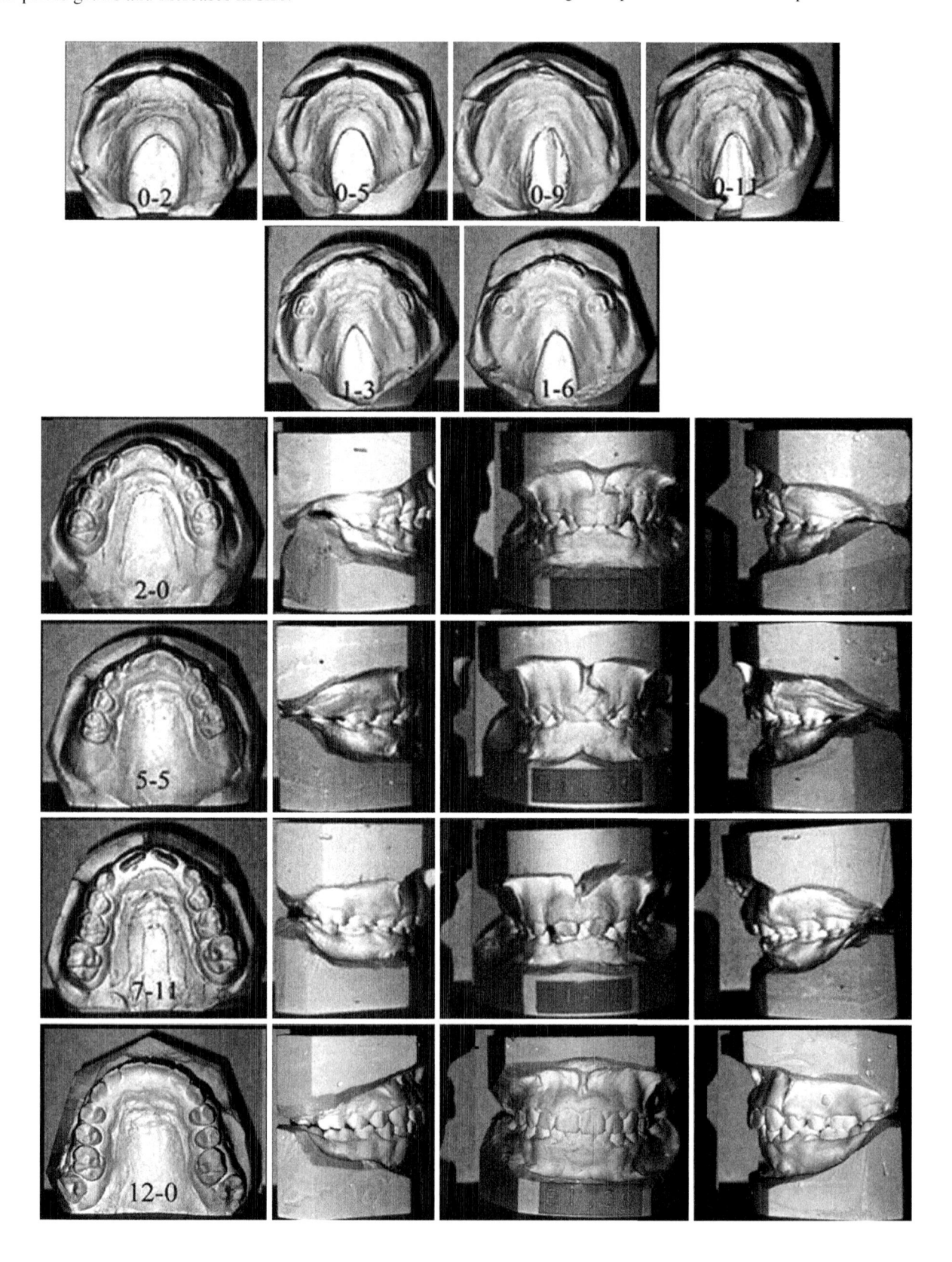

## 7.6 CASE SM XX-53

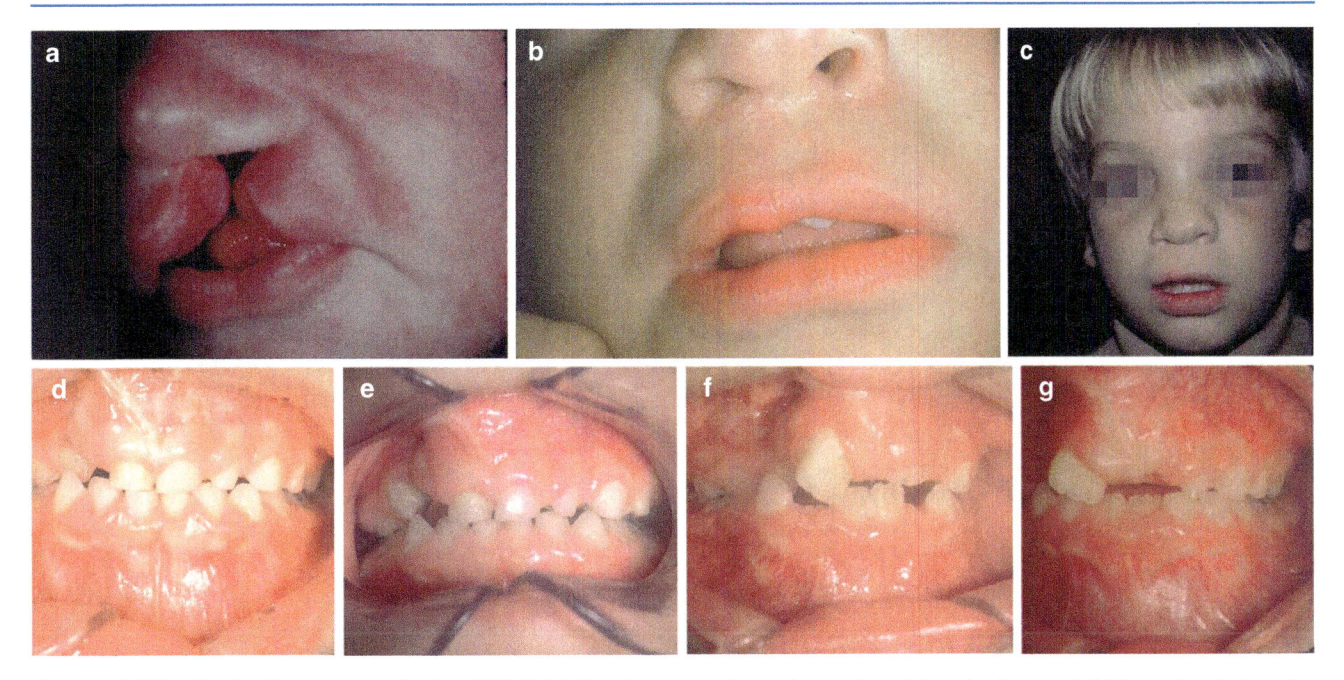

**Case BB (WW–62). Maxillary protraction in a UCLP.** (a) Complete unilateral cleft lip and palate. (b) and (c) Lip and nose after surgery. (d) Cuspid crossbite of the lateral cleft segment at 5 years of age due to mesioangular rotation of the palatal segment. (e) Buccal occlusion after expansion using a quad helix expander. (f) and (g) 6 years of age. Note relapse of cuspid crossbite due to failure of using a palatal arch retainer.

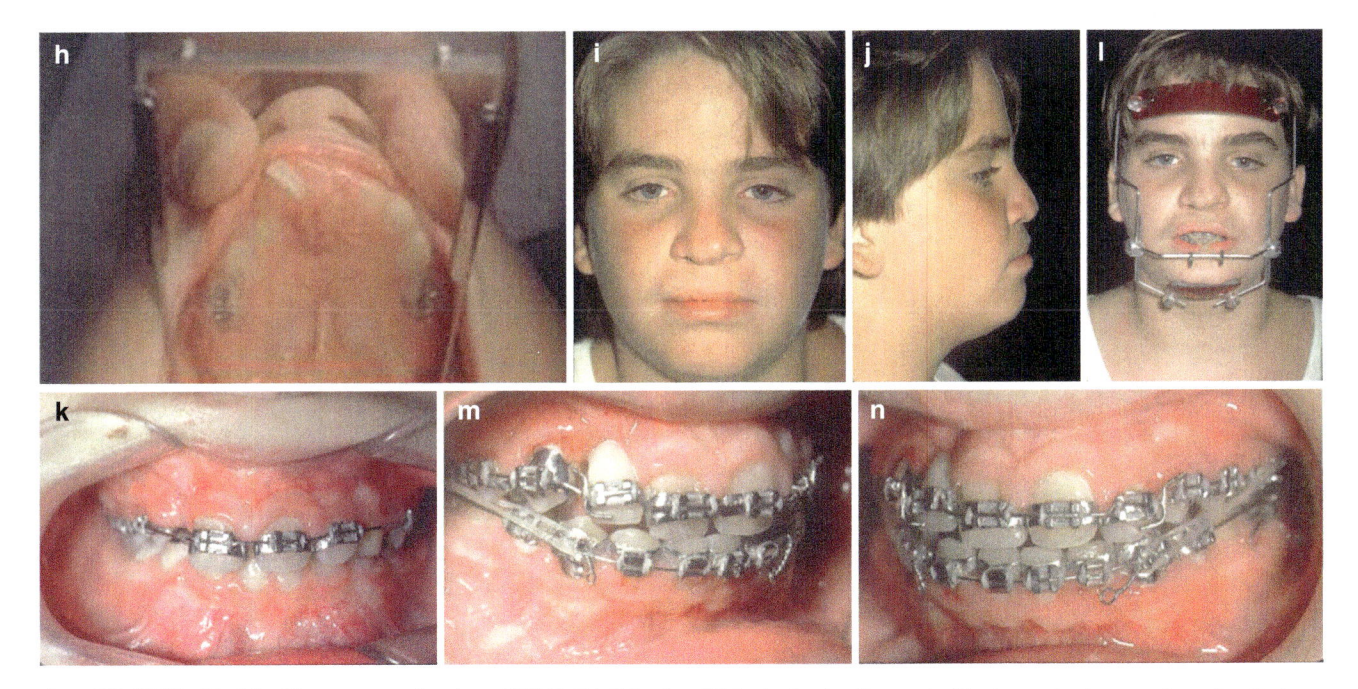

**Case BB (WW–62). Maxillary protraction in a UCLP.** (h) Palatal view showing good arch form. (i) and (j). Facial photographs at 8 years. (k) Orthodontic alignment of incisors prior to secondary alveolar bone graft. (l) Protraction facial mask with elastics (m) and (n).

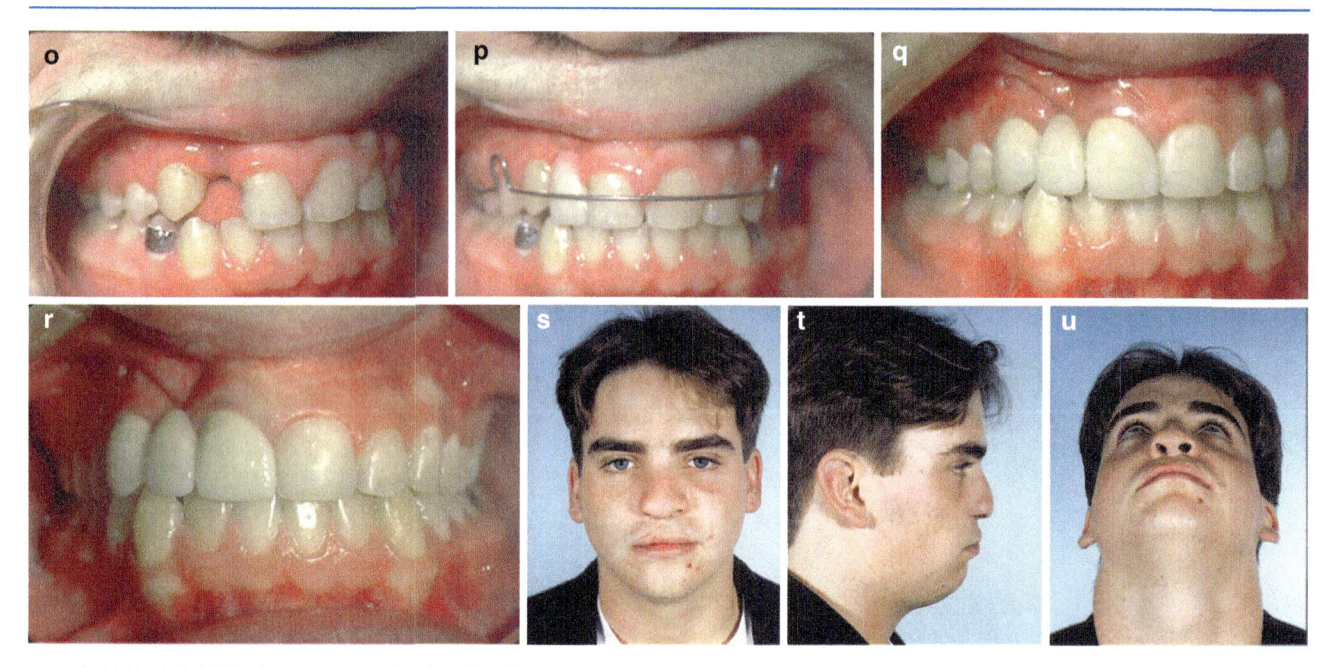

**Case BB (WW–62). Maxillary protraction in a UCLP.** Class III elastics used to maintain tension at circummaxillary suture during the time not wearing protraction forces. (**o**) Occlusion after orthopedic-orthodontic forces. Lateral incisor space regained. (**p**) Removable retainer with lateral incisor pontic. Fig 10–3. (**q**) and (**r**) Fixed bridge at 18 years of age replacing missing lateral incisor and stabilizing maxillary arch form (**s**), (**t**), and (**u**).

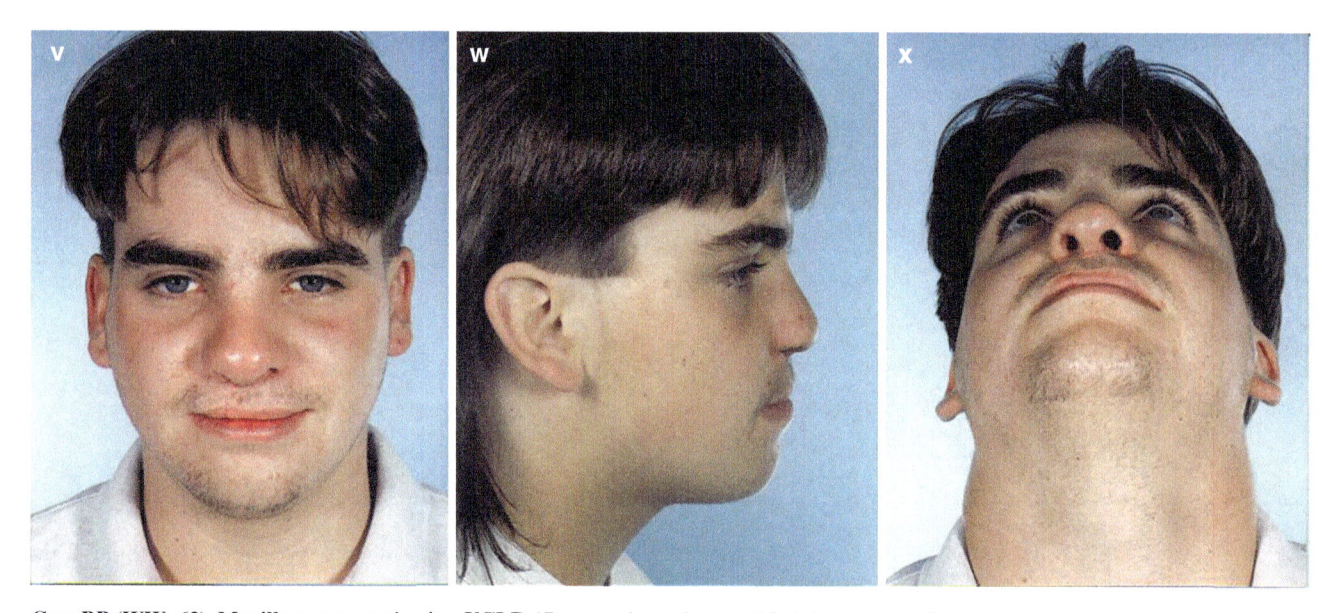

**Case BB (WW–62). Maxillary protraction in a UCLP.** 17 years prior to nose–lip revision. (**v**), (**w**), and (**x**). Facial photos at 19 years, showing good facial symmetry after revision.

## 7.6 CASE SM XX-53

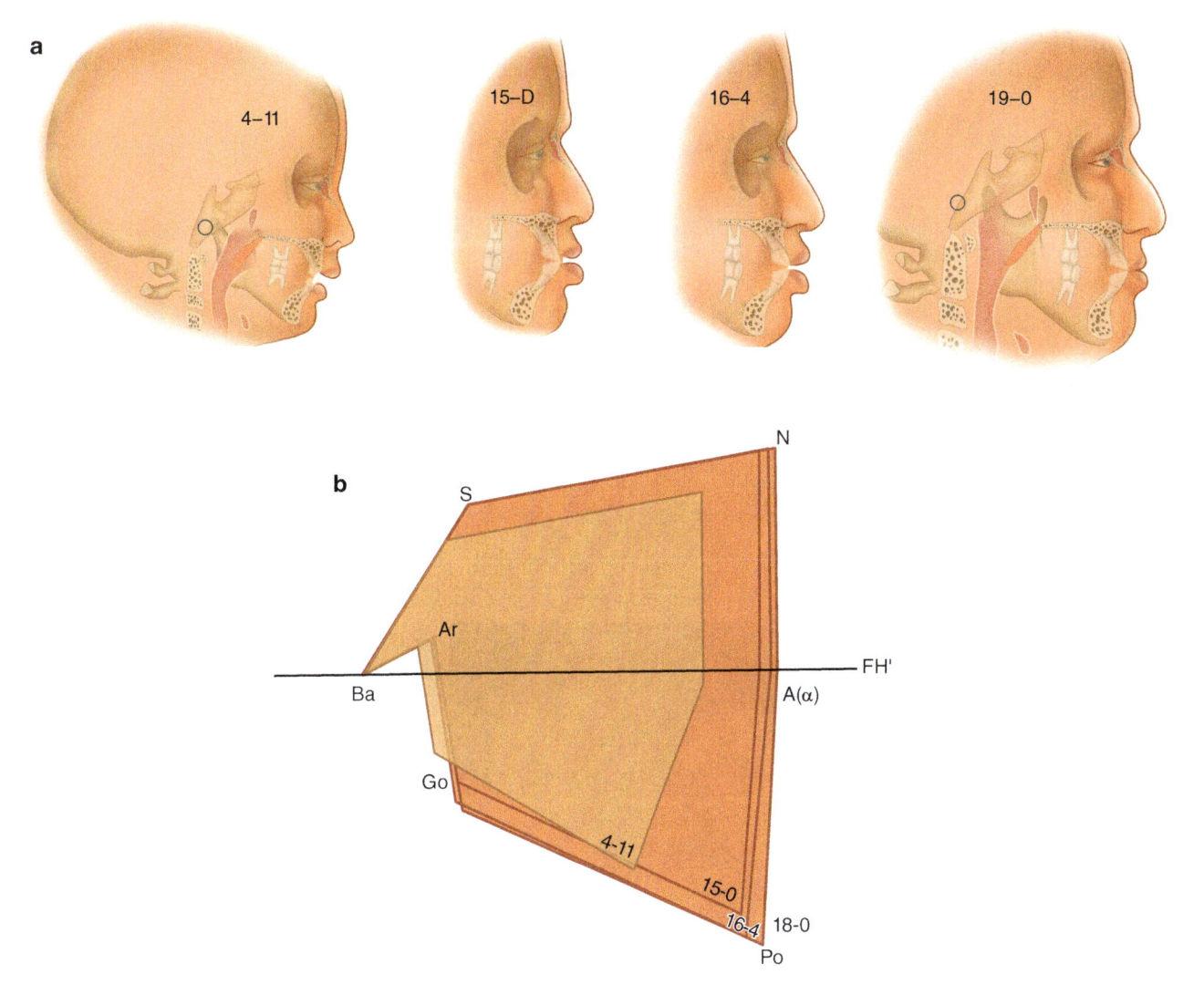

(**a**) Lateral cephalometric tracings and superimposed polygons (Basion Horizontal Method) for case BB (WW-62) show an excellent facial growth pattern. (**b**) The midfacial growth increment between 15 to 16.3 years, when the protraction facial mast was used, increased midfacial protrusion to a greater degree than would have occurred normally—enough movement to avoid surgery.

62　　7　Complete Unilateral Cleft Lip and Palate Conservative Treatment (Non-presurgical Orthopedics)

## 7.7 Complete Unilateral Cleft Lip and Palate

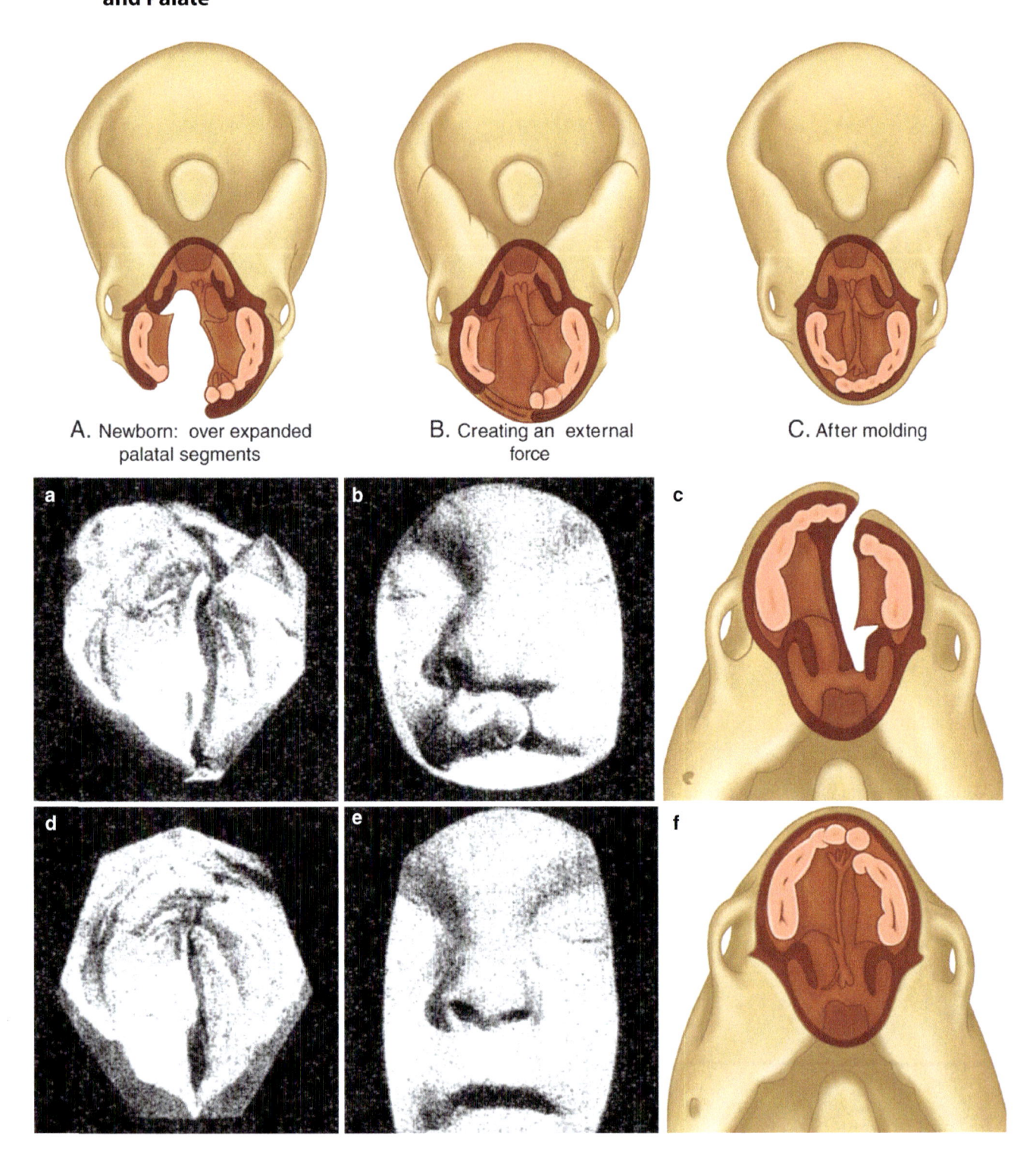

A. Newborn: over expanded palatal segments

B. Creating an external force

C. After molding

## 7.8 Molding Geometric Relationships

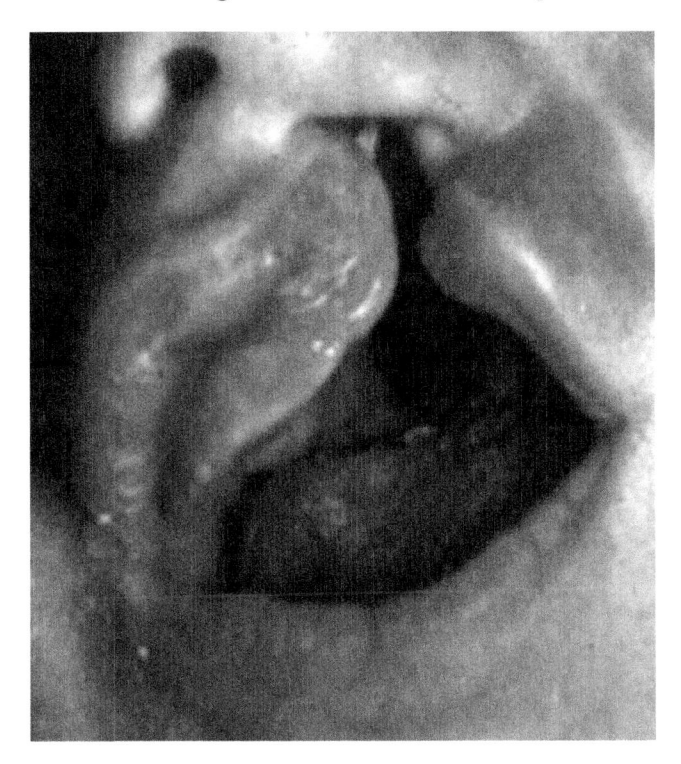

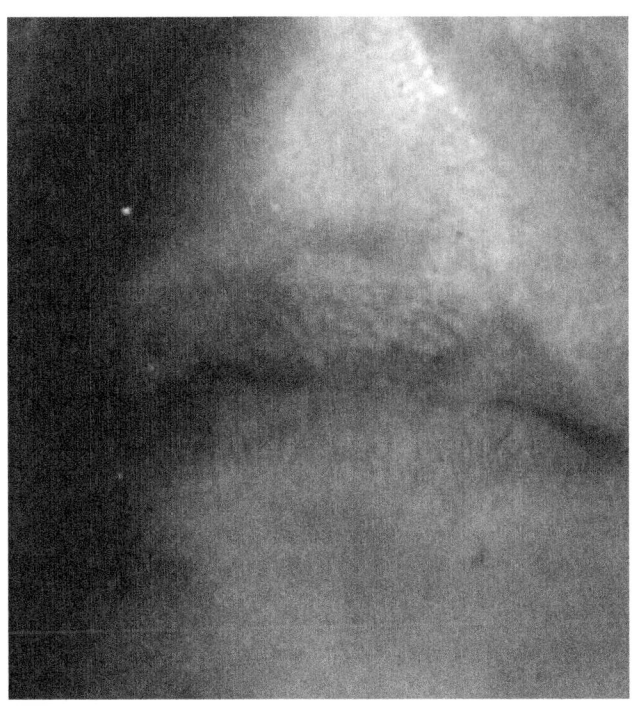

Newborn

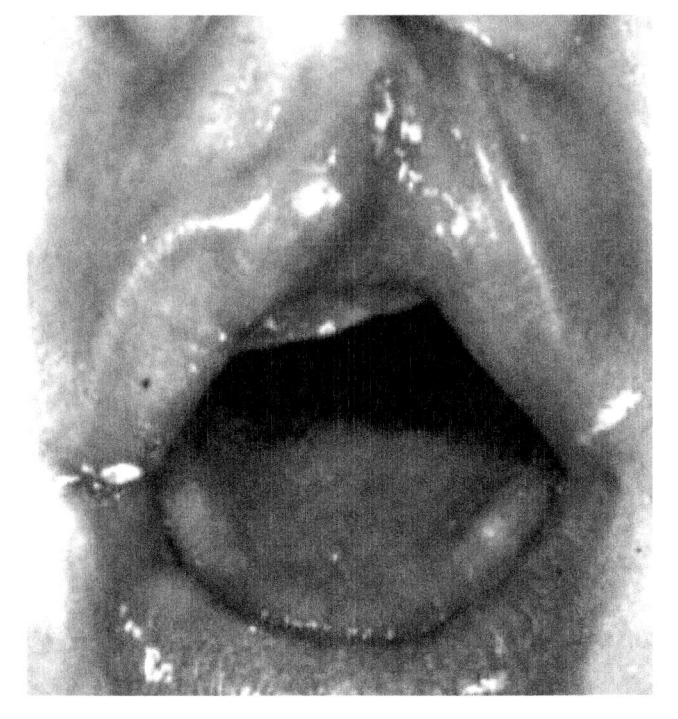

6 Months—definitive lip surgery

3 Months—lip adhesion

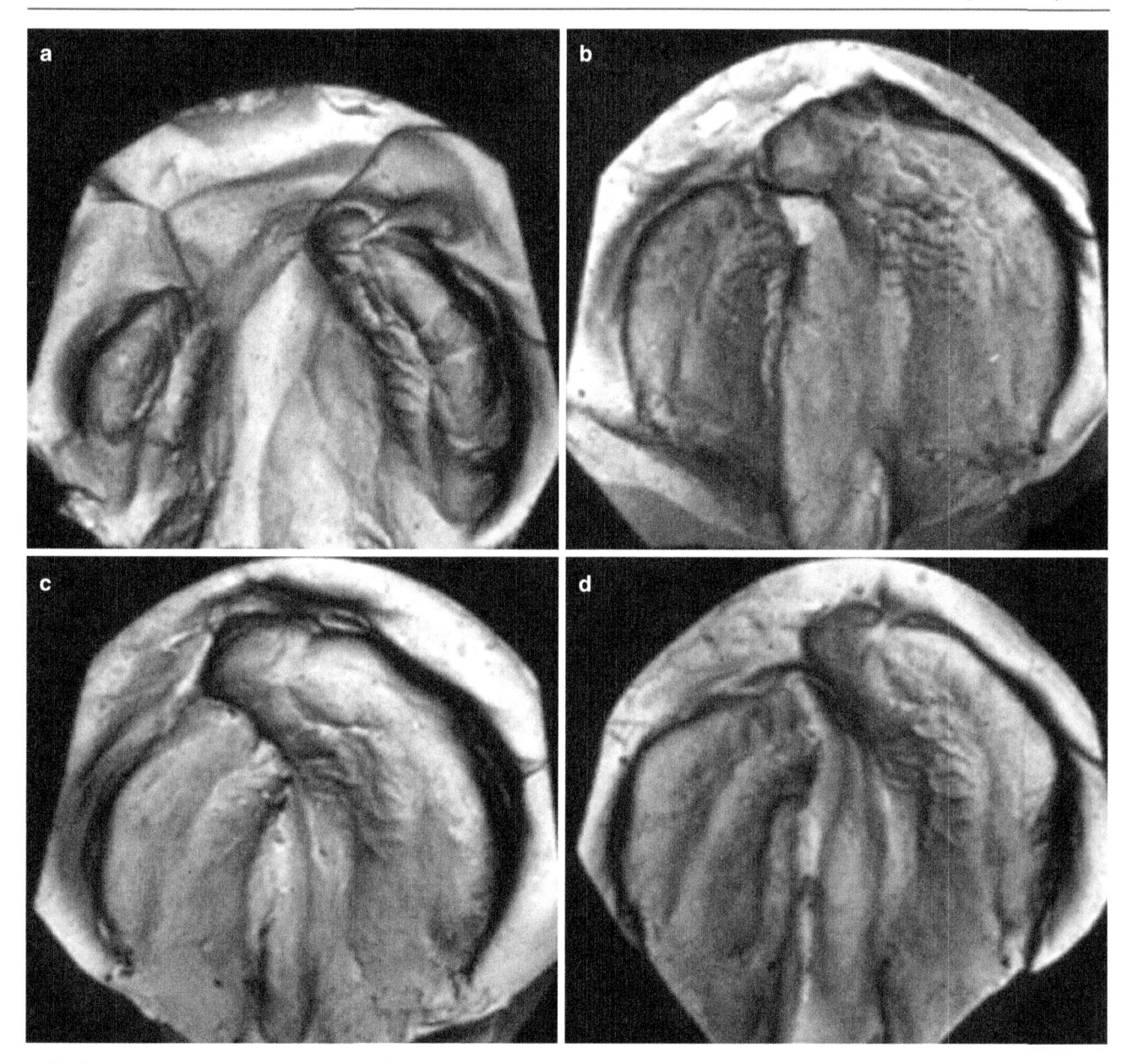

A. Newborn: overexpanded segments. B. Butt joint relationships. C. Overlapping segments. D. No contact of segments

7.8 Molding Geometric Relationships

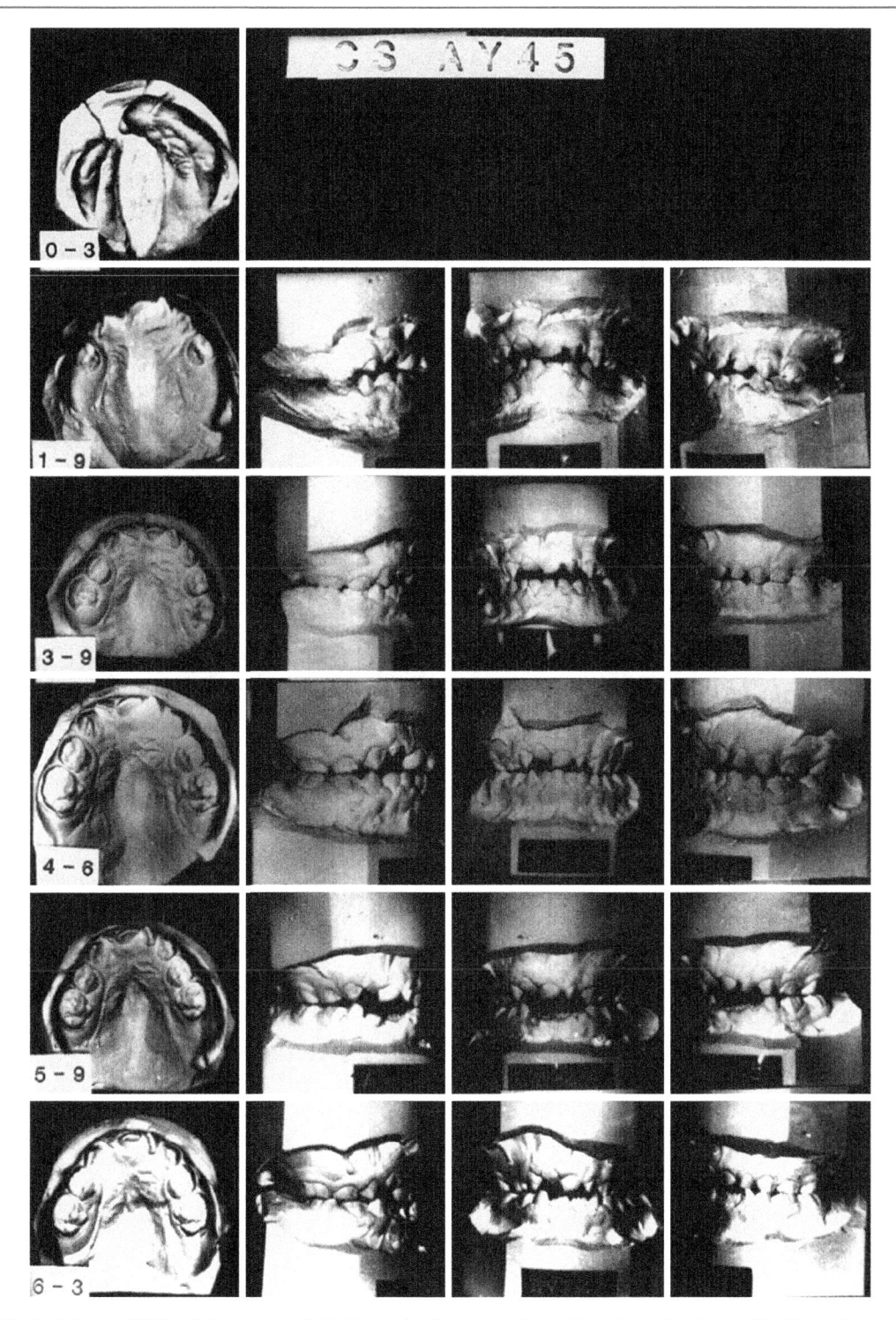

**Case CS (AY-45).** Serial casts CUCLP. **0-3**. newborn. **1-9**. After palatal segments were brought together with PSOT. Teeth are slightly in an open bite and in a tip-to-tip relationship. The right lateral incisor space is closed. **3-9, 4-6, 5-9, 6-3** Show the same occlusal relationship

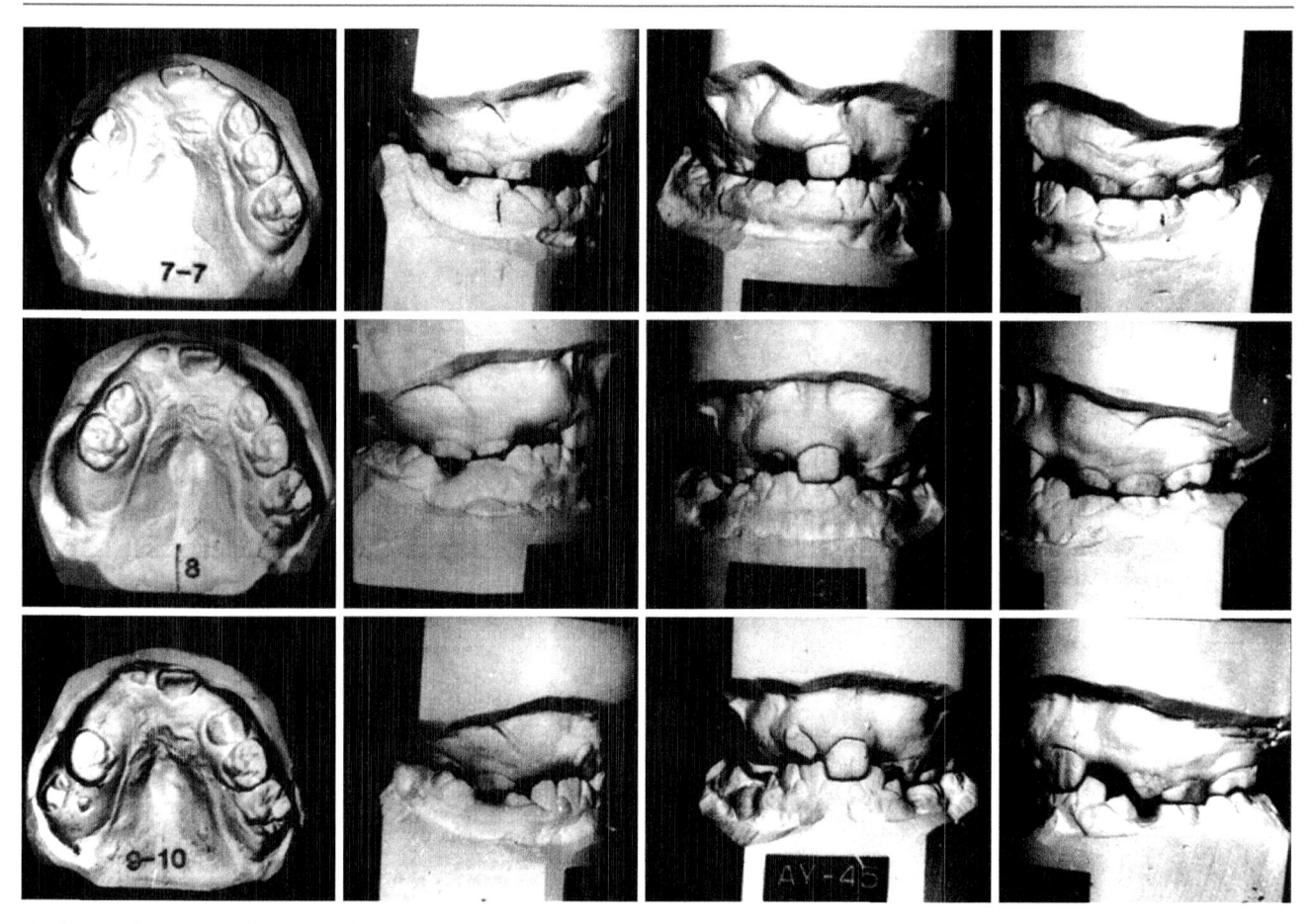

At **7 years, 8 years, and 9 years**: The permanent central incisors are erupting in good overjet-overbite relationship; however, the closure of the right lateral incisor space is due to the maxillary incisors being displaced to the left.

## 7.9 Berkowitz Palatal Growth Analysis

Palatal casts superimposed on rugae and registered on vomer point.

There is good three dimensional growth, most of which occurs posteriorly to accommodate the developing molars. Very little growth occurs anteriorly in all cases whether unilateral or bilateral clefts.

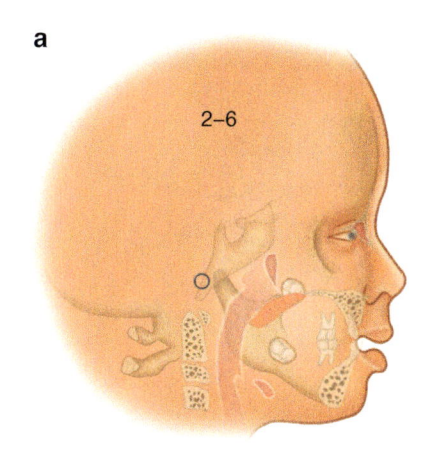

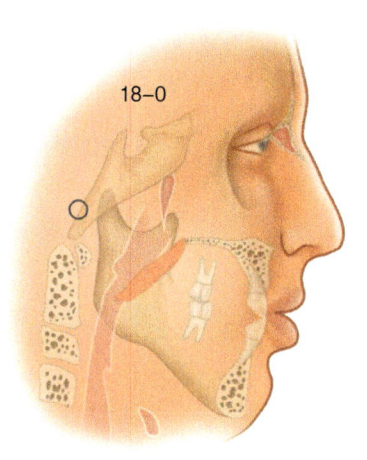

(left) Normal pharyngeal architecture. Good velar length. (right) Flat face is maintained through growth periods. The early anterior crossbite is corrected

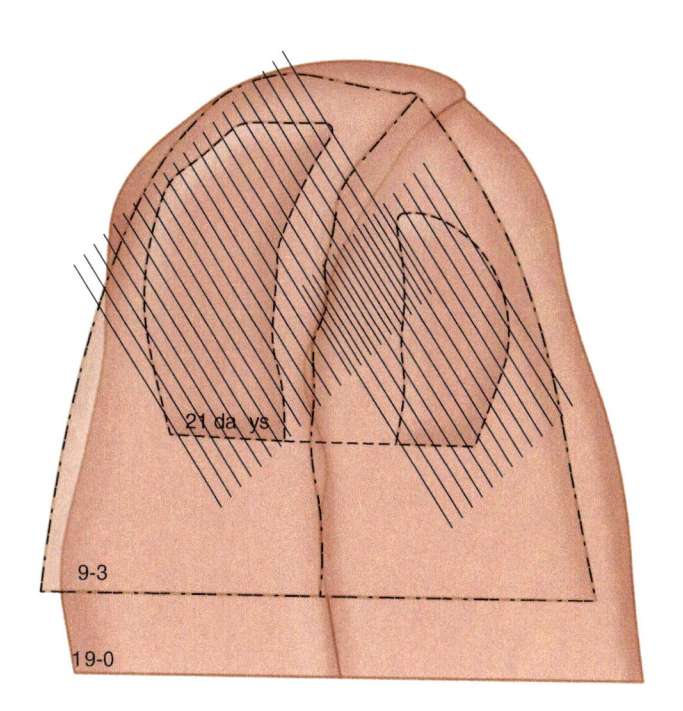

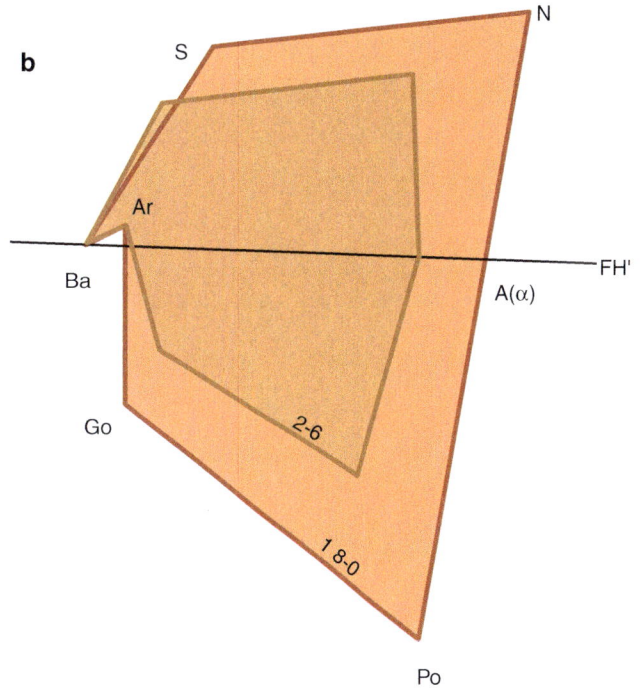

**COBEN CEPHALOMETRIC ANALYSIS:** shows entire maxillary complex growing and being carried forward relative to the spine.

## 7.10 Rapid Closure of the Palatal Cleft Space

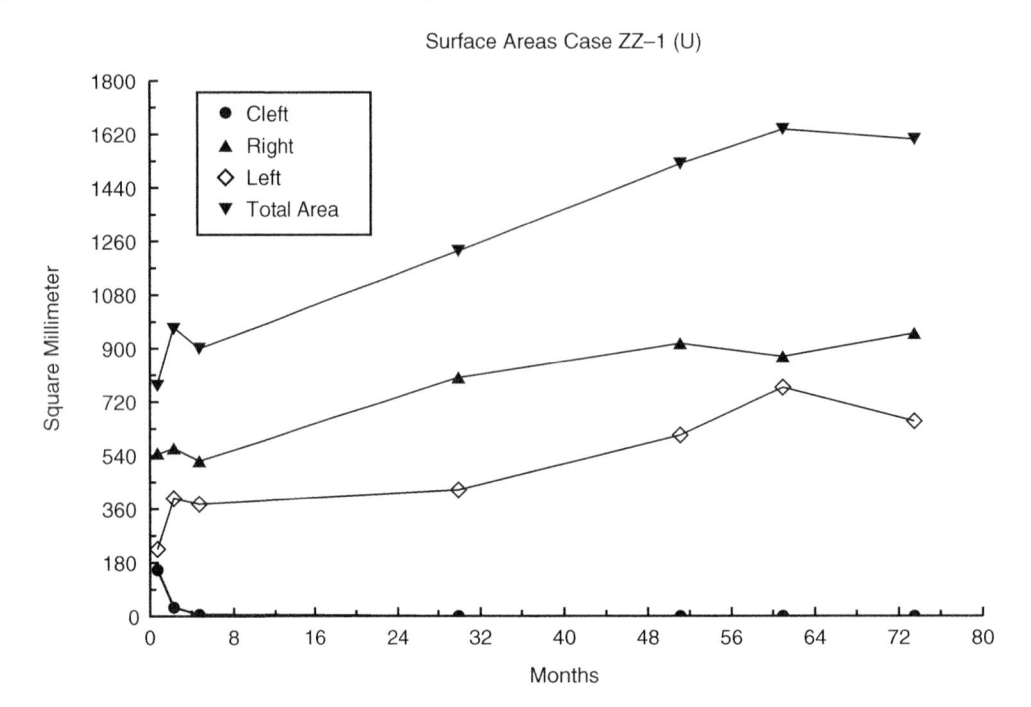

## 7.11 Rolf Tindlund Bergen Norway

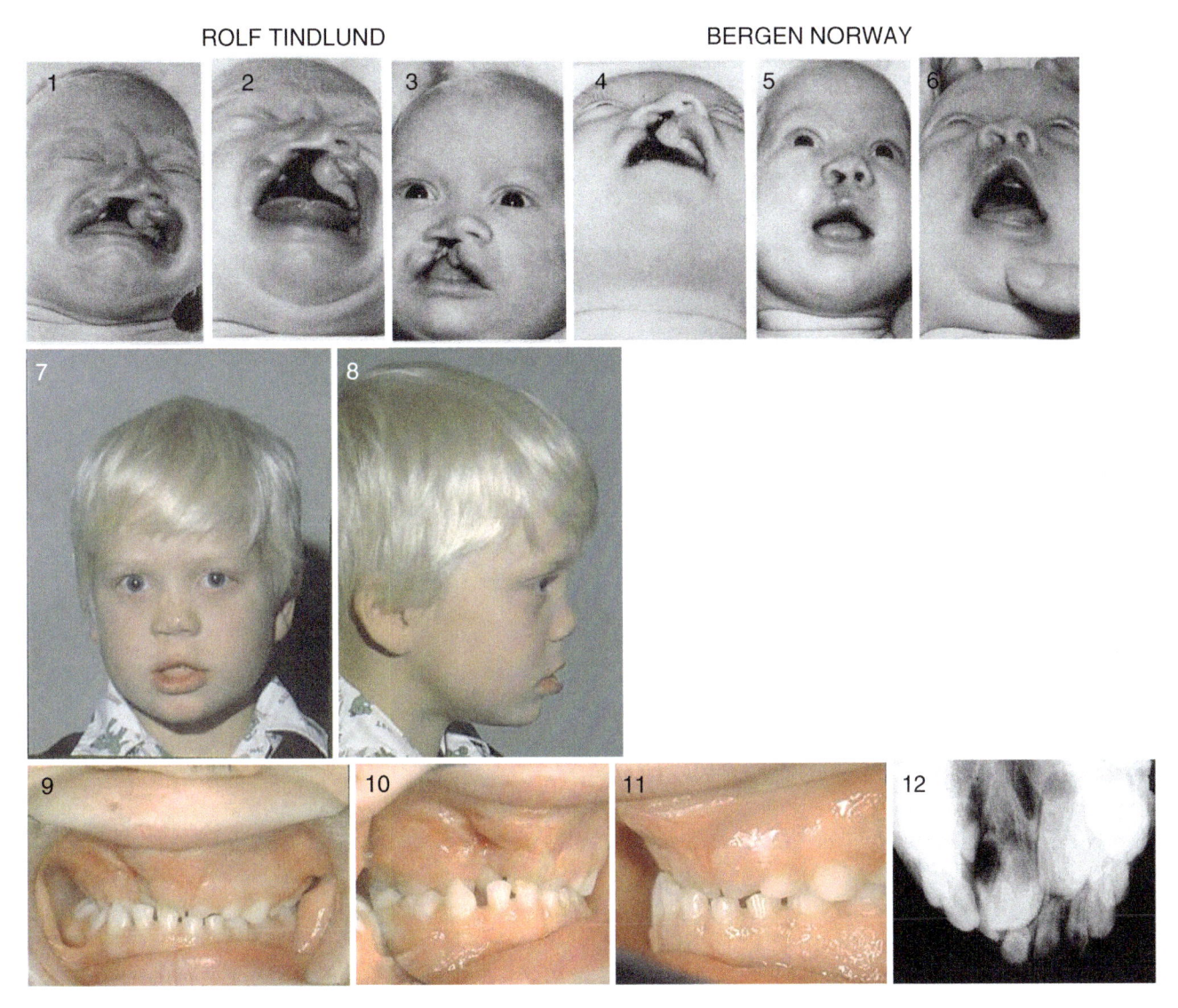

Complete UCLP, category 2A. (1–2) At birth, January 1975, (3–4) After presurgical orthopedics; (5–6) Lip closure at age 3 months; (7–12) At 6 years moderate anterior and unilateral posterior crossbites with a slight concave profile

Secondary alveolar bone grafts between seven-nine years of age. Conservative orthodontics will follow which may include a protraction facial mask or maxillary surgery.

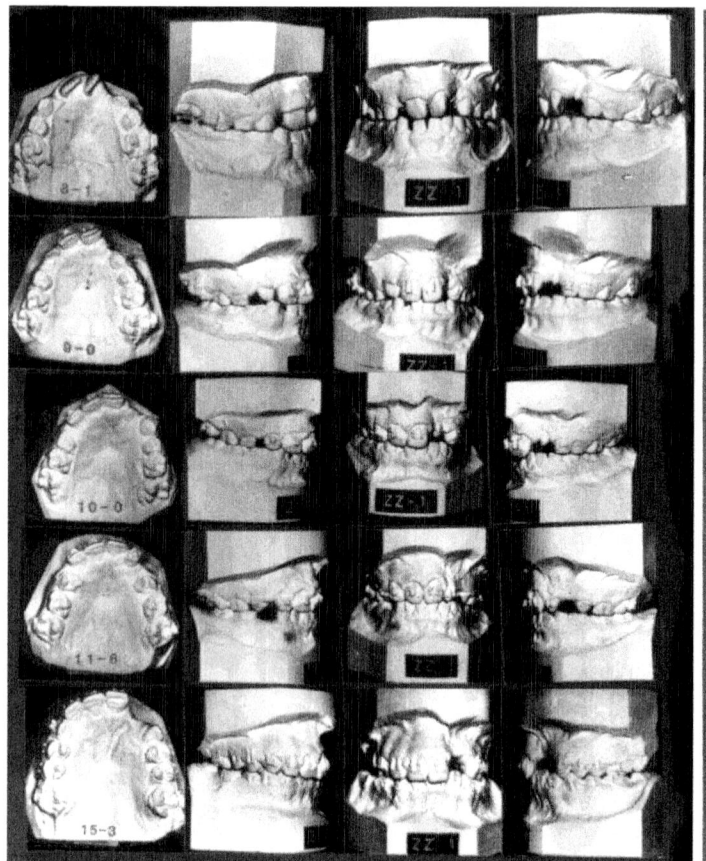

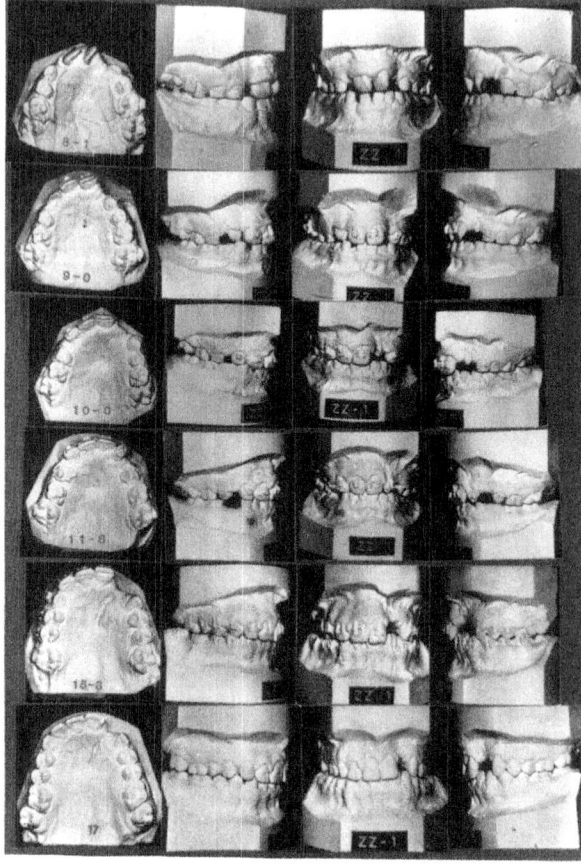

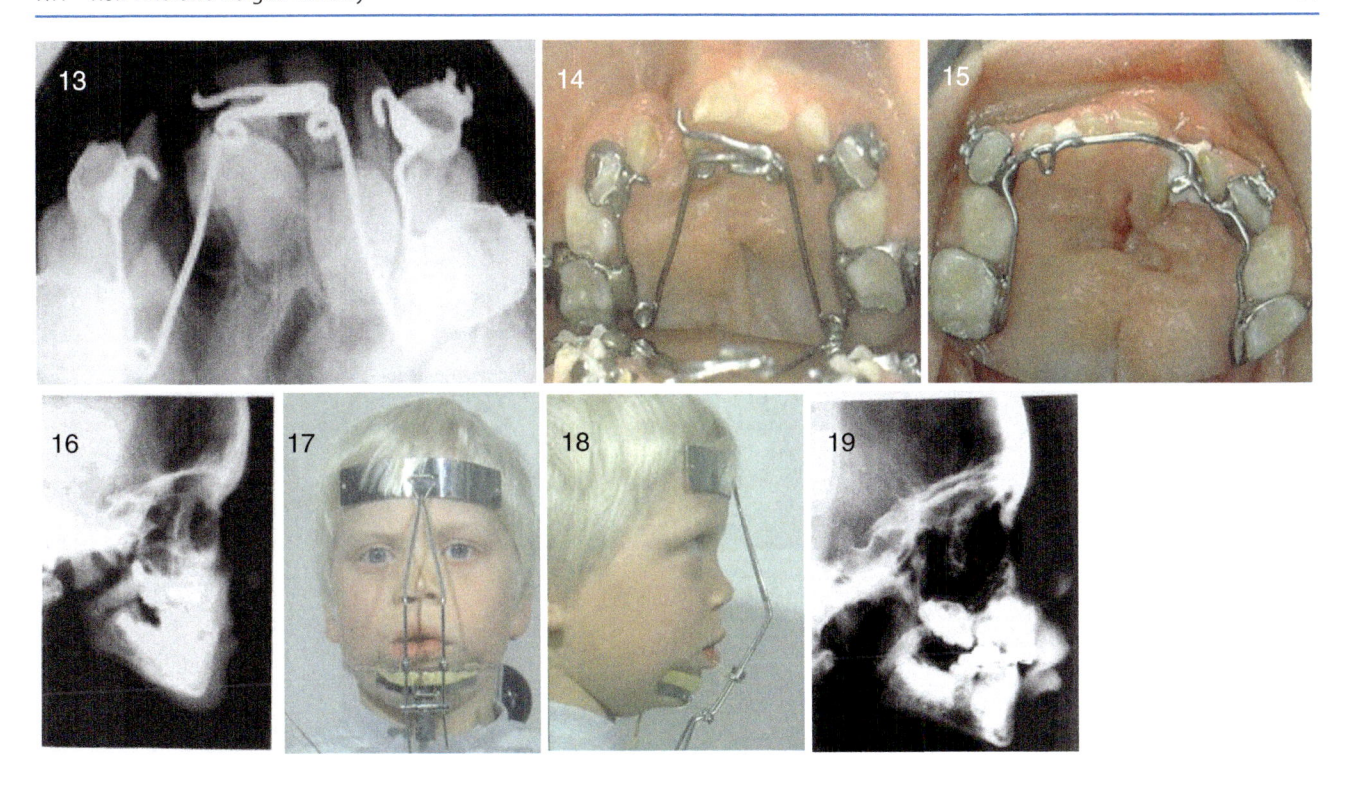

## 7.11 Rolf Tindlund Bergen Norway

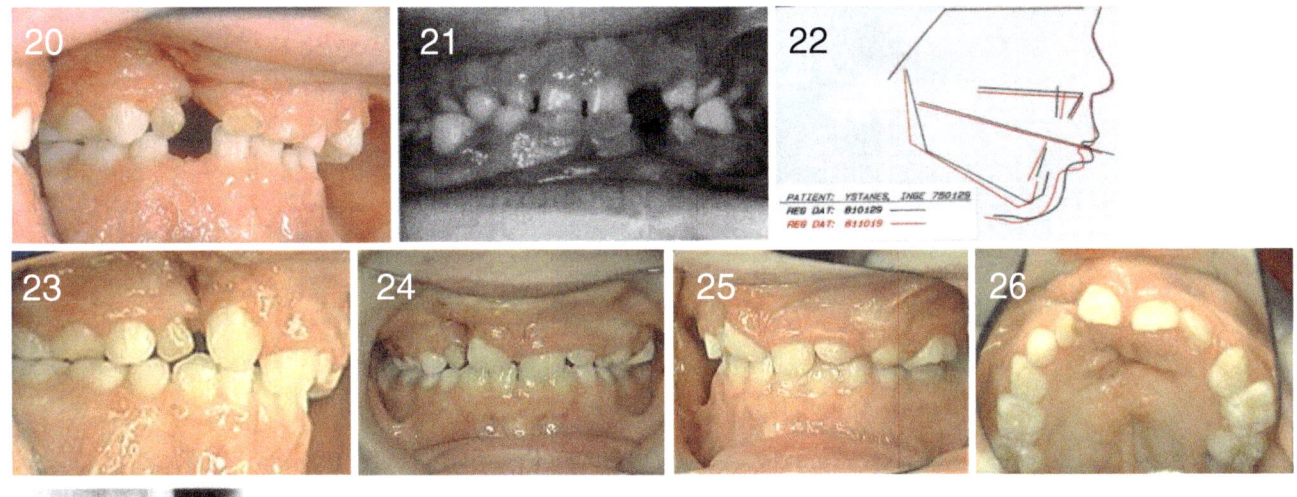

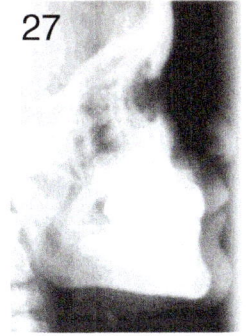

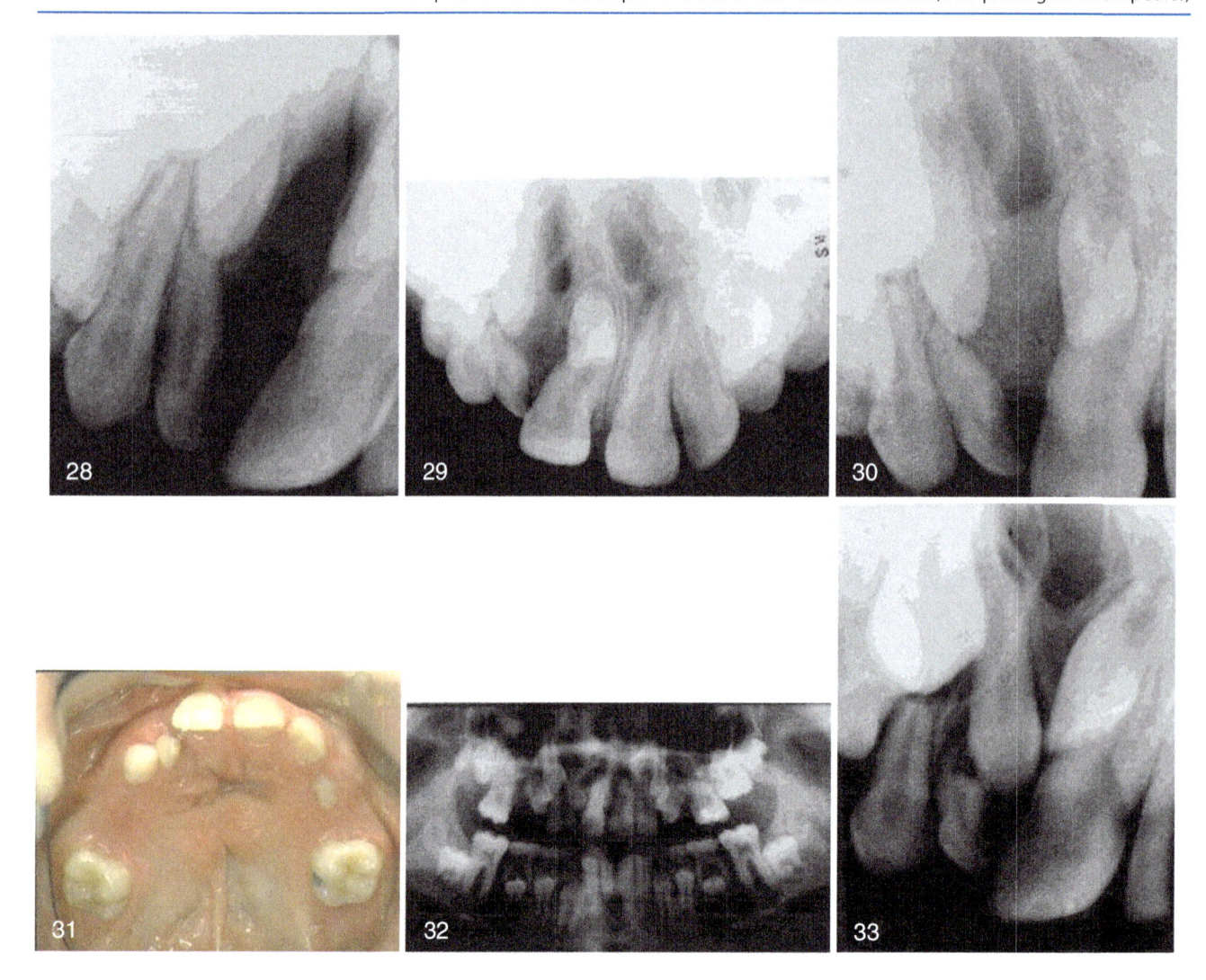

72     7   Complete Unilateral Cleft Lip and Palate Conservative Treatment (Non-presurgical Orthopedics)

## 7.11 Rolf Tindlund Bergen Norway

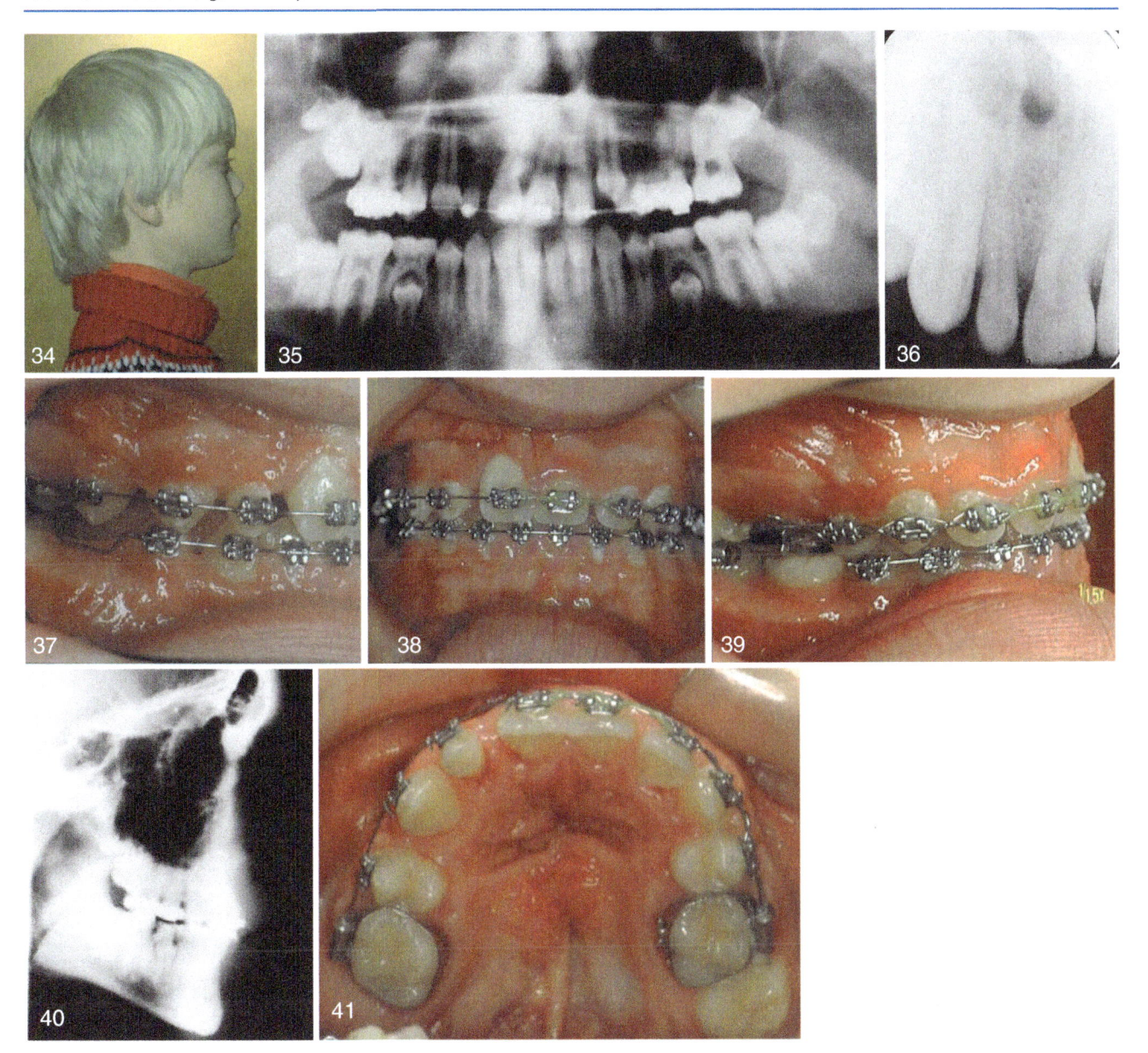

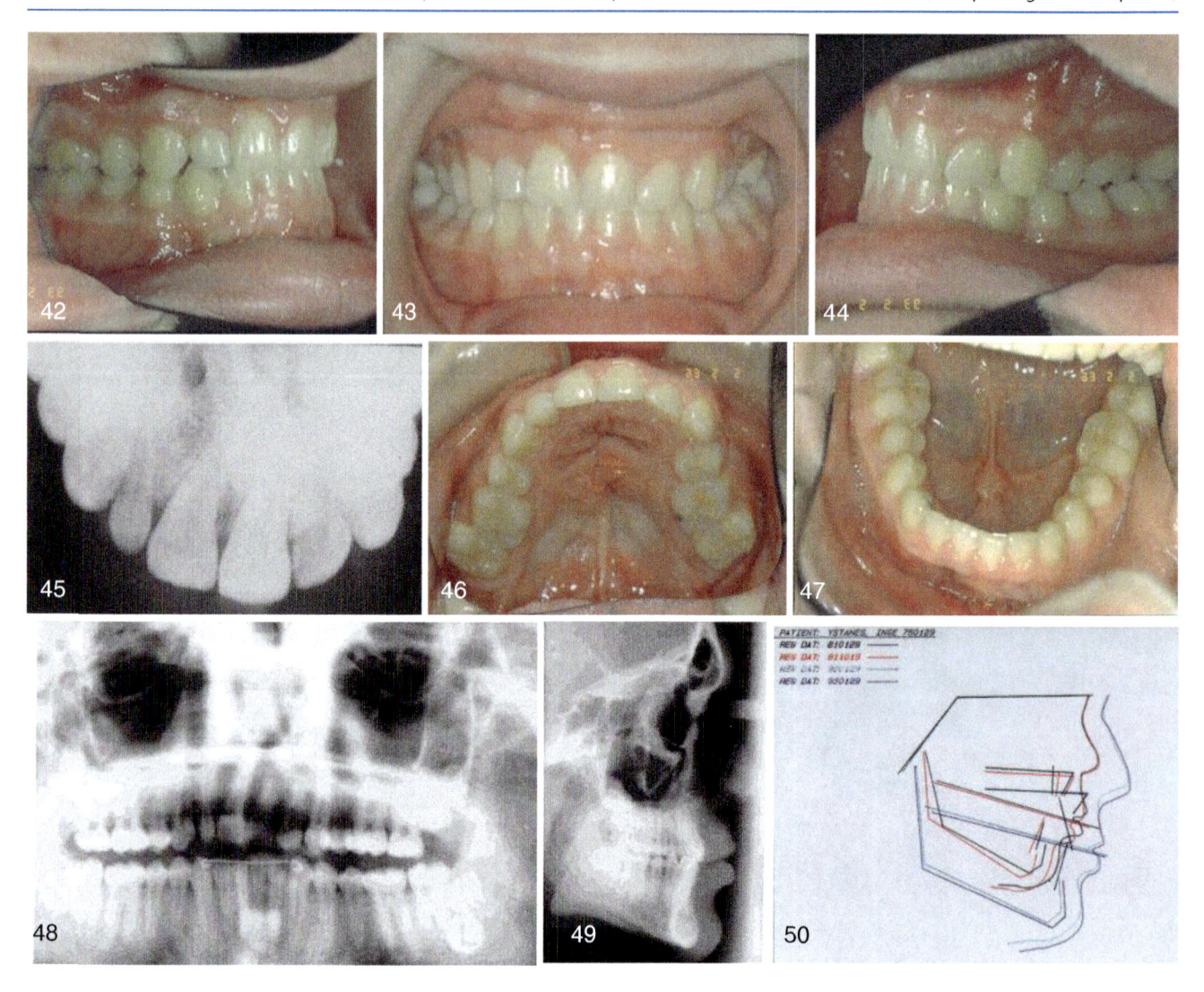

74 | 7 Complete Unilateral Cleft Lip and Palate Conservative Treatment (Non-presurgical Orthopedics)

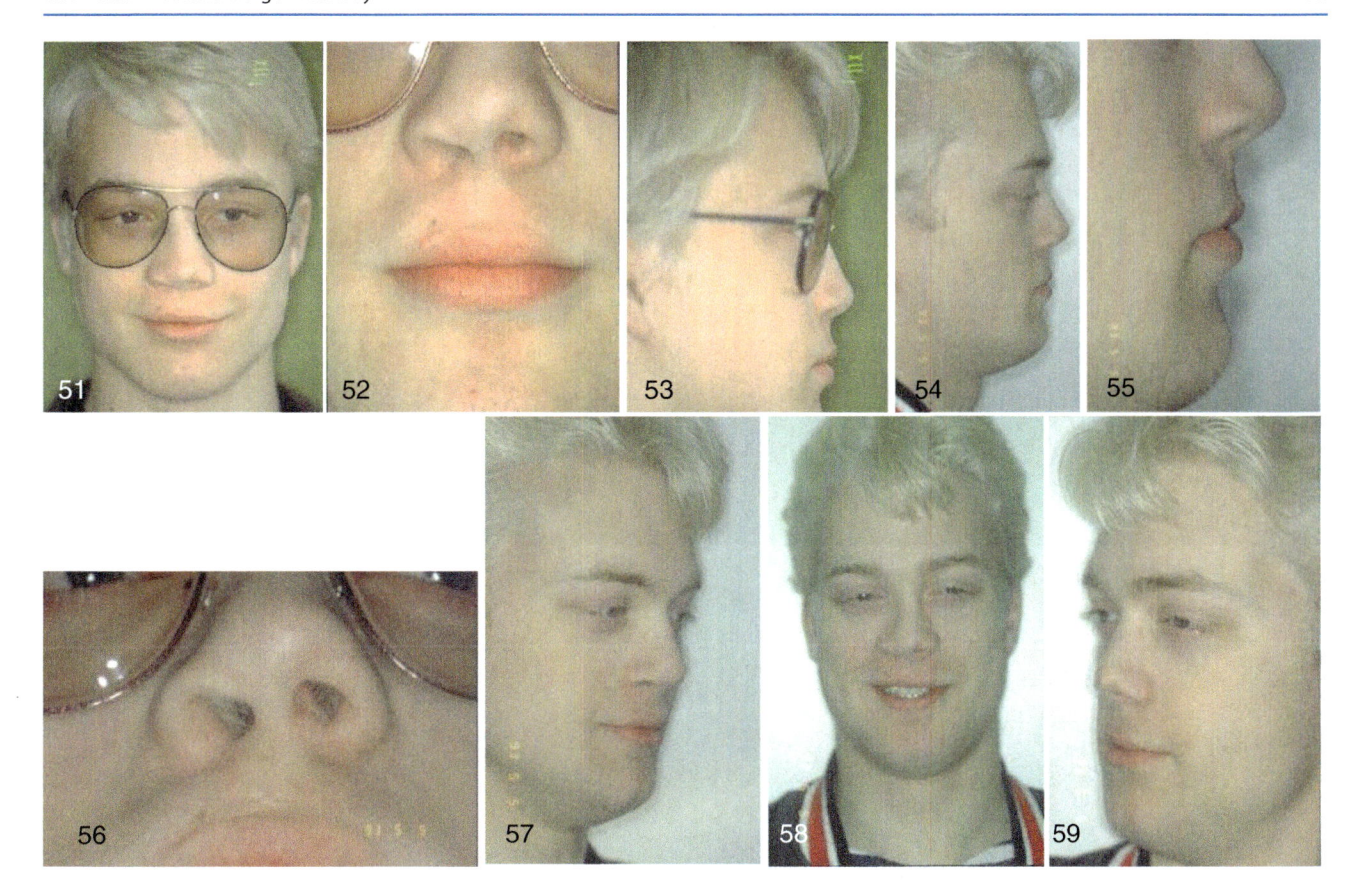

(13–27) Interceptive orthopedics from 6.0 years includes transverse expansion for 3 months using a quad helix, (14) followed by protraction for 6 months using a facial mask, (17–18) and retention using a fixed palatal arch wire (15) to encourage spontaneous eruption of upper permanent incisors into normal position. A nice dental smile was achieved without early orthodontic alignment of the upper incisors (28–33) Alveolar bone grafting at 10.5 years. Two right upper lateral permanent incisors erupted into the cleft area (34) Facial profile at 12 years (35–41) Conventional orthodontics at 13.5 years lasting for 18 months. The two upper second bicuspids were missing and the supernumerary right upper lateral permanent incisor was removed. (42–48) Dental occlusion at 18.5 years; (49–50) Cephalometric graphic analysis at 6, after interceptive orthopedics, and at 15, and 18 years (51–53) Facial appearance at 15 years; (54–59) Facial appearance at 18.5 years.

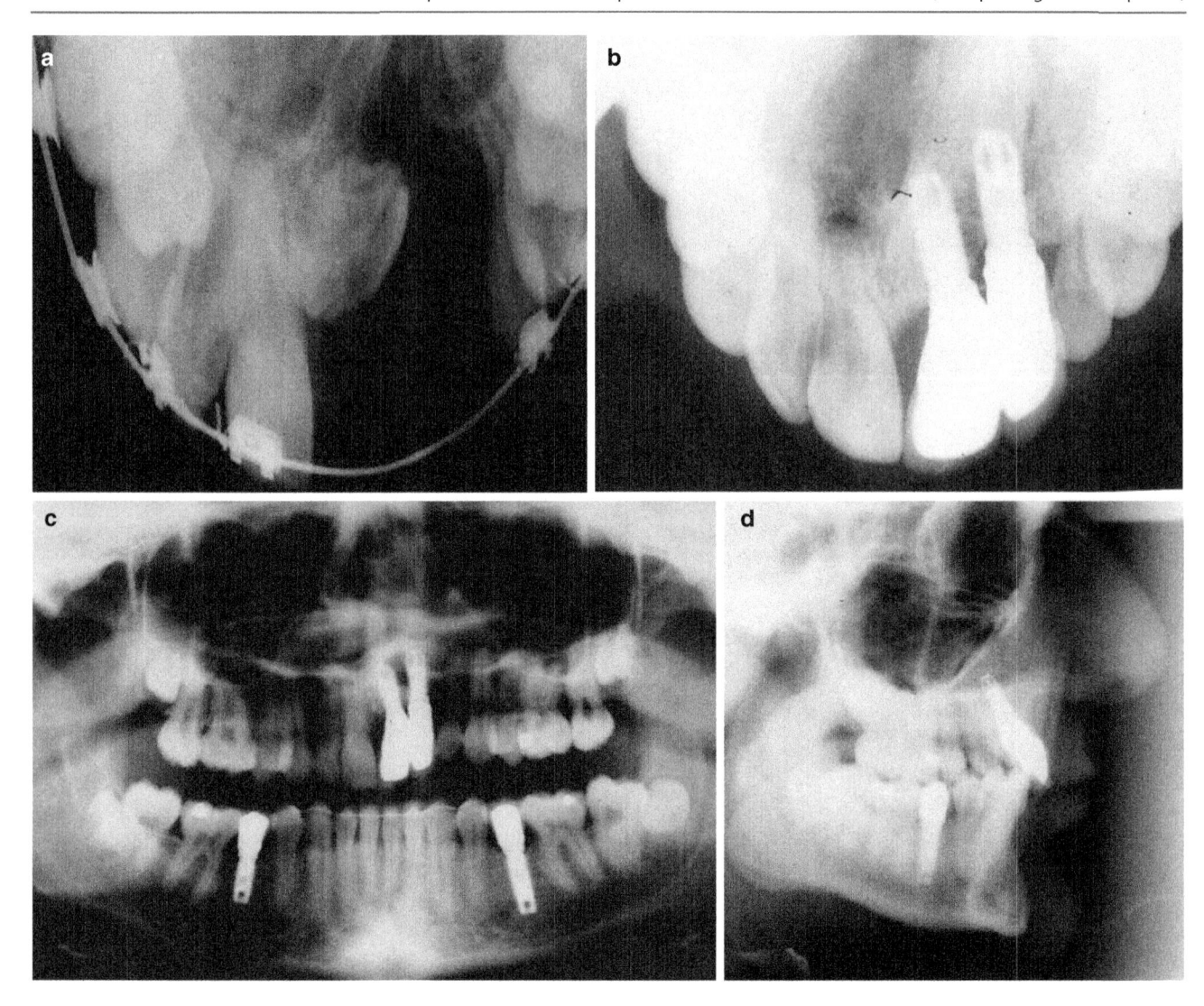

Complete UCLP, category 2A, born 1974. (**a**) At 15 years during the period of conventional orthodontics the severely malformed left permanent central incisor was removed at the time of secondary alveolar bone grafting. (**b**), (**c**), and (**d**) Radiograph at 18.5 years showing dental implants for the replacement of left upper central and lateral incisors and both lower second bicuspids.

## 7.11 Rolf Tindlund Bergen Norway

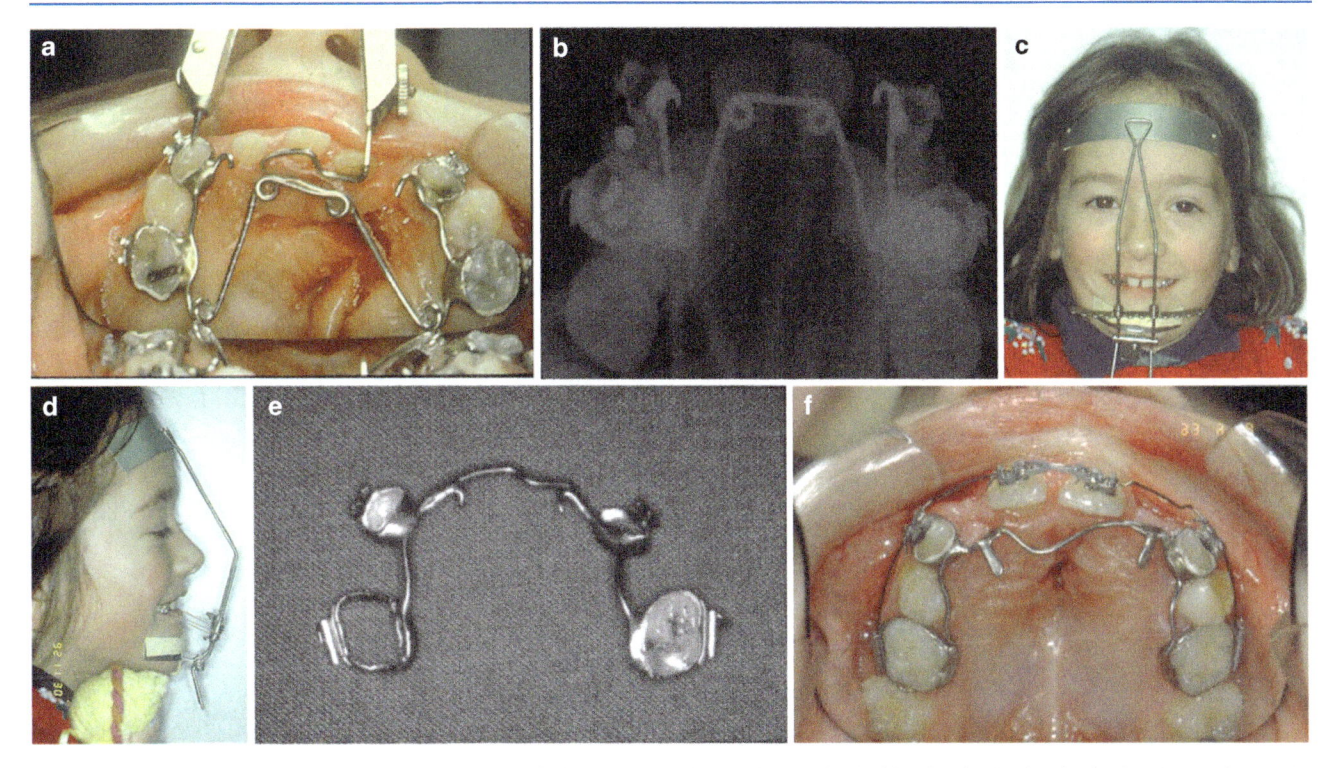

**Interceptive orthopedics (Bergen rationale).** (**a**) and (**b**) Transverse maxillary widening using a modified quad helix appliance. (**c**) and (**d**) Followed by maxillary protraction with a facial mask. (**e**) and (**f**) Correction retained with a fixed palatal arch with brackets and tubes for early alignment of the upper incisors. Retention is utilized until deciduous anchor teeth are shed.

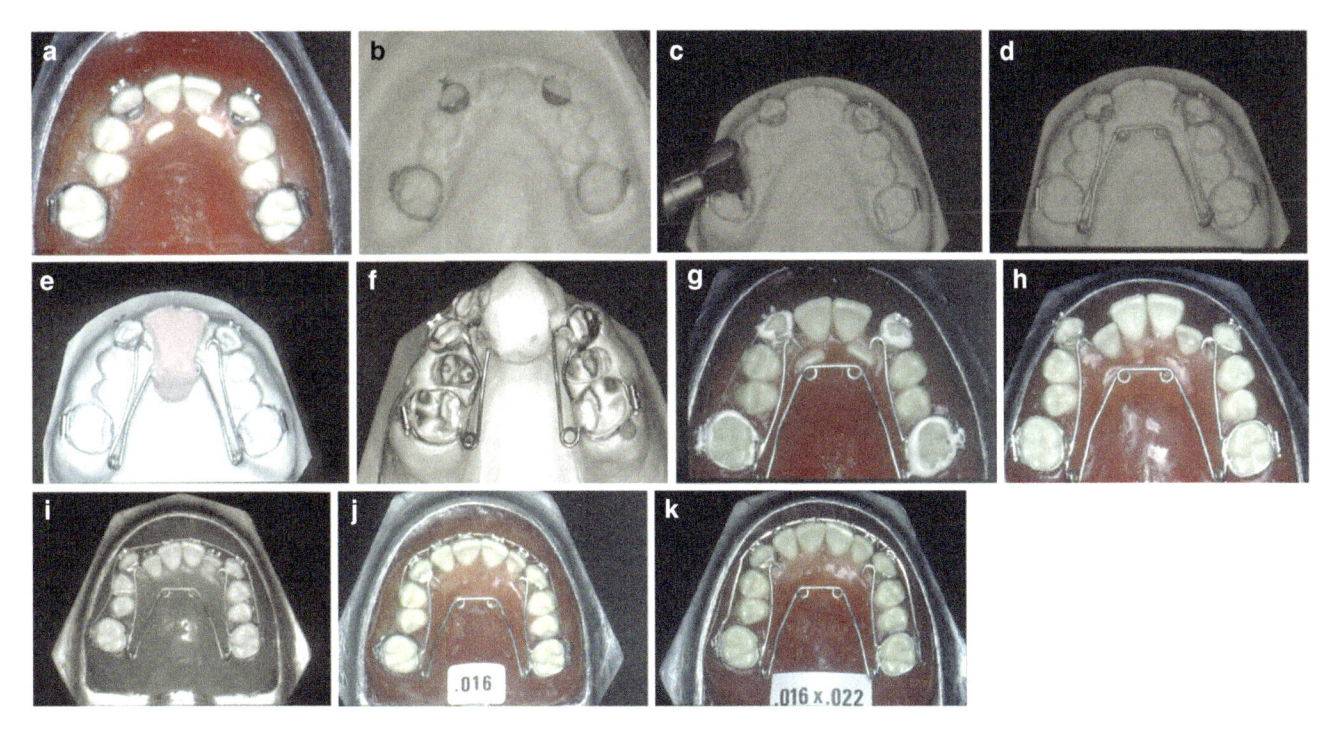

Fabricating a modified quad helix appliance. (a) and (b) Bilateral posterior crossbite with lack of space for erupting lateral permanent incisors. Bands with brackets or tubes are fitted to the upper deciduous cuspids and deciduous second molars and carefully replaced into an alginate impression. (c) Plaster removed underneath soldering zones. (d) Quad helix arms are precisely adjusted. (e) and (f) Quad helix arms are soldered to all four bands. (g) Each arm is individually activated. (h) Cemented. (i), (j), and (k) Combined with round labial arches for alignment of incisors. l. Labial incisor root-torque with rectangular archwire.

3 weeks

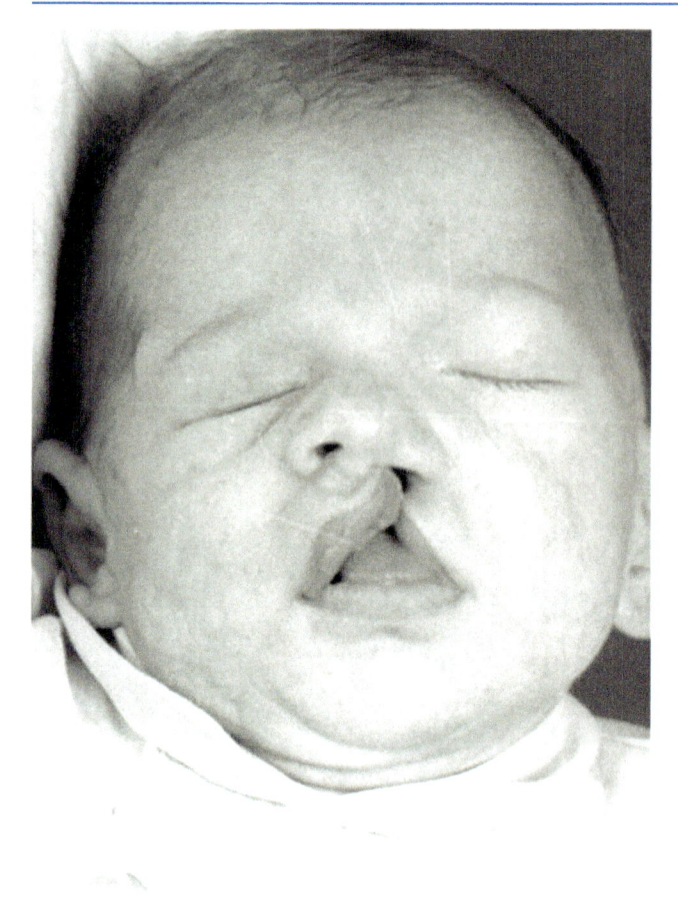

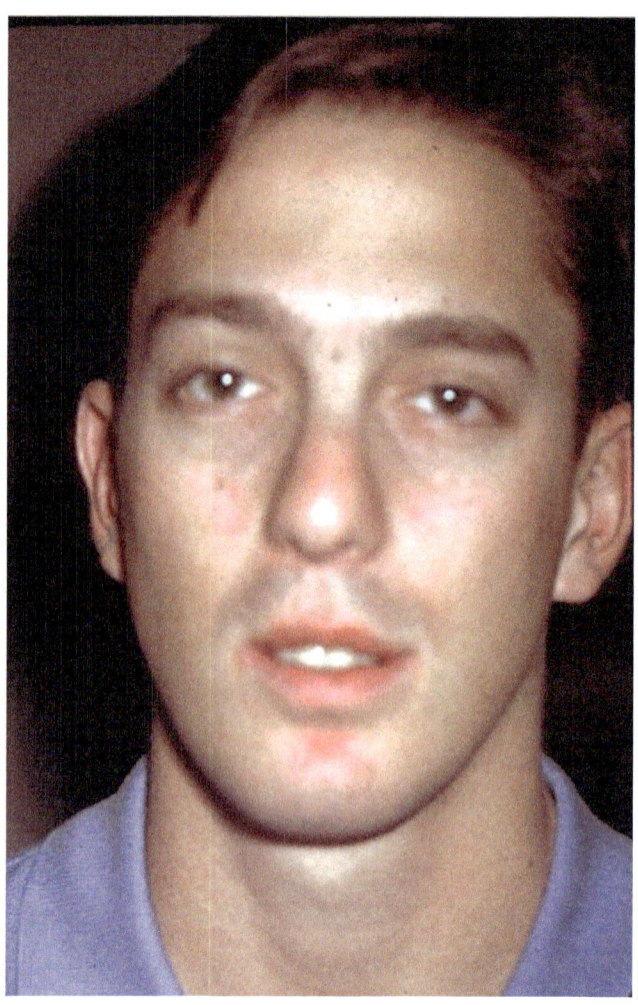

23 years

## 7.12 Complete Unilateral Cleft Lip and Palate

### 7.12.1 Minor Orthodontics

**Newborn**

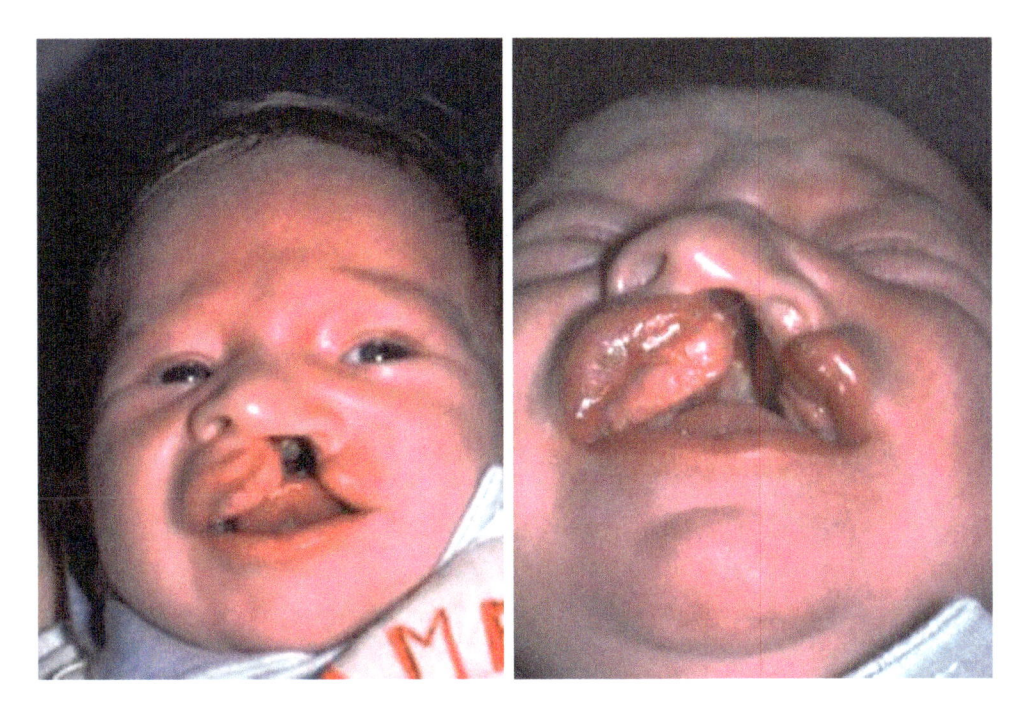

Lip adhesion → Rotation Advancement.
 Palatal Closure at 18 months → Excellent Occlusion.
 **2 years**
 Rotation Advancement

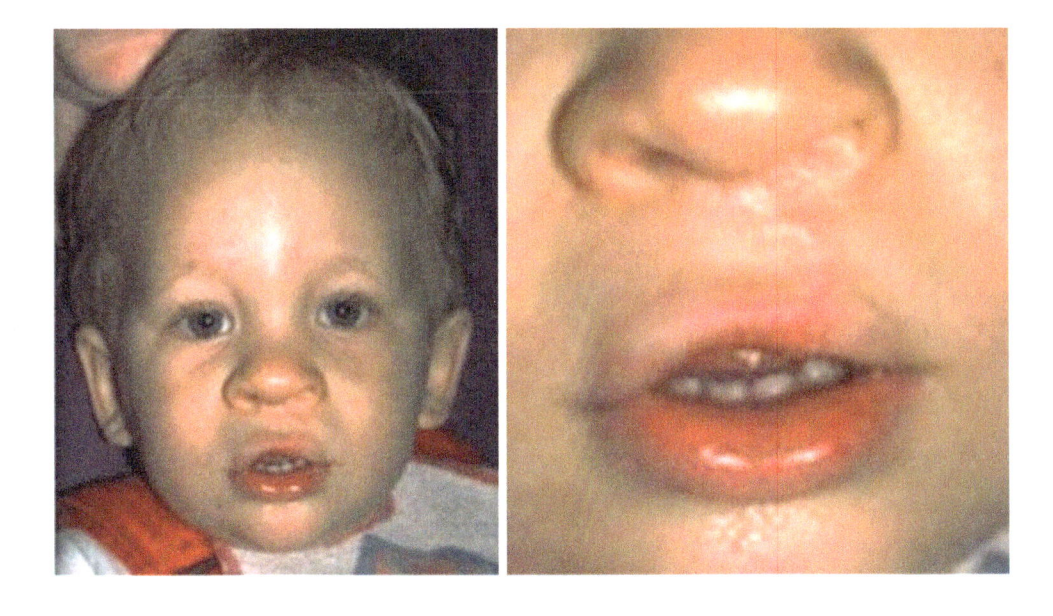

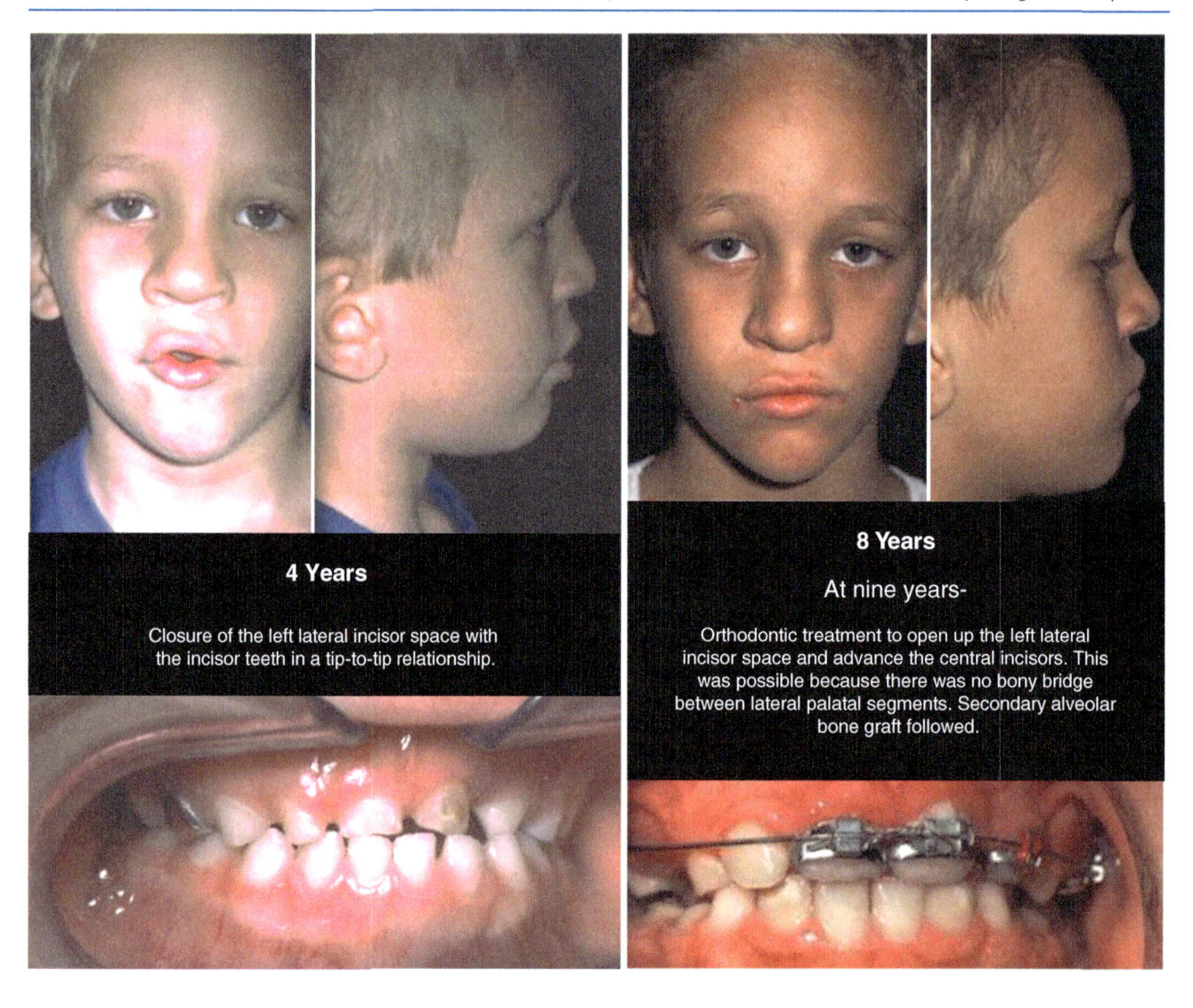

**4 Years**

Closure of the left lateral incisor space with the incisor teeth in a tip-to-tip relationship.

**8 Years**

At nine years-

Orthodontic treatment to open up the left lateral incisor space and advance the central incisors. This was possible because there was no bony bridge between lateral palatal segments. Secondary alveolar bone graft followed.

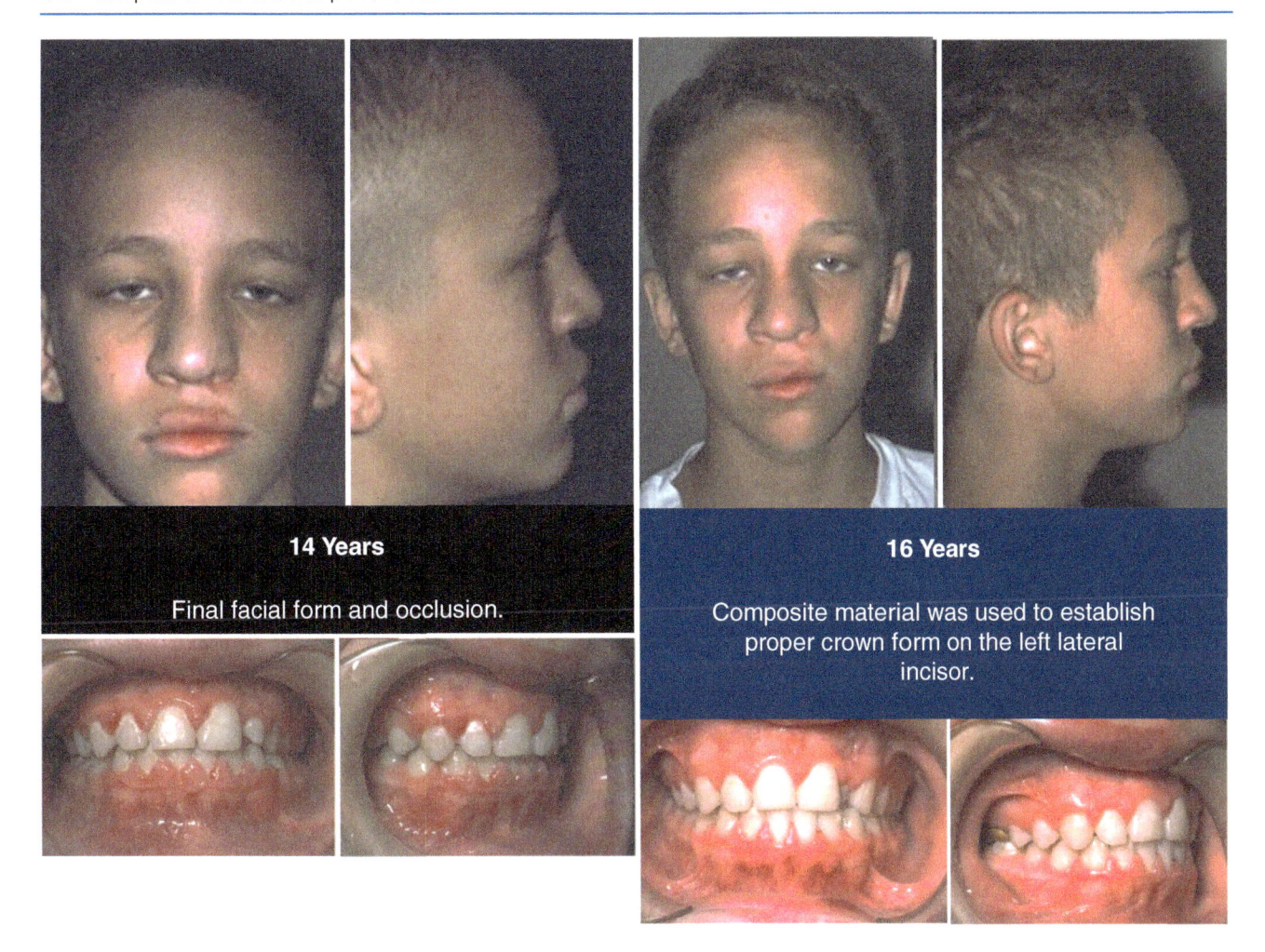

## 7.12 Complete Unilateral Cleft Lip and Palate

**14 Years**

Final facial form and occlusion.

**16 Years**

Composite material was used to establish proper crown form on the left lateral incisor.

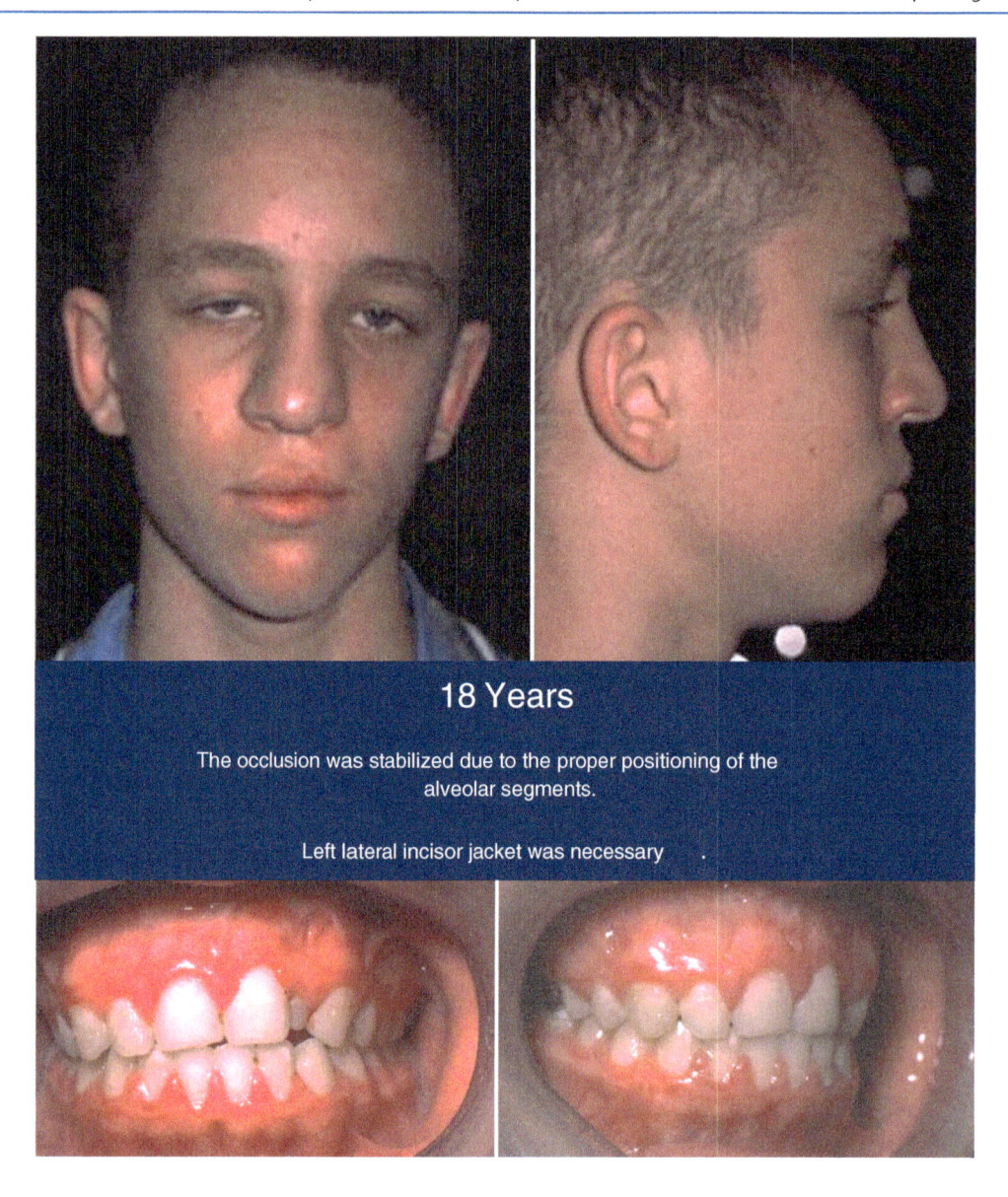

## 18 Years

The occlusion was stabilized due to the proper positioning of the alveolar segments.

Left lateral incisor jacket was necessary.

## 7.12 Complete Unilateral Cleft Lip and Palate

### 7.12.2 Failure of Advancing Teeth with Protraction Facial Mask

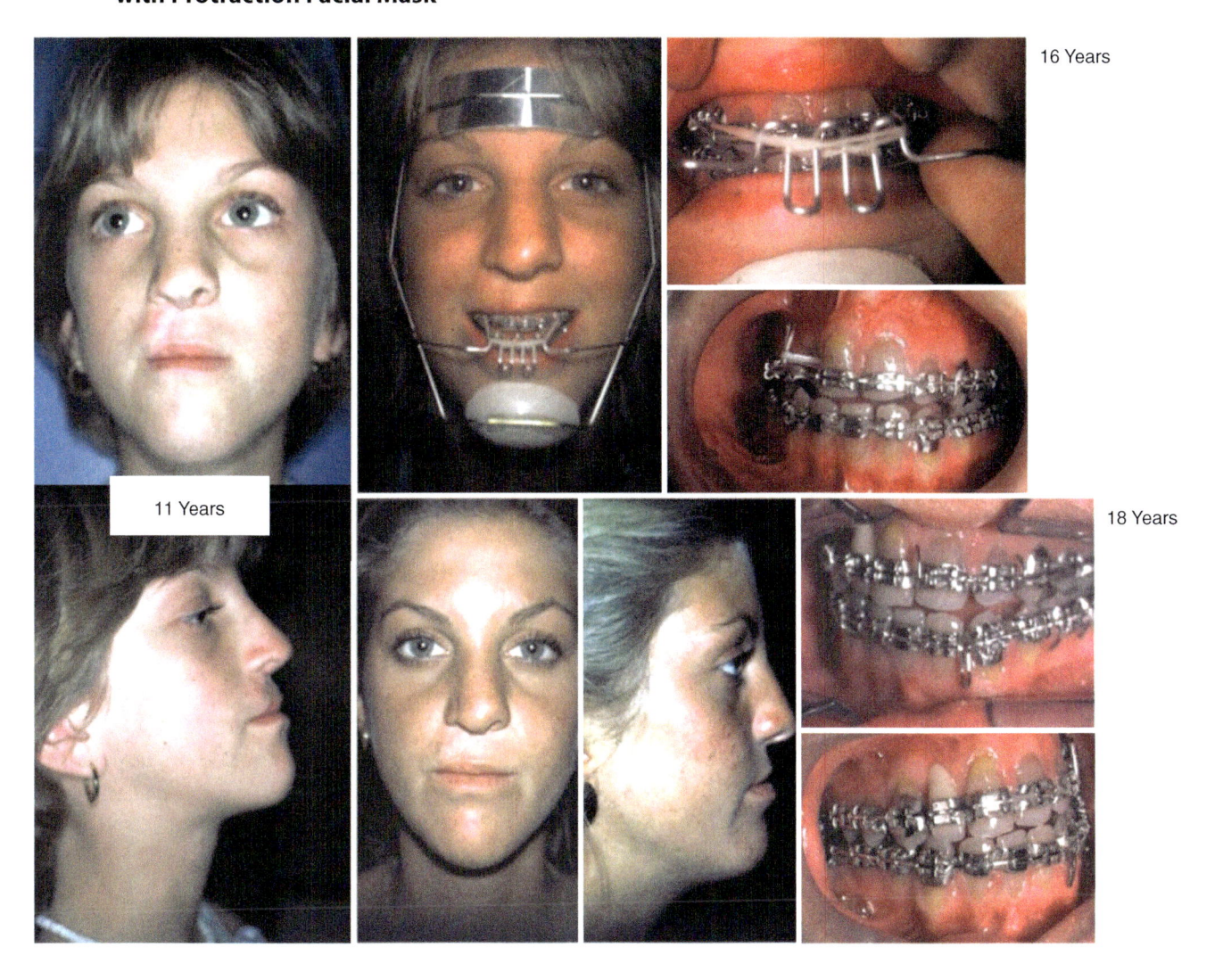

11 Years

16 Years

18 Years

## 7.13 Complete Unilateral Cleft Lip and Palate

Early blockage of the lateral incisor space necessitating premaxillary advancement

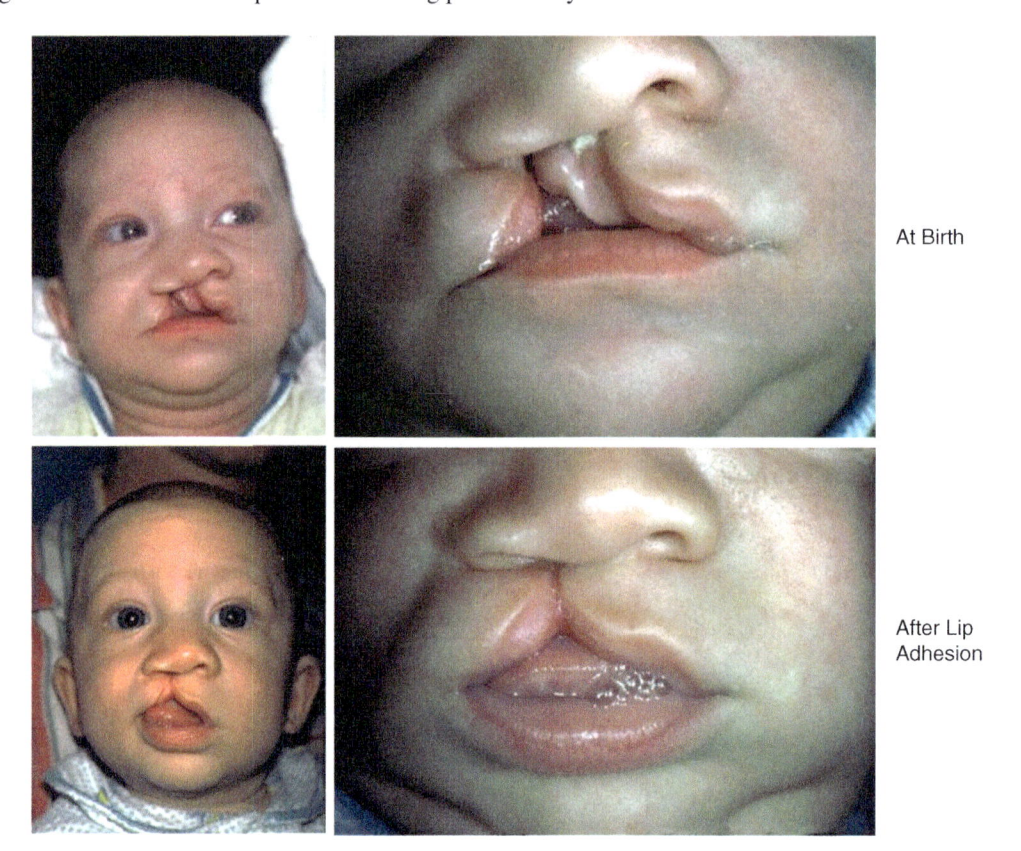

At Birth

After Lip Adhesion

## 7.13 Complete Unilateral Cleft Lip and Palate

Overlapping premaxillary segment

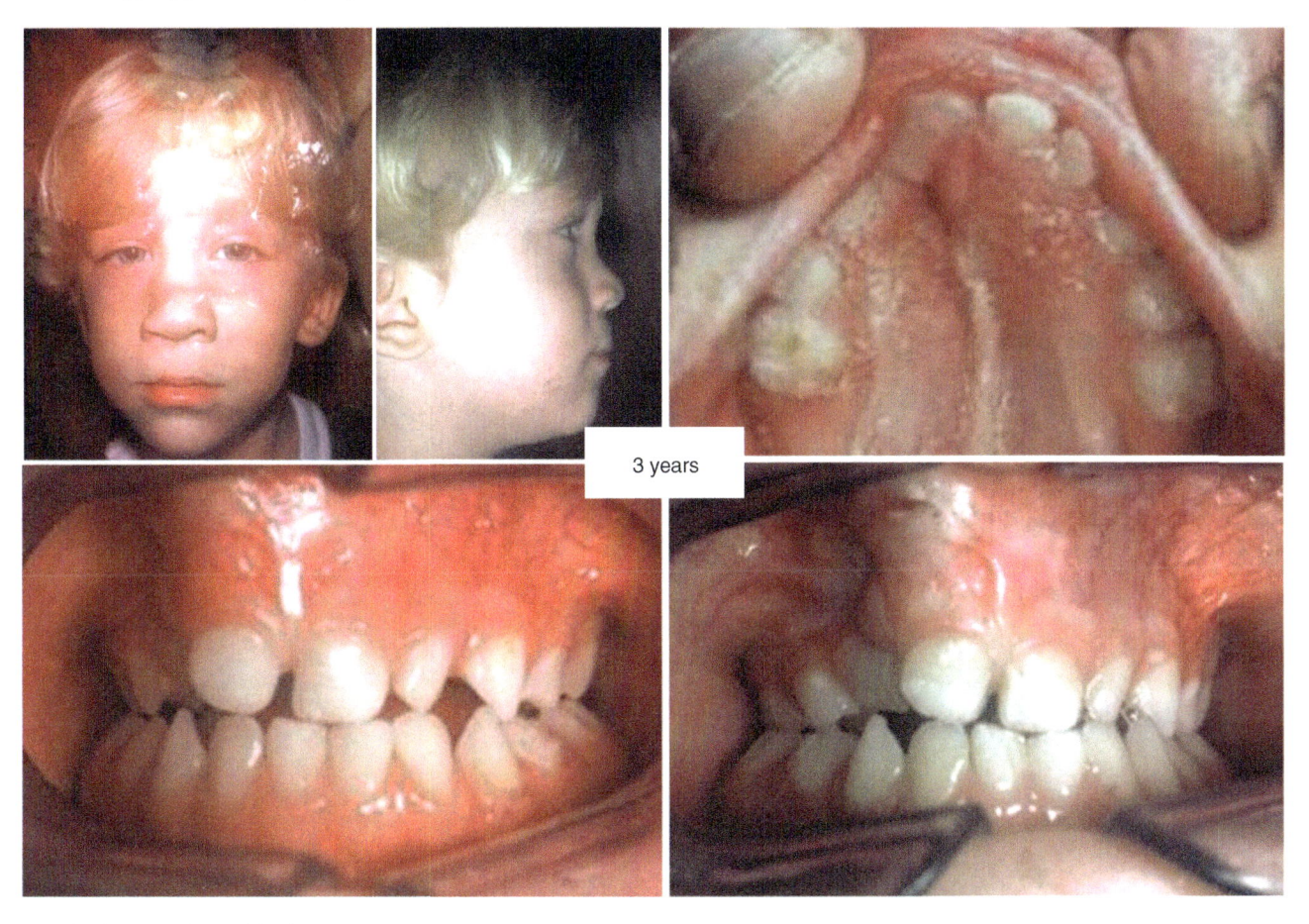

3 years

Blocked-out lateral incisor

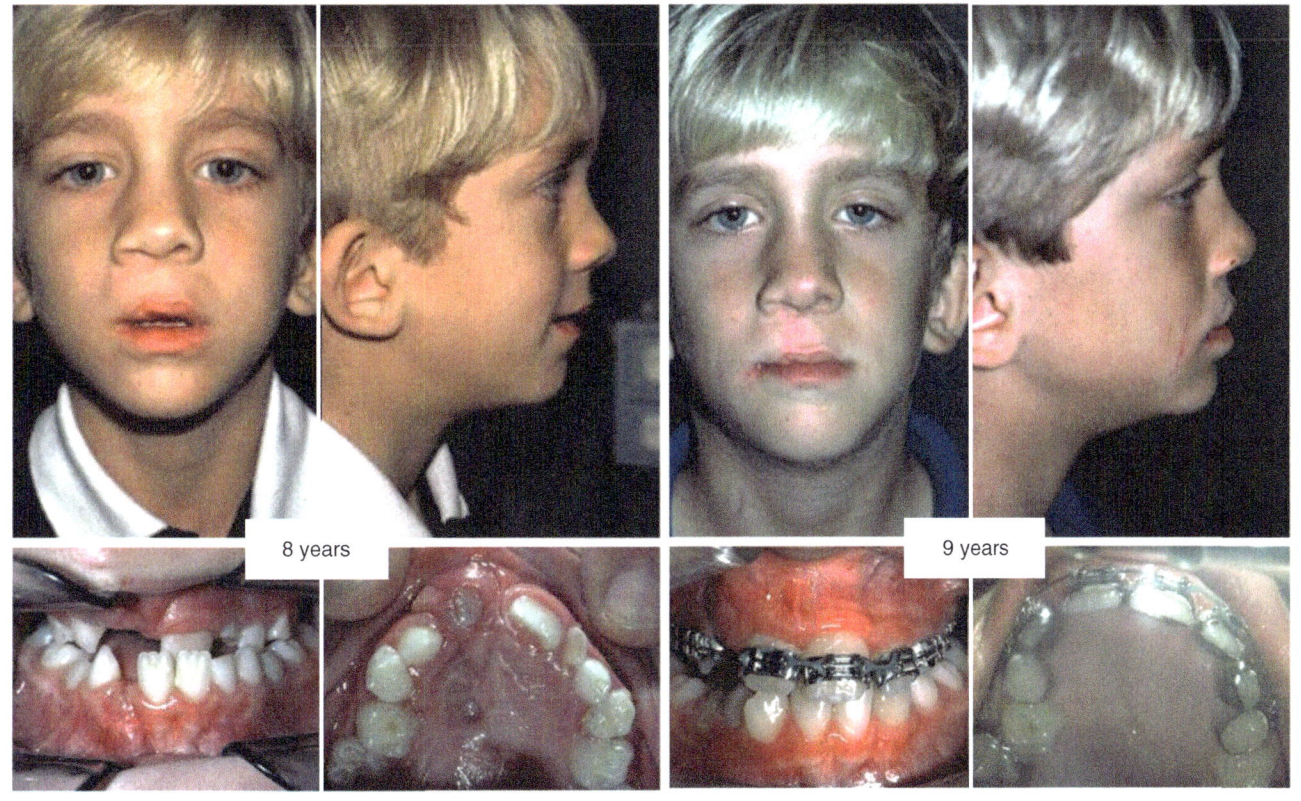

8 years

9 years

Anterior crossbite

Making room for the lateral incisor

10 years

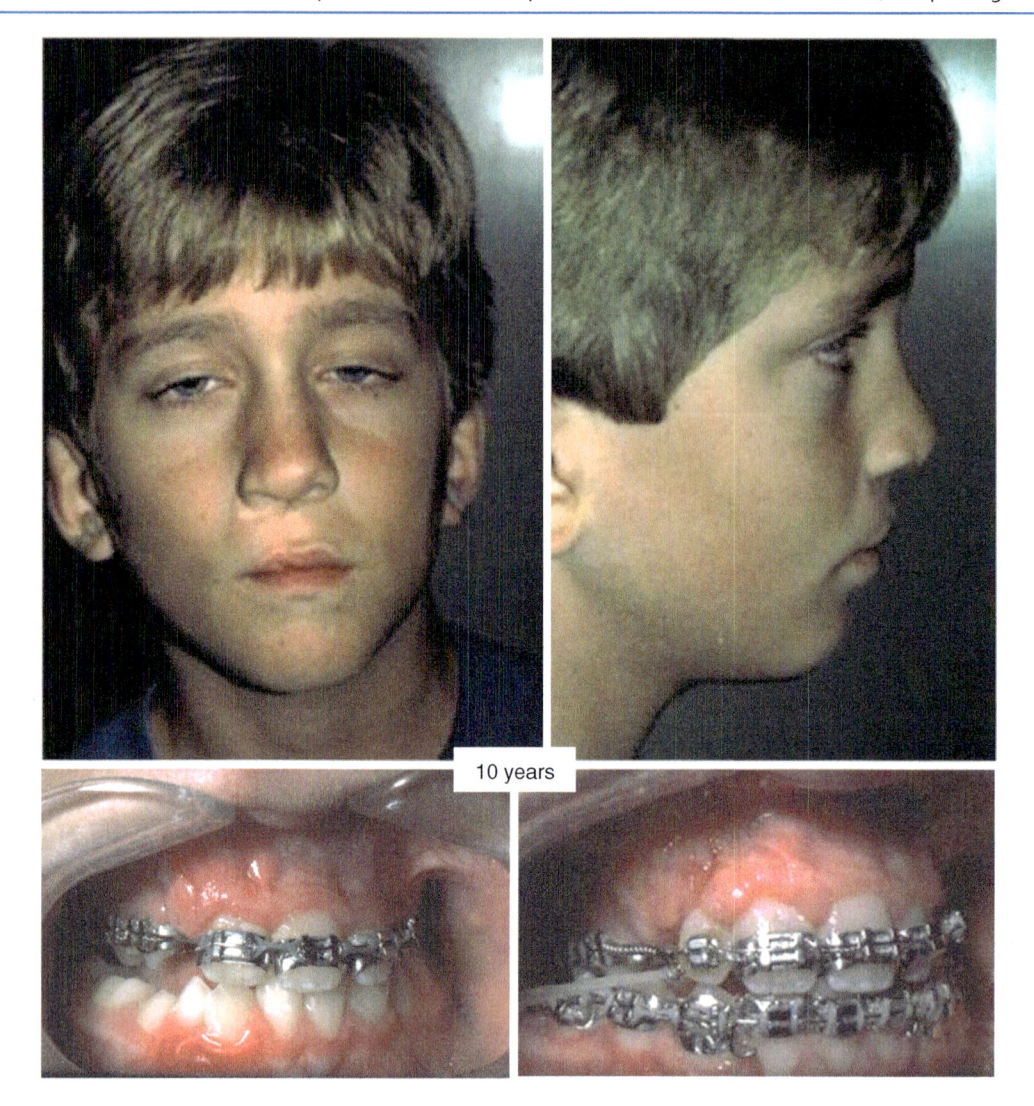

## 7.13 Complete Unilateral Cleft Lip and Palate

Mid-lines corrected allow for room to erupt lateral incisor

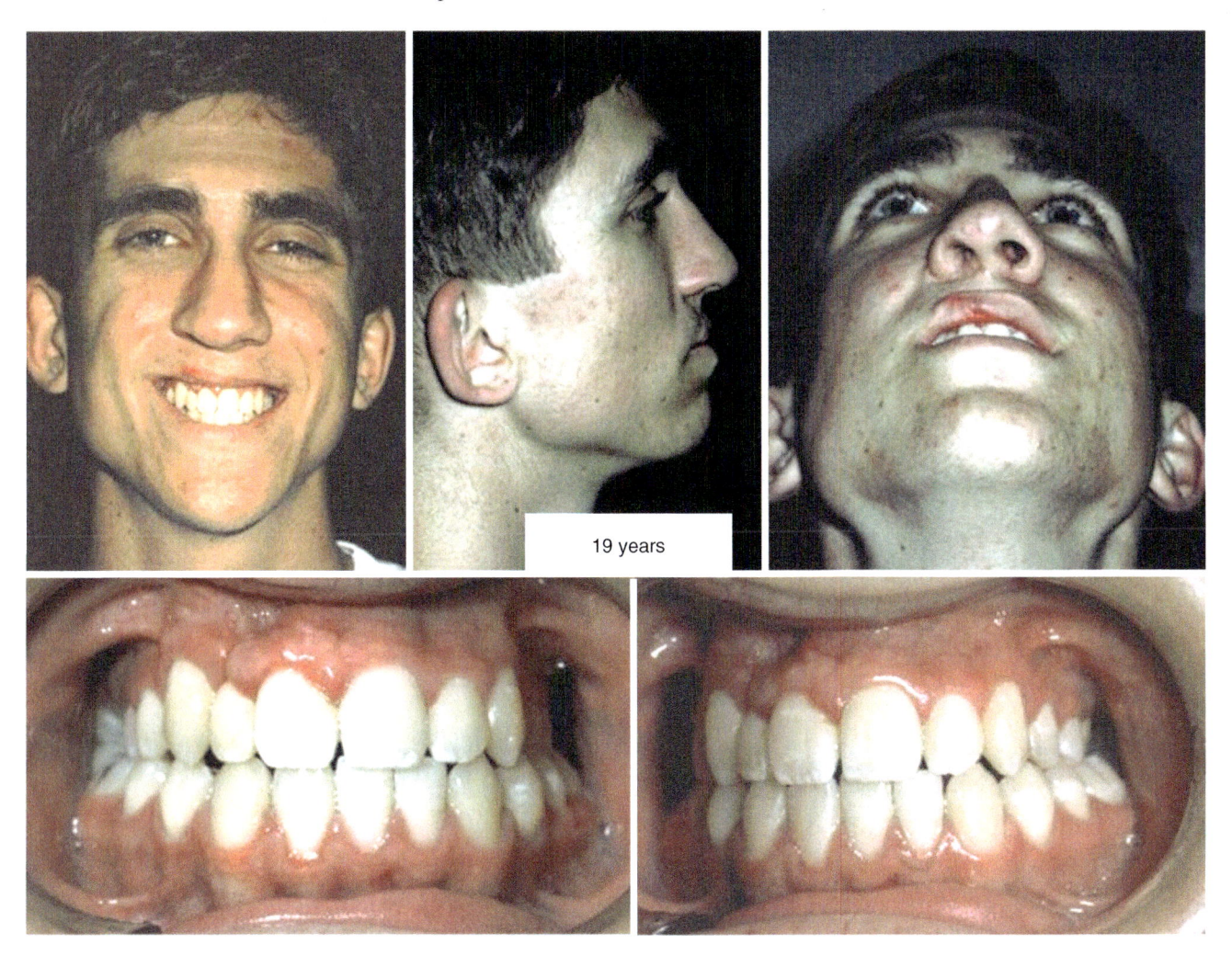

19 years

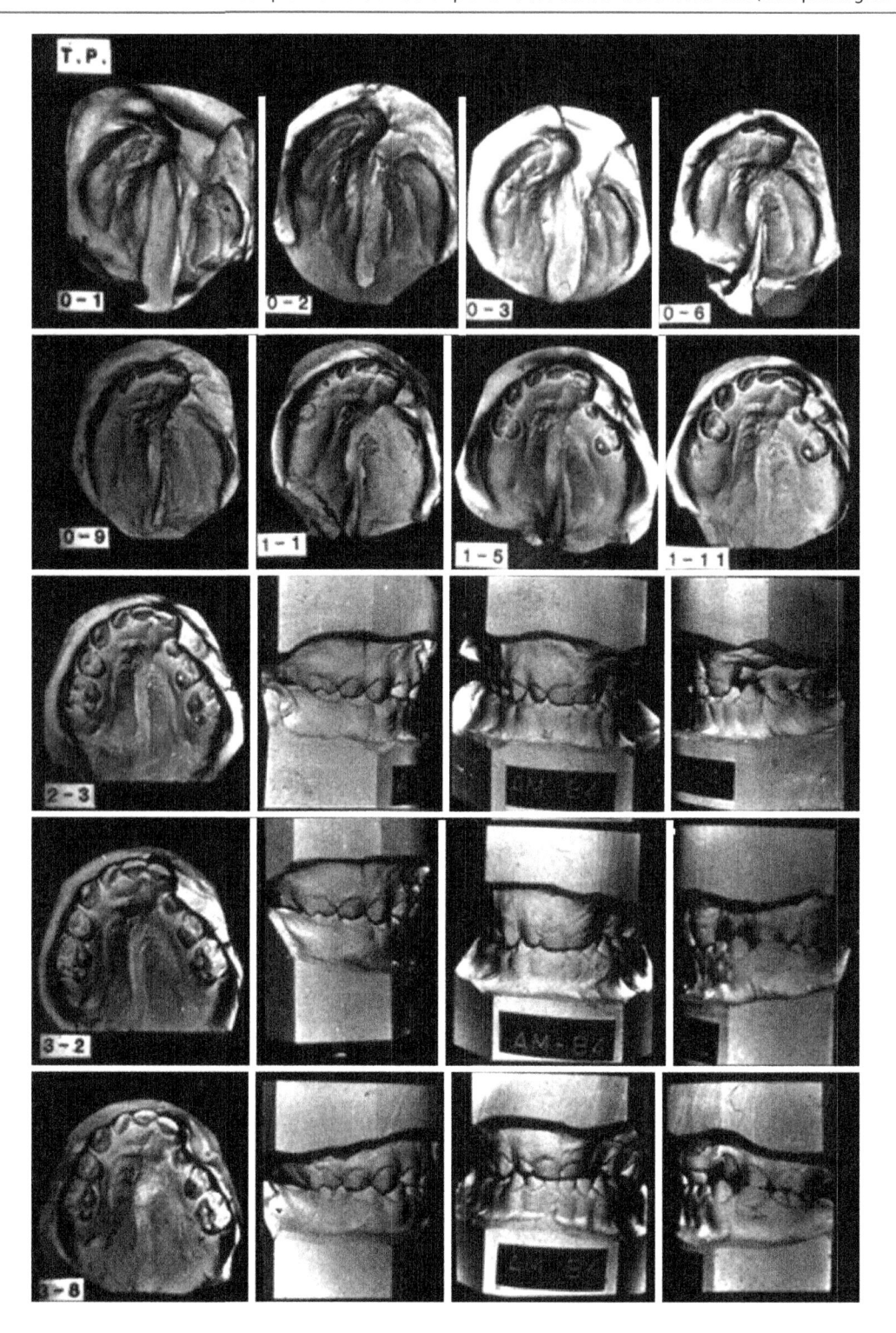

7 Complete Unilateral Cleft Lip and Palate Conservative Treatment (Non-presurgical Orthopedics)

The following serial casts depict changes in arch form and size due to growth and development.

Changes in arch form:

- Molding due to change in lip muscle forces. Pressure against the palatal segments brings them together.

- The segments unequally increase in size at all surfaces. The arch form could vary after lip adhesion. Either:

  (a) Butt joint
  (b) Overlapping premaxillary segments
  (c) No contact of segments

## 7.13 Complete Unilateral Cleft Lip and Palate

In all of the serial cast images, the relative size of images to each other are not true—but the size of cleft space to palatal size medial to the alveolar ridges are correct.

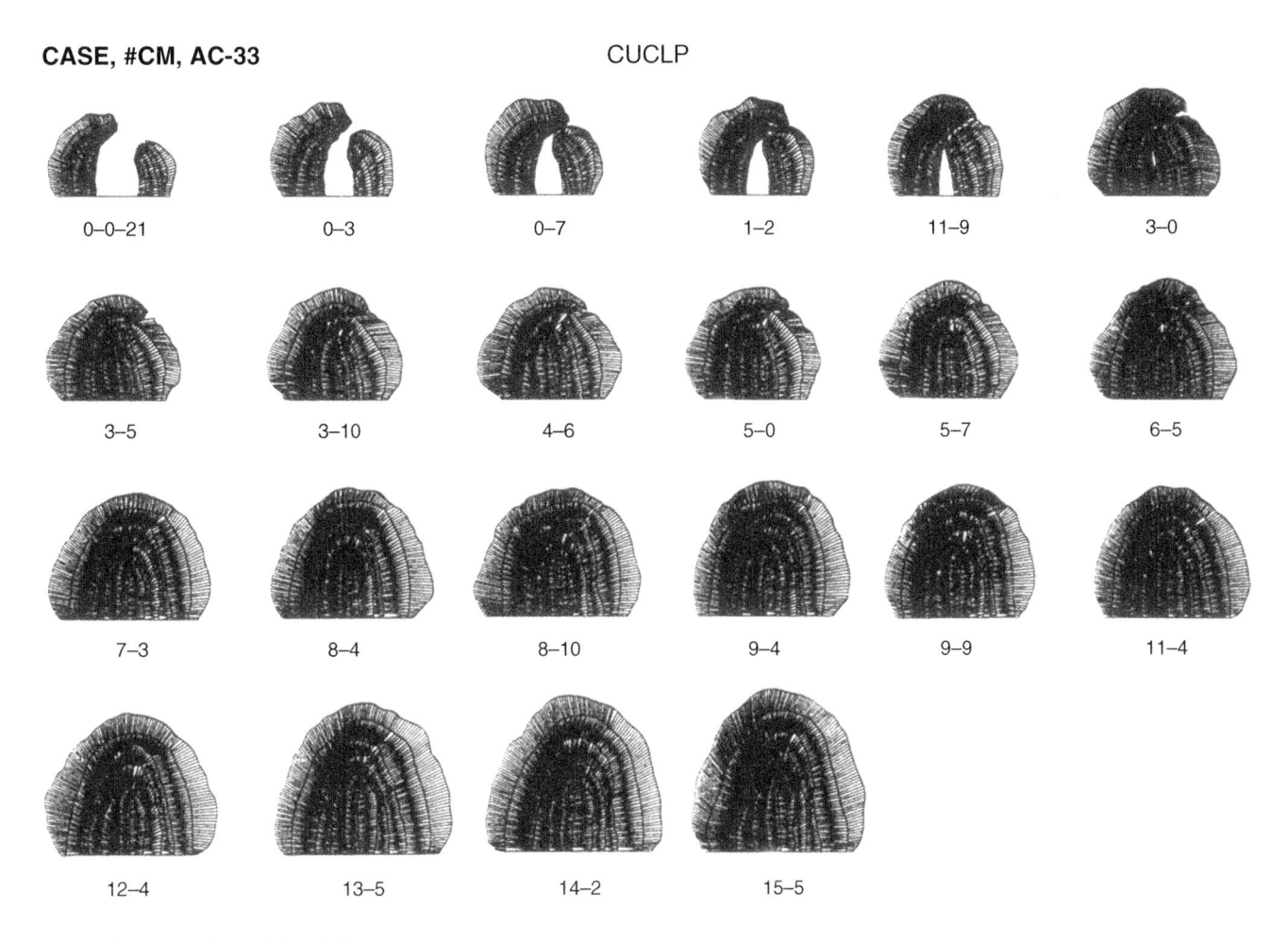

**CASE, #CM, AC-33**  CUCLP

0–0–21   0–3   0–7   1–2   11–9   3–0

3–5   3–10   4–6   5–0   5–7   6–5

7–3   8–4   8–10   9–4   9–9   11–4

12–4   13–5   14–2   15–5

Rapid narrowing of the cleft space

## 7.14 Various Facial Growth Patterns Coben Analysis: Basion Horizontal

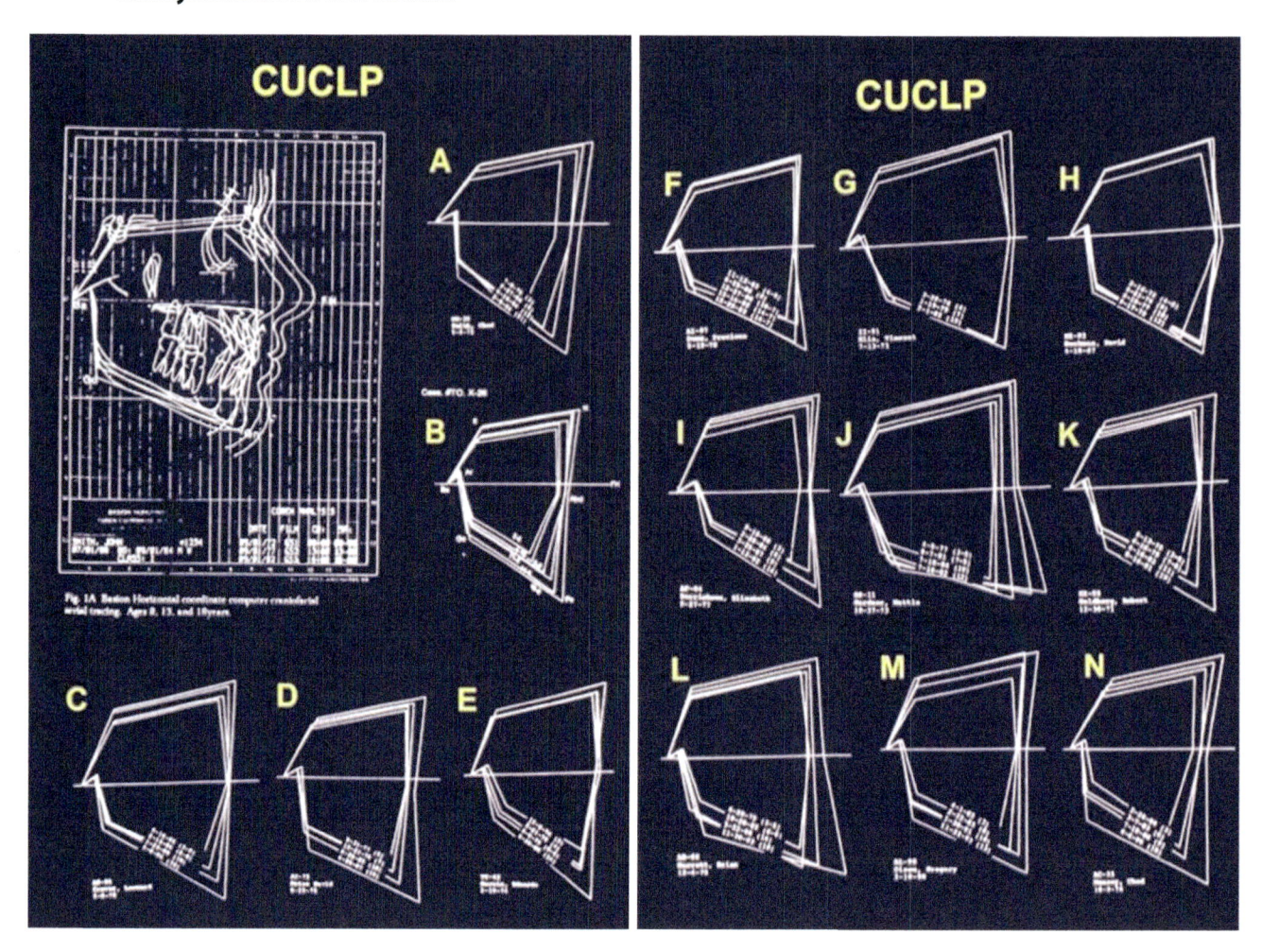

## 7.15 Complete Unilateral Cleft Lip/Palate

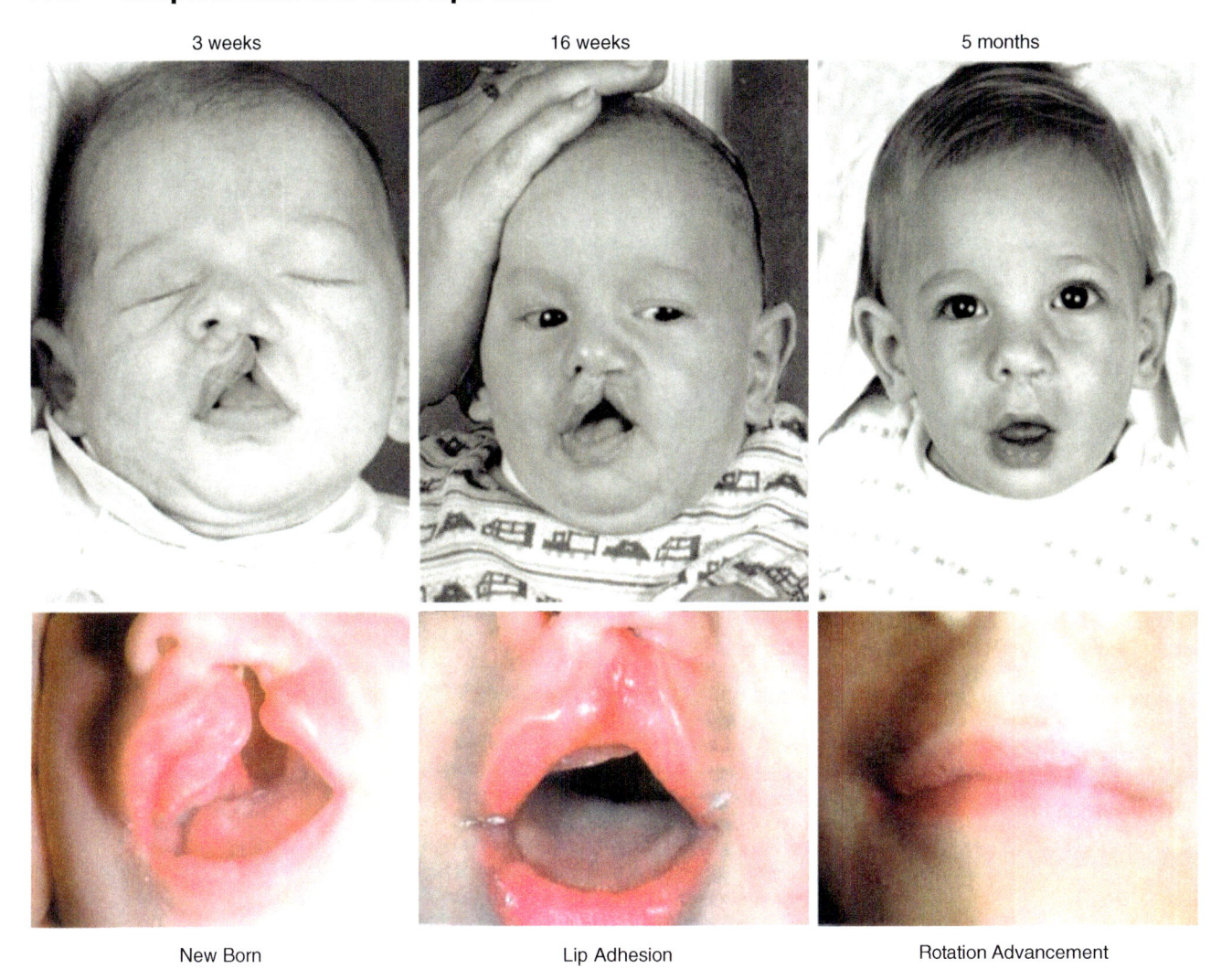

3 weeks        16 weeks        5 months

New Born        Lip Adhesion        Rotation Advancement

6 years					8 years

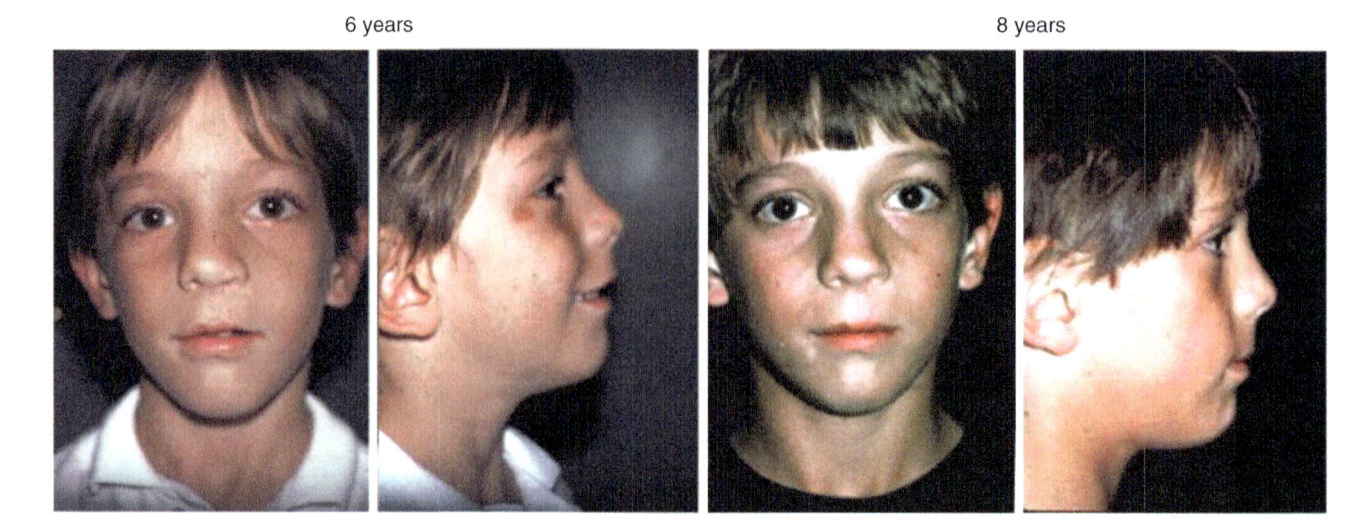

Good Facial Aesthetics

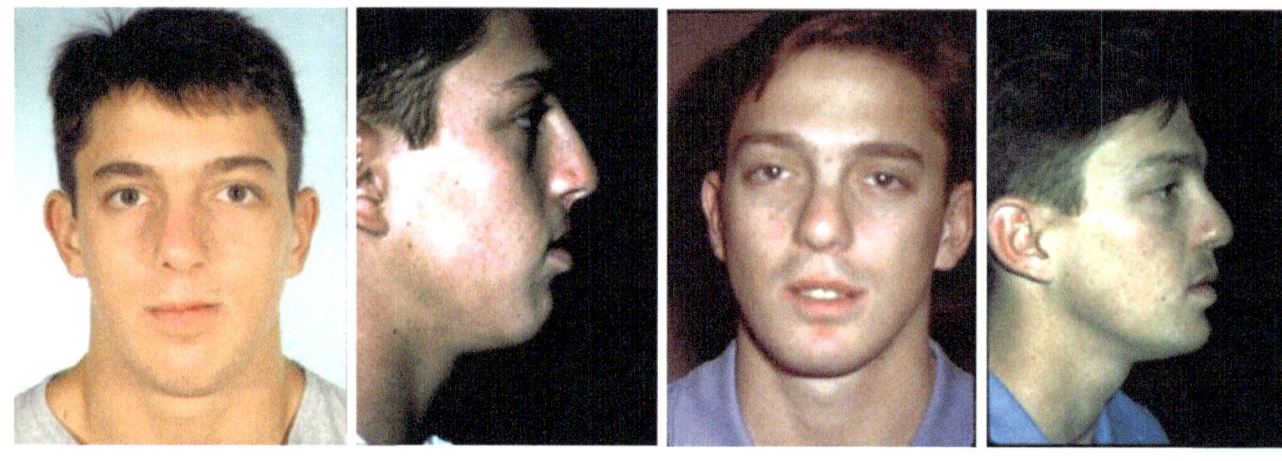

18 years					23 years

7.15 Complete Unilateral Cleft Lip/Palate

**4 years**

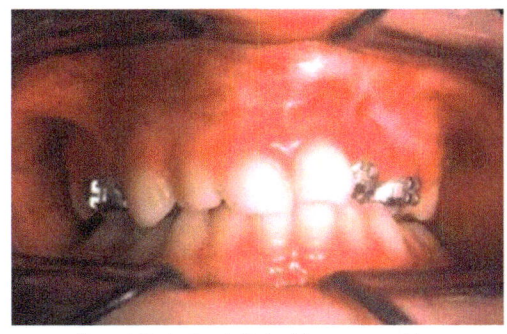

Crossbite in the left deciduous cuspid

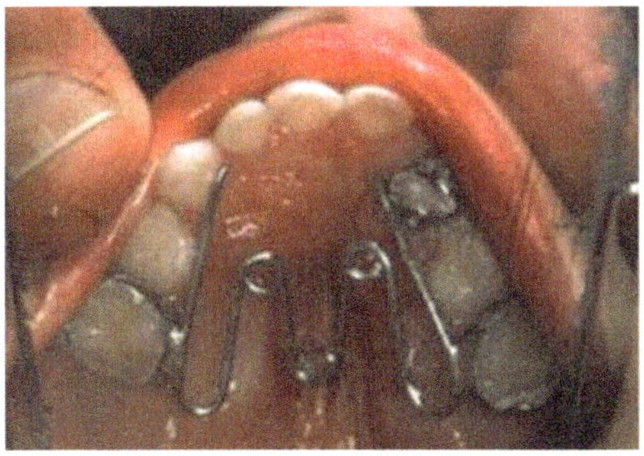

Fixed Palatal Expander

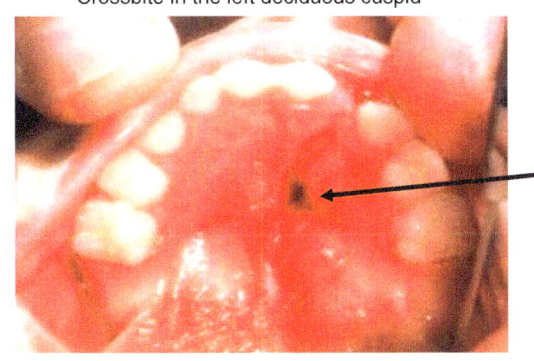

**5 years**

Palate expanded revealing a small fistula.

Left lateral incisor space is open.

**8 years**

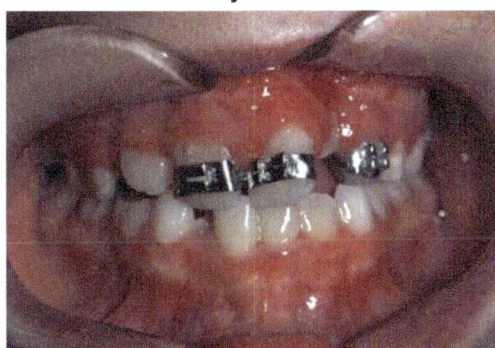

**8 years:**
Maxillary central incisors brought together prior to secondary alveolar bone grafting.

**13 years:**
Teeth in ideal occlusion. Large palatal fistula: No speech problem was reported due to fistula. It was closed after orthodontics was completed.

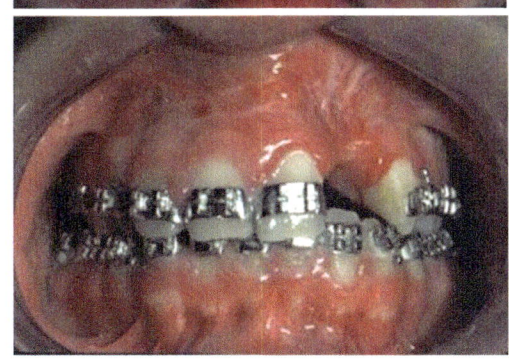

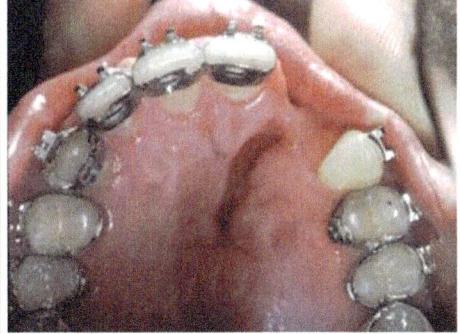

**13 years**

## 22 Years

Anterior bridge with false tooth in left lateral incisor space.

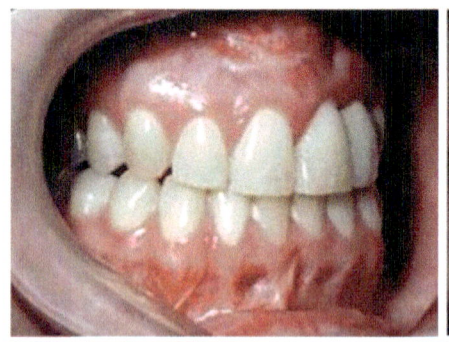

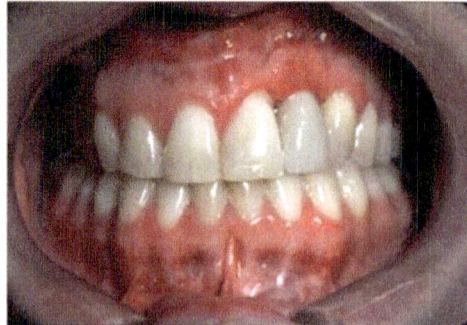

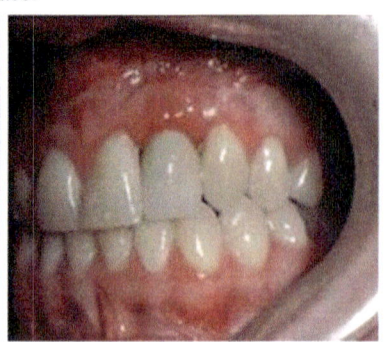

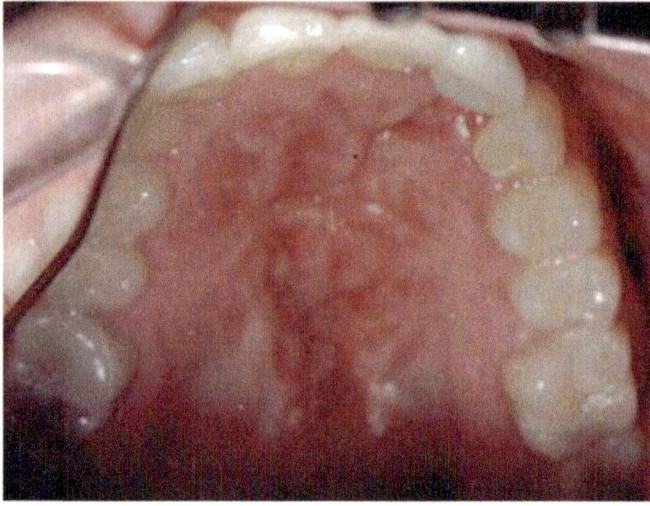

Fistula closed

## 7.16 Median Cleft of the Premaxilla

### 7.16.1 Cleft of the Alveolus only with Missing Central and Lateral Incisors

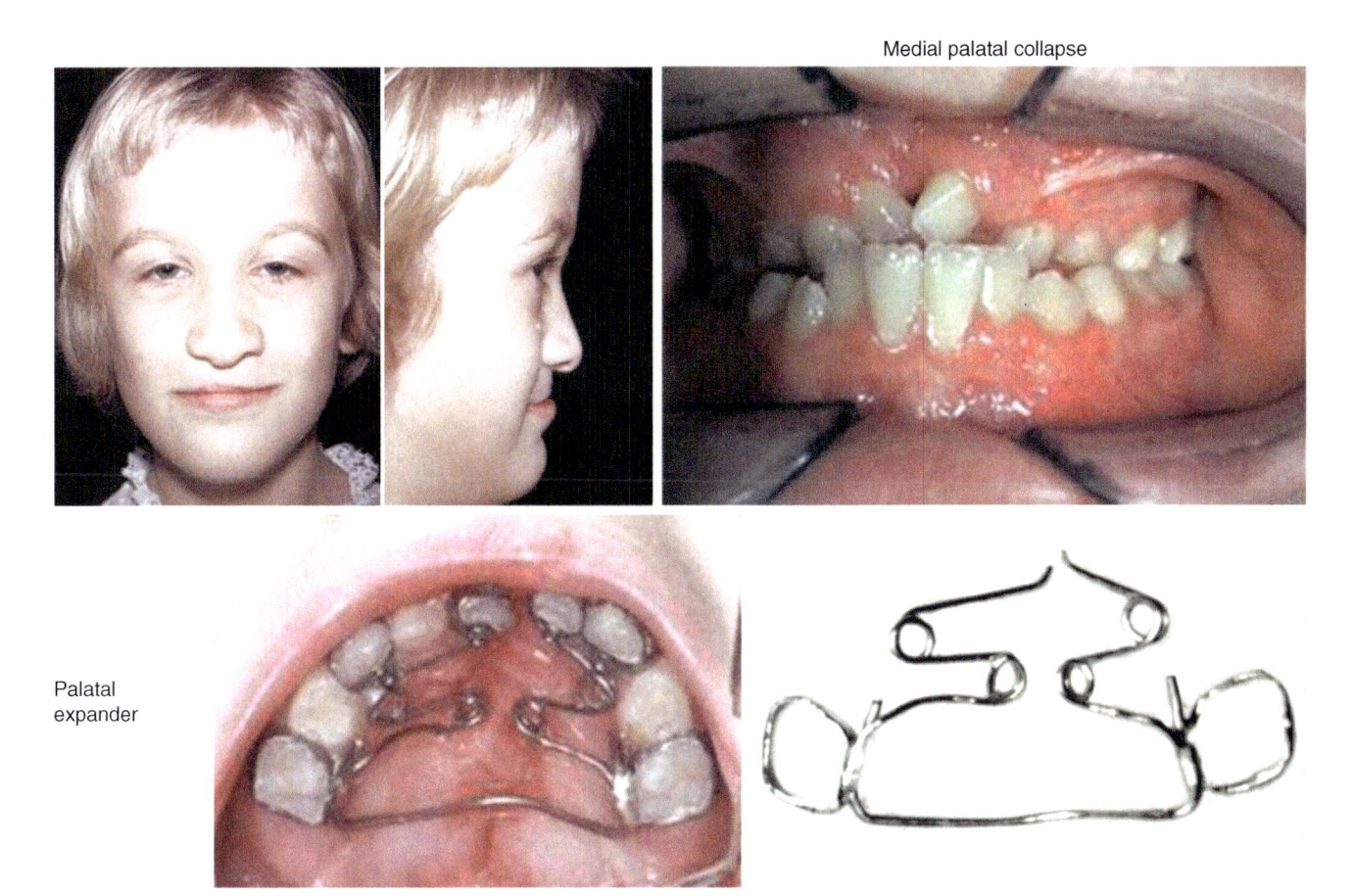

Medial palatal collapse

Palatal expander

First and Second Stage of Expansion/Advancement

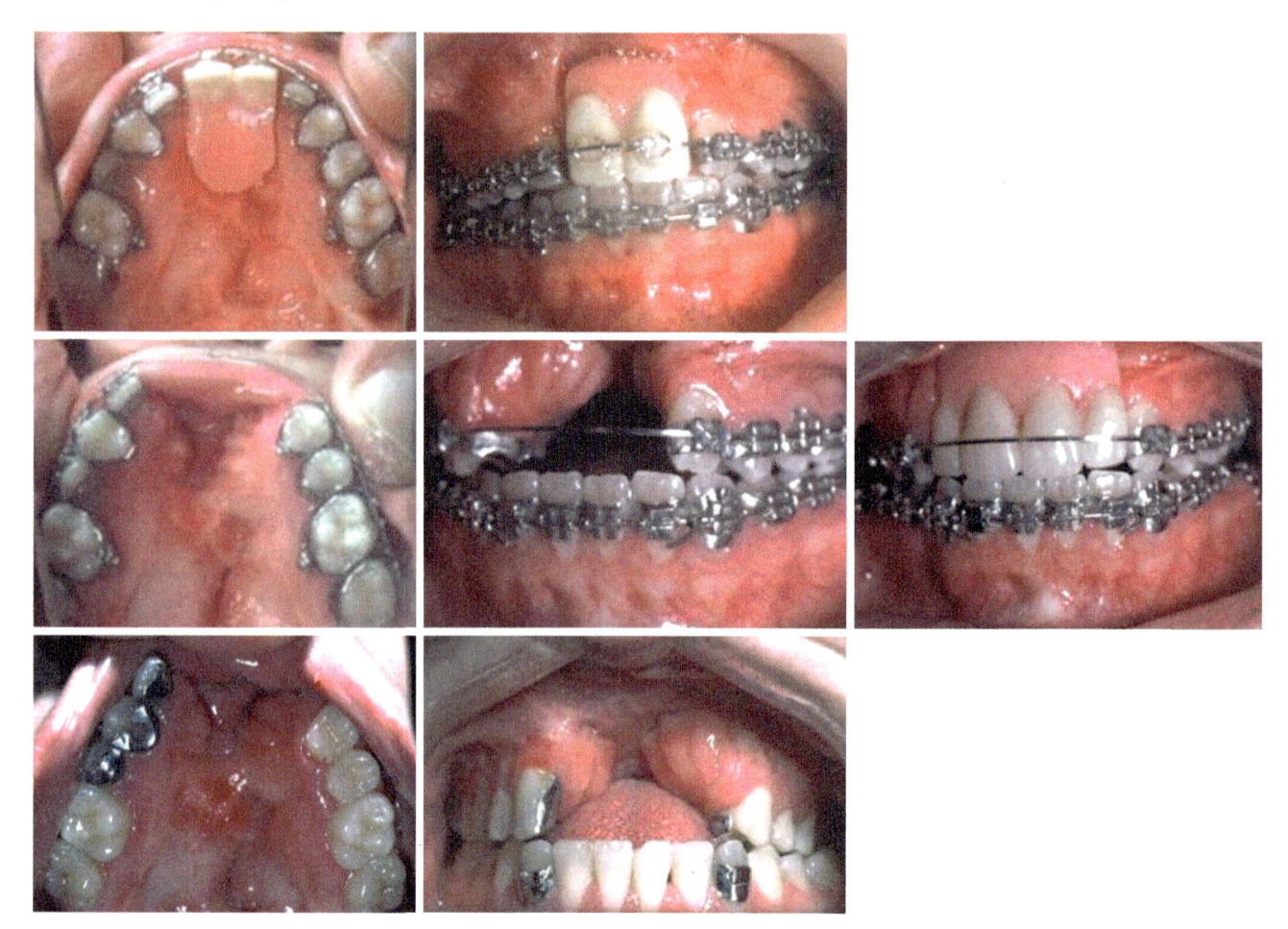

# Protraction Facial Mask

## 8.1 Protraction Facial Mask Orthopedics

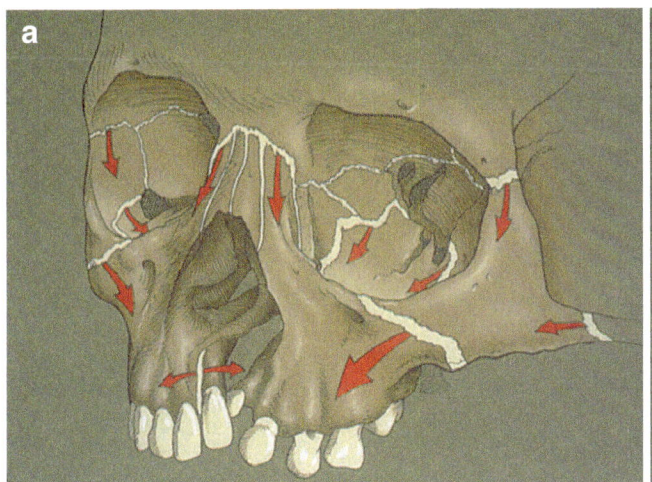

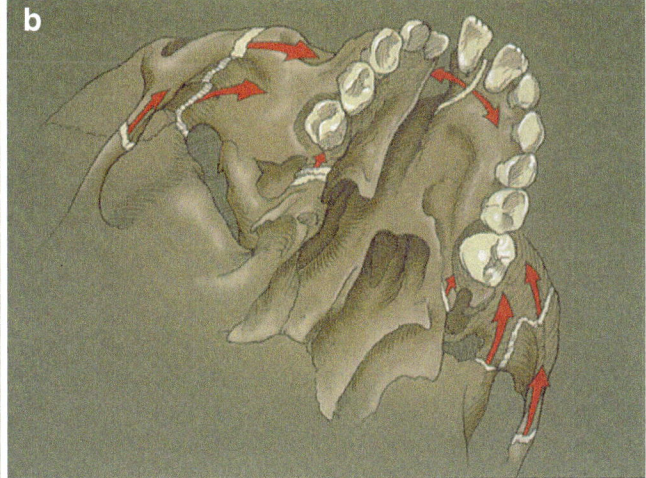

**Protraction of the maxillary complex using orthopedic forces.** The maxilla articulates with nine bones: two of the cranium, the frontal and ethmoid, and seven of the face, viz., the nasal, zygoma, lacrimal, inferior and medial concha, palatine, vomer and its fellow on the opposite side. Sometimes it articulates with the orbital surface, and sometimes with the lateral pterygoid plate of the sphenoid. Illustration showing how protraction forces applied to the maxilla depend on the disarticulation and growth of all the dependent sutures. (Courtesy of *Edward Genecov*)

## 8.2 Distraction Osteogenesis

### 8.2.1 The Rigid External Distraction (RED II) System: Polley and Figuroa

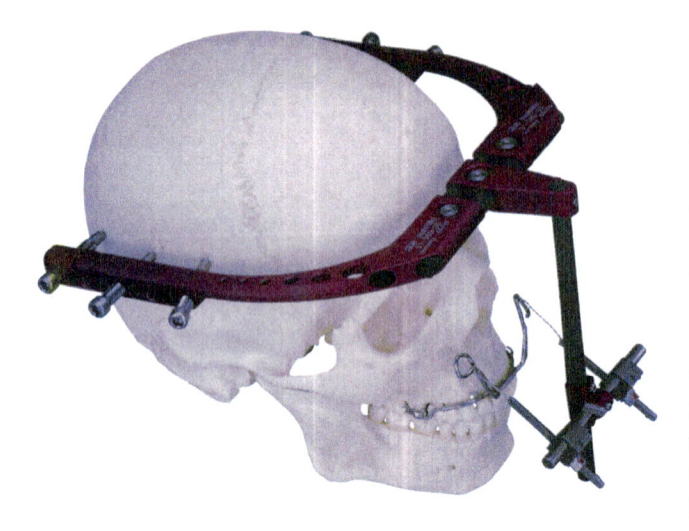

Distraction osteogenesis has become an essential treatment modality for patients with craniomaxillofacial anomalies. The incredible success of the RED (rigid external distractor) for the treatment of severe maxillary hypoplasia associated with cleft palate patients has led to the application of the device to treat many more complex craniofacial anomalies. With the introduction of the RED II, the craniomaxillofacial patients with maxillary and midface skeletal hypoplasia can be effectively treated utilizing the principles of distraction osteogenesis. This technique has unique advantages over traditional surgical methods for the treatment of patients with severe maxillary and midface deficiencies. Some of these important advantages include:

- Ability to successfully treat patients at any age including childhood.
- Ability to treat patients with severe skeletal deficiencies who are not amenable to, or would receive compromised results with, conventional orthognathic surgery.
- Ability to focus treatment on only the affected skeletal region.
- Ability to treat severe deformities with minimal associated morbidity and at reduced cost.
- No bone grafting or internal fixation devices required.

The KLS-Martin rigid external distraction (RED II) system provides the means to obtain predictable and consistent results in maxillary and midface distraction. This system was designed to provide the surgeon the ability to deliver controlled rigid distraction forces without the need for internal hardware. The advantages of this Rigid External Distraction (RED II) system are multiple and include:

- Allows rigid distraction forces.
- Allows multidirectional, accurate distraction.
- Allows for multiplanar adjustability of distraction forces at any time during the distraction procedure.
- Is easily and quickly placed at the time of osteotomy.
- Is easily and quickly removed in the office or clinical setting.
- Allows for predictable results.
- Assures patient compliance during the distraction procedure.

8.2 Distraction Osteogenesis

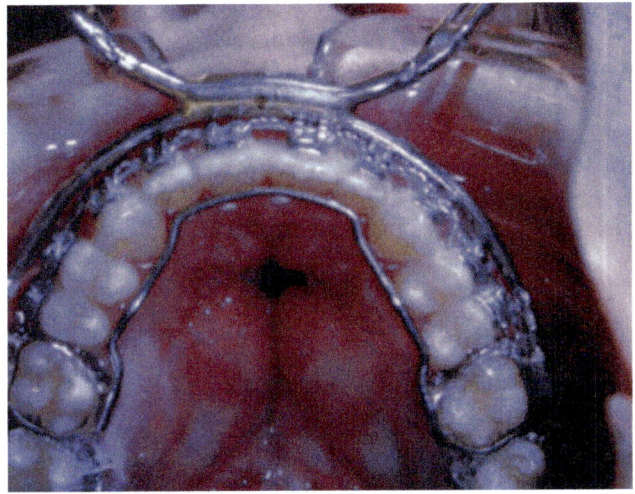

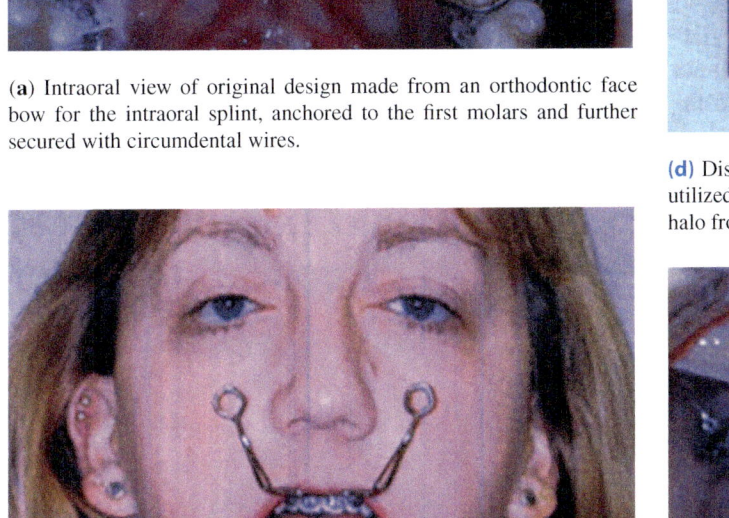

(a) Intraoral view of original design made from an orthodontic face bow for the intraoral splint, anchored to the first molars and further secured with circumdental wires.

(b) Facial view of patient wearing the device prior to surgery and demonstrating the external traction hooks.

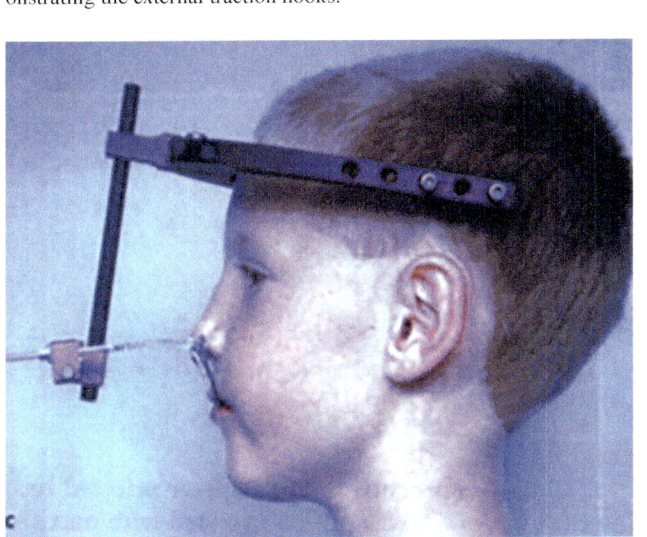

(c) Patient wearing the rigid external distraction system. Note the wires connecting the traction hooks from the intraoral splint to the traction screws from the rigid external distraction device.

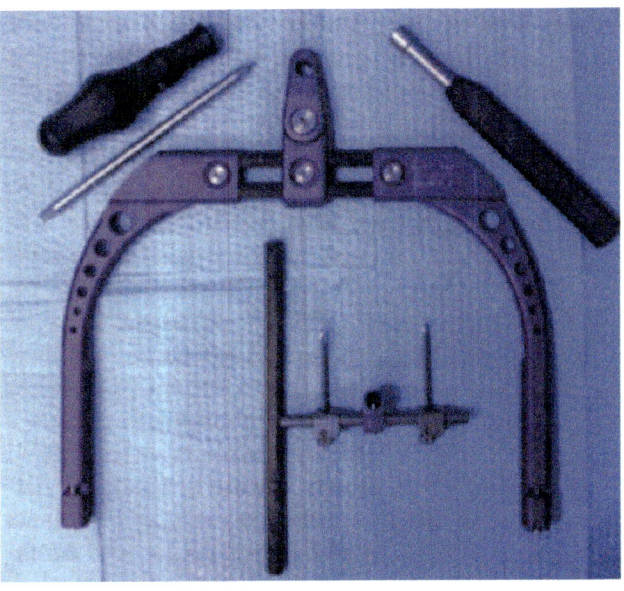

(d) Disassembled distraction device. Note posterior screws on the halo, utilized during midfacial advancement to clear the anterior part of the halo from forehead.

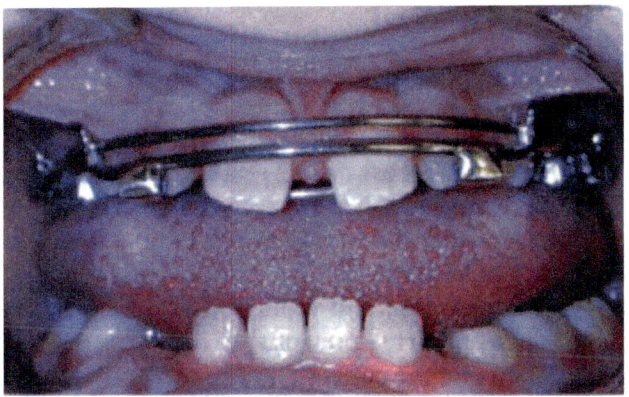

(e) Intraoral view of newly designed intraoral splint with removable external distraction hooks. Designed in this fashion to avoid the presence of hooks at surgery.

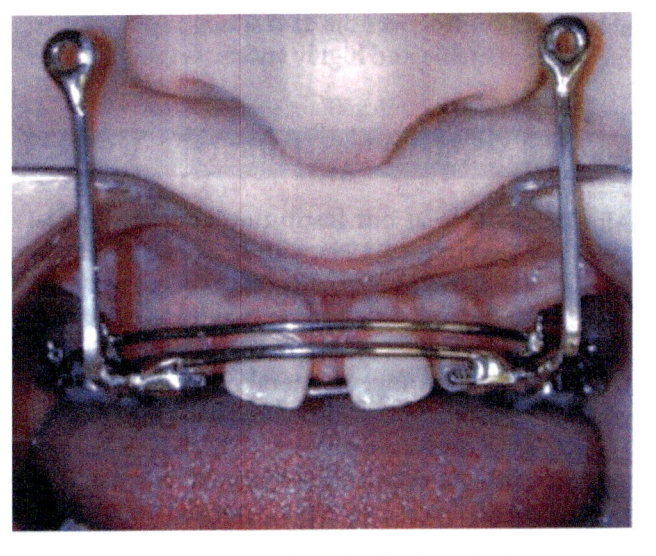

(f) Intraoral splint with removable distraction hooks in place.

### 8.2.2 Before and After: Results of Using the Rigid External Distraction (RED II) System

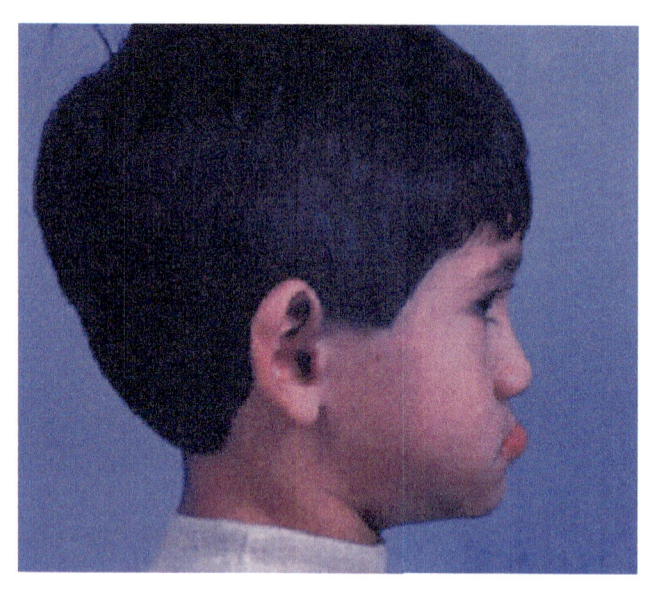

5-year-old patient prior to Rigid External Distraction (RED) treatment

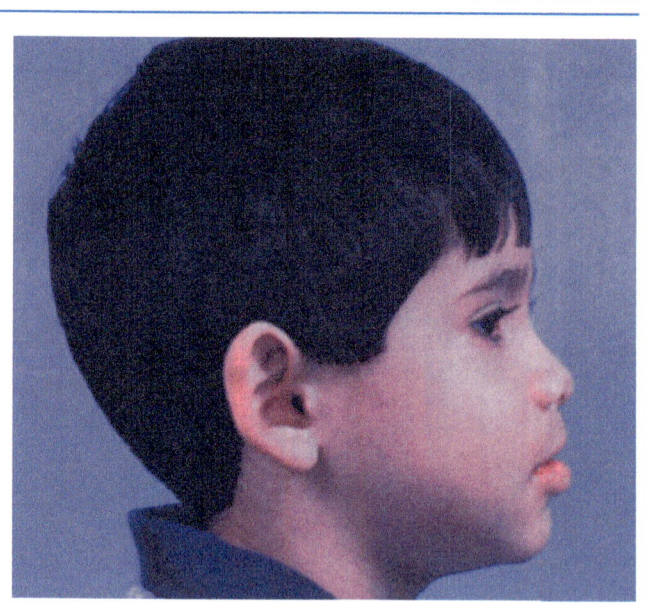

5-year-old patient after Rigid External Distraction (RED) treatment

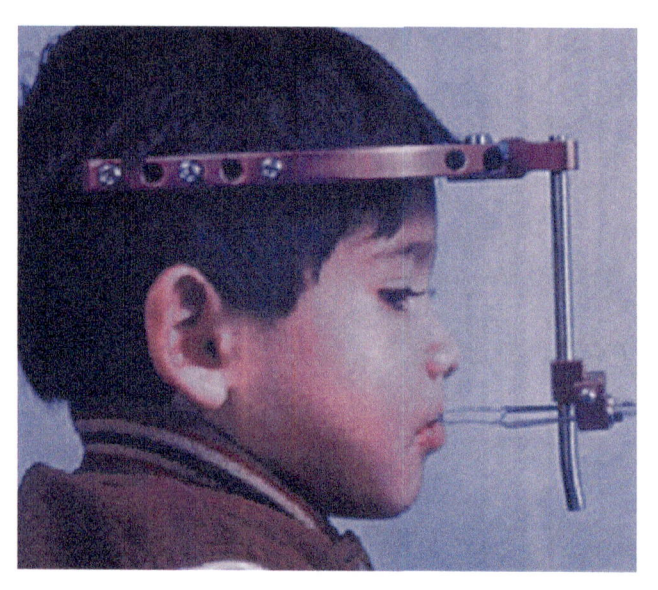

Patient fitted with a rigid external distractor during treatment

## 8.2 Distraction Osteogenesis

Predistraction (solid line) and postdistractions (broken line) average tracings for rigid external distraction group. Note the significant maxillary advancement (effective incisor advancement 11.6 mm) with correction of overjet, improvement of skeletal convexity, and minimal changes in mandibular position. Note the significant soft tissue changes including the significant degree of lip and nasal tip advancement.

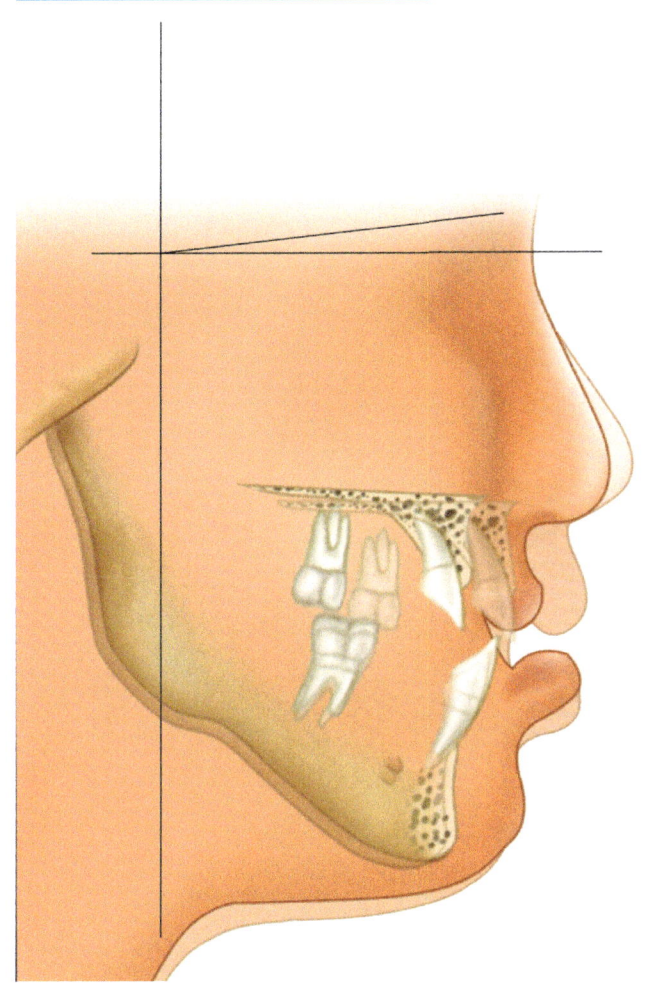

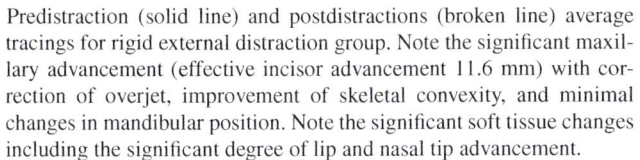

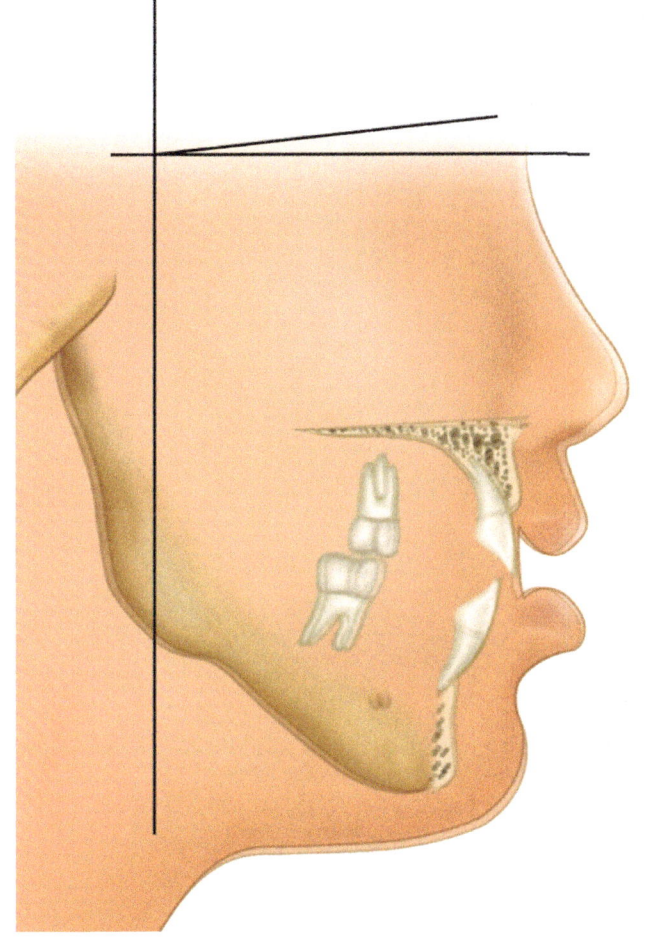

Postdistraction (solid line) and 1 year (broken line) after distraction average tracings of the cleft sample treated with the rigid external distraction system. Note excellent stability of the advanced maxilla.

## 8.3 Distraction Osteogenesis to the Mandible: F. Molina

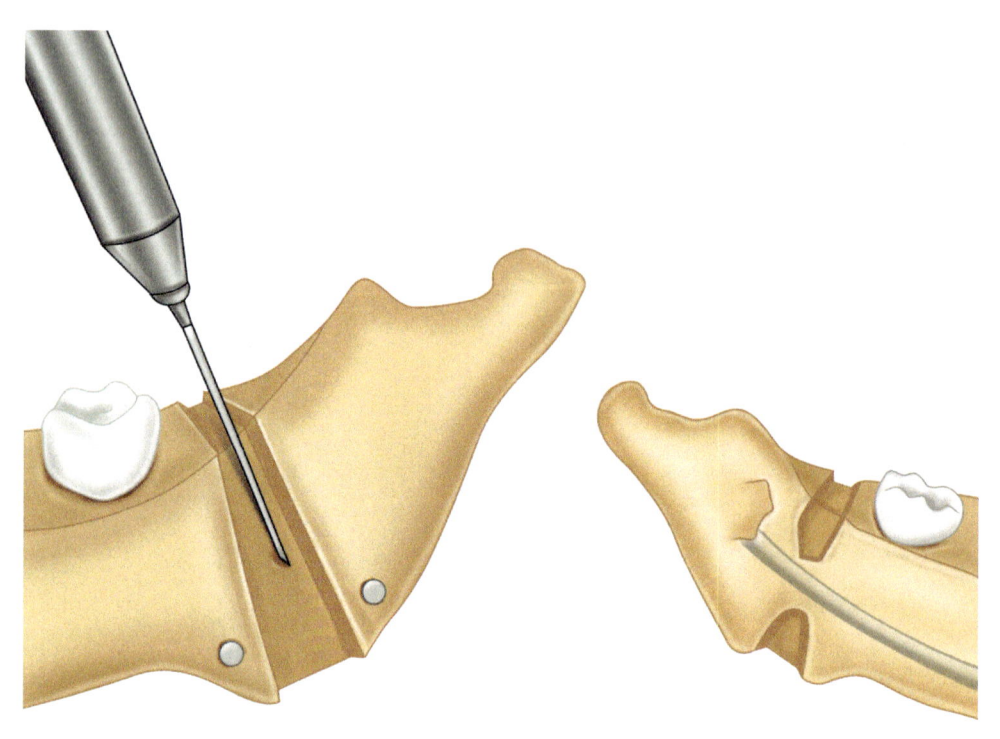

(a) and (b) Side-cutting burr and the external-extended corticotomy from the free mandibular border to the gonial angle. The corticotomy is interrupted as soon as the cancellous bone is visible. (b) At the lingual cortex, the bone cut is incomplete, preserving 6–7 mm of the internal cortical flayer at the site of the neurovascular bundle.

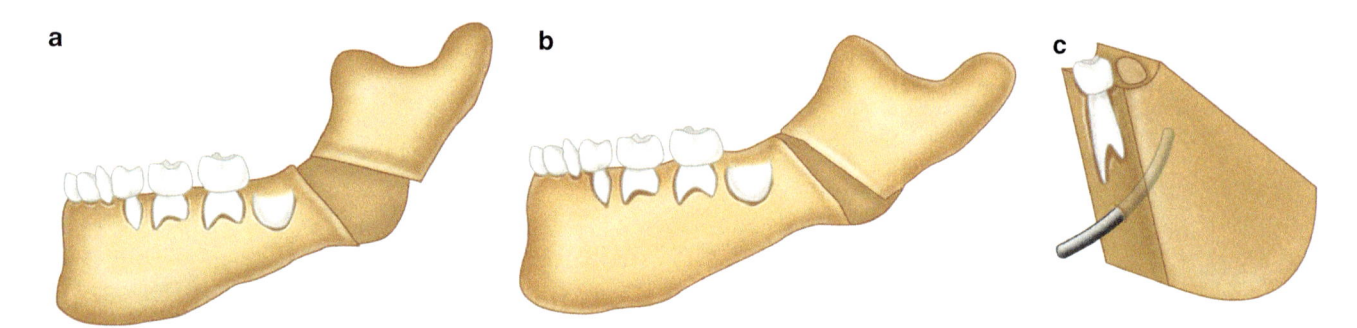

(a) Location of the corticotomy in a Grade II-A hemifacial microsomia. (b) Using an oblique vector, the new bone formation production is larger at the angle and minor at the alveolar ridge, also at the initial portion of the ascending ramus. (c) Tridimensional diagram of the regenerate bone. The new volumetric bone formation corrects the height, the length, and position of the mandible. The tooth buds and neurovascular elements have been preserved.

## 8.4 Hemifacial Microsomia: Distraction Osteogenesis: F. Molina

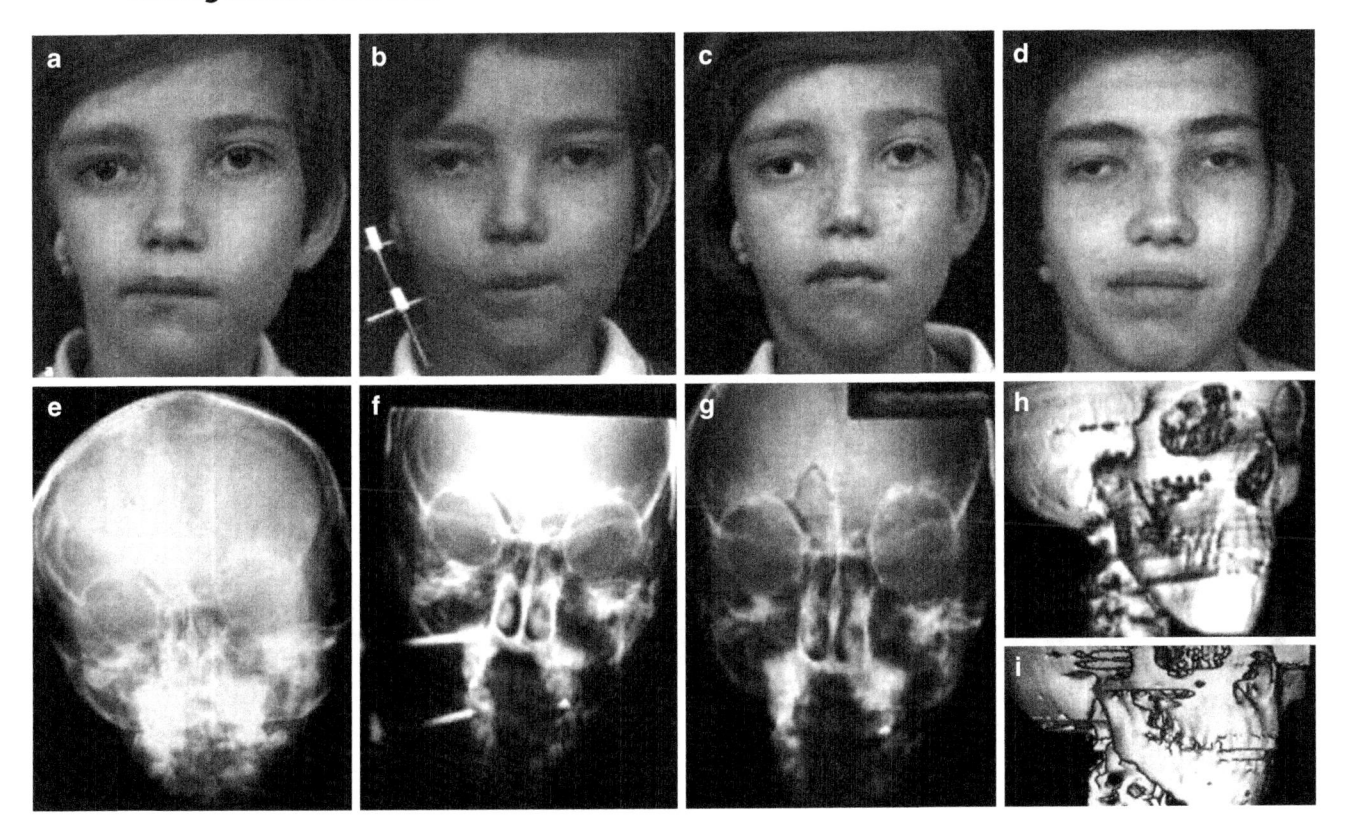

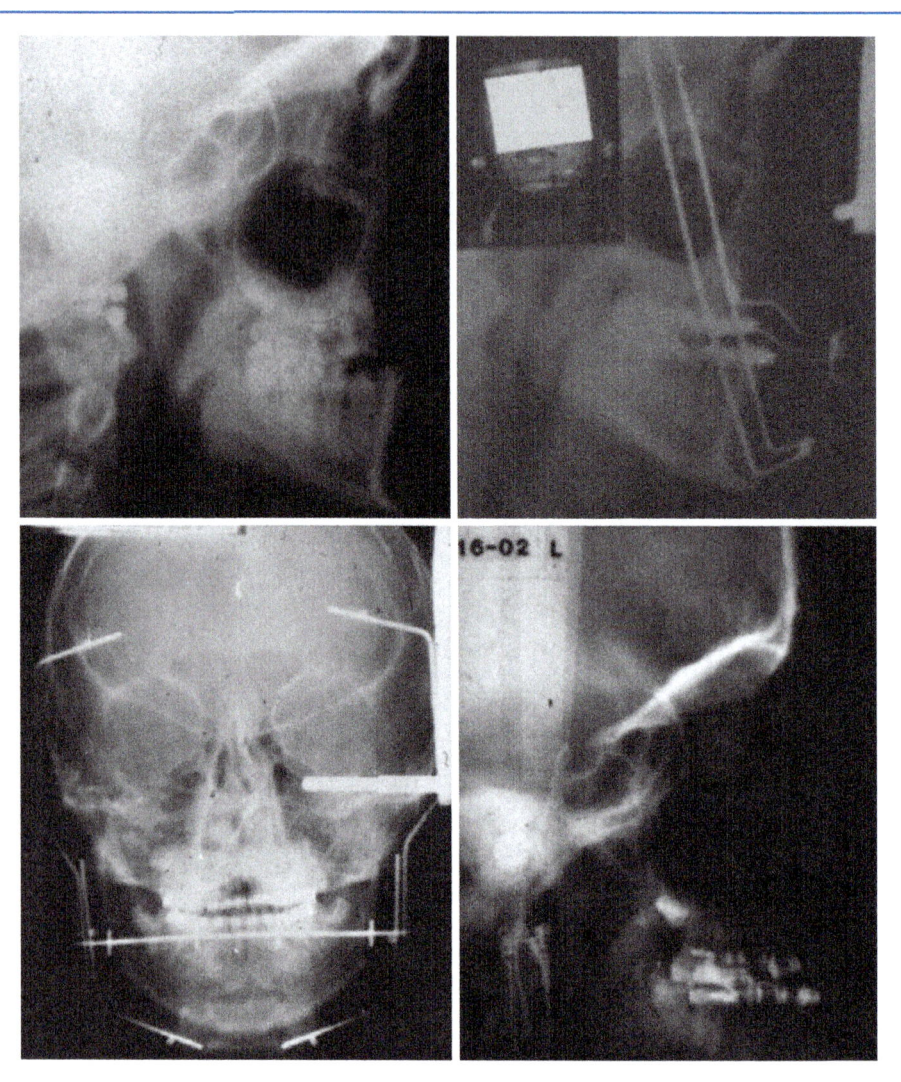

Use of an orthopedic protraction facial mask to advance the maxilla

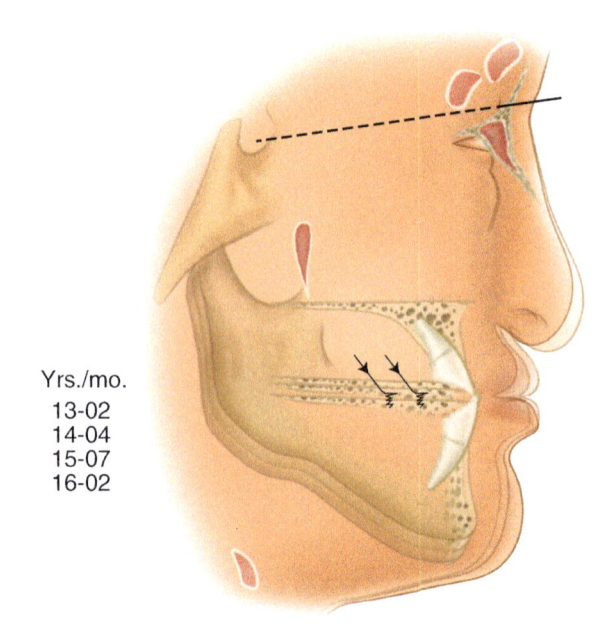

Yrs./mo.
13-02
14-04
15-07
16-02

Forward movement of the maxillary complex using a protraction facial mask

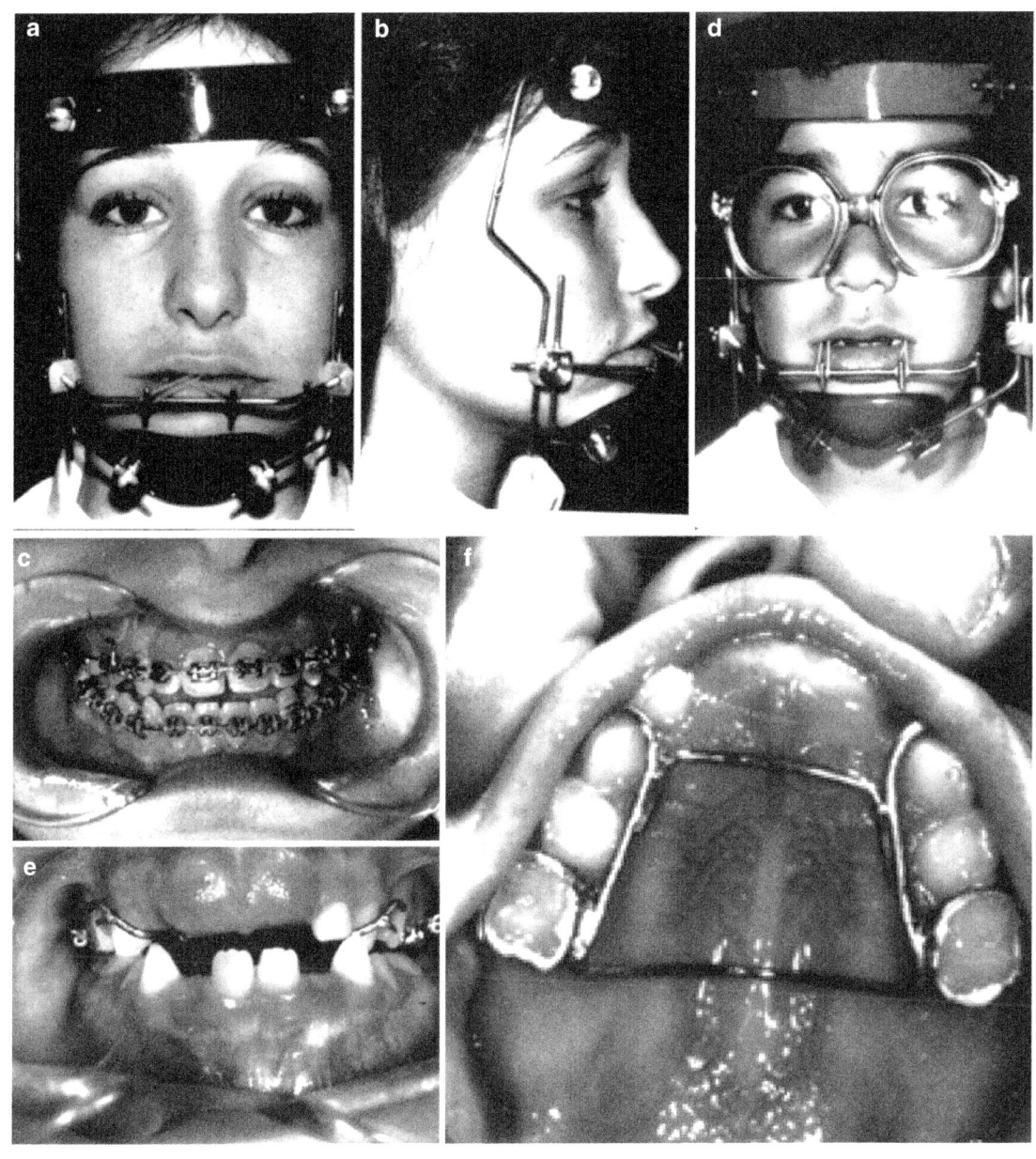

A. Orthodontics

For tooth advancement forces to be directed anteriorly from the cuspids parallel to the occlusal plane. Movement limited to 2-3 mm.

B. Orthopedics (bone movement) is dependent upon forces being applied downward and forward at the cuspid and at least 350 - 400 g/side.

(a) Frontal and (b) lateral views of a Delaire-style protraction facial mask. Padded chin and forehead rests distribute reaction forces of 350–400 g per side equally to both areas. Elastics are attached to hooks placed on the arch wire between the cuspids and lateral incisor. (c) Intraoral view of edgewise-rectangular arch with hooks for protraction elastics. (d), (e), and (f) Delaire-style protraction facial mask used with a fixed labial-palatal wire framework. Elastic forces of 350–400 g per side can still be used with this intraoral framework.

### 8.5　A.S. Case# AY-46 Vertical Growth Pattern

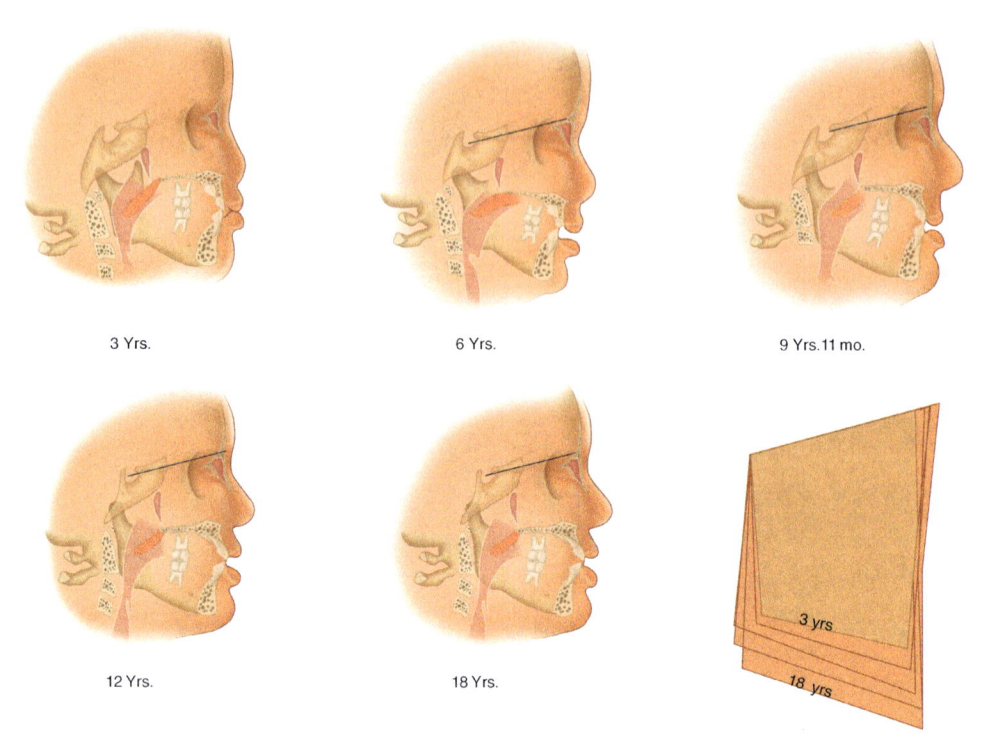

3 Yrs.　　　　6 Yrs.　　　　9 Yrs.11 mo.

12 Yrs.　　　　18 Yrs.　　　　3 yrs / 18 yrs

**Fig 9–24. Case AS (AY-46).** (**a**) Serial lateral cephalometric tracings and (**b**) Serial superimposed polygons (Basion Horizontal method) show slightly retarded midfacial growth. Fortunately, the vertical mandibular growth pattern compliments a reduced midfacial growth preventing the creation of an anterior crossbite. Comments: Protraction orthopedic forces was initiated when more permanent teeth have erupted at 10-9.

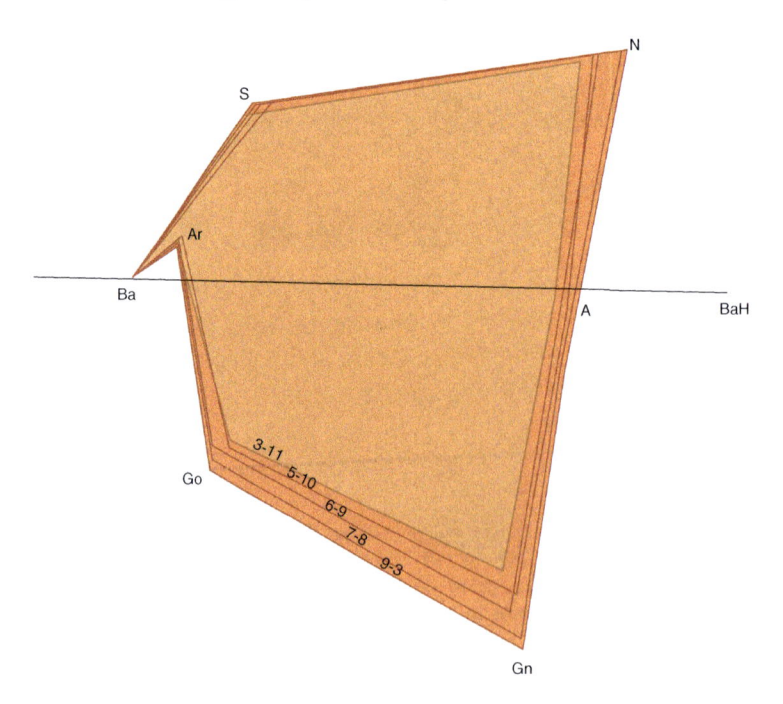

### 8.6　Vertical Growth Pattern

This case demonstrates why it was possible to establish good facial aesthetics and occlusion without the need to surgically advance the midface or retract the mandible. Although a slight facial concavity exist, it was still aesthetically acceptable.

# Complete Bilateral Cleft Lip and Palate

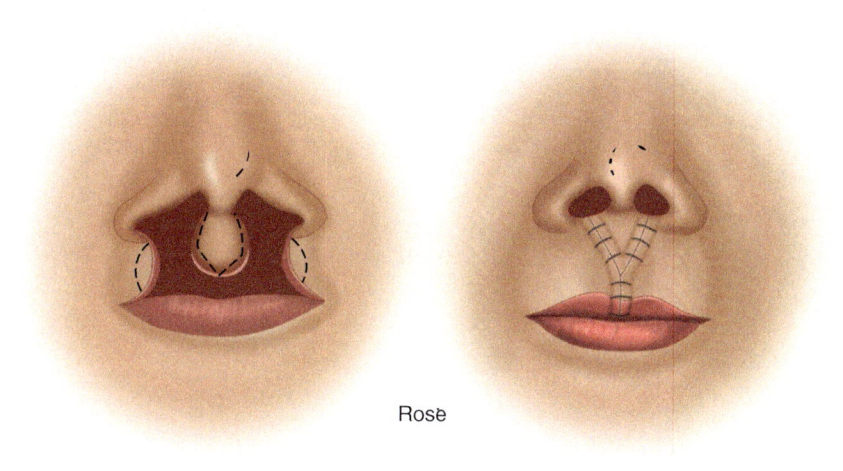

9

Rose

Various surgical techniques used to unite the lip in BCLP. Experience has shown that the best results are obtained when the prolabium is used to construct the entire midportion of the lip.

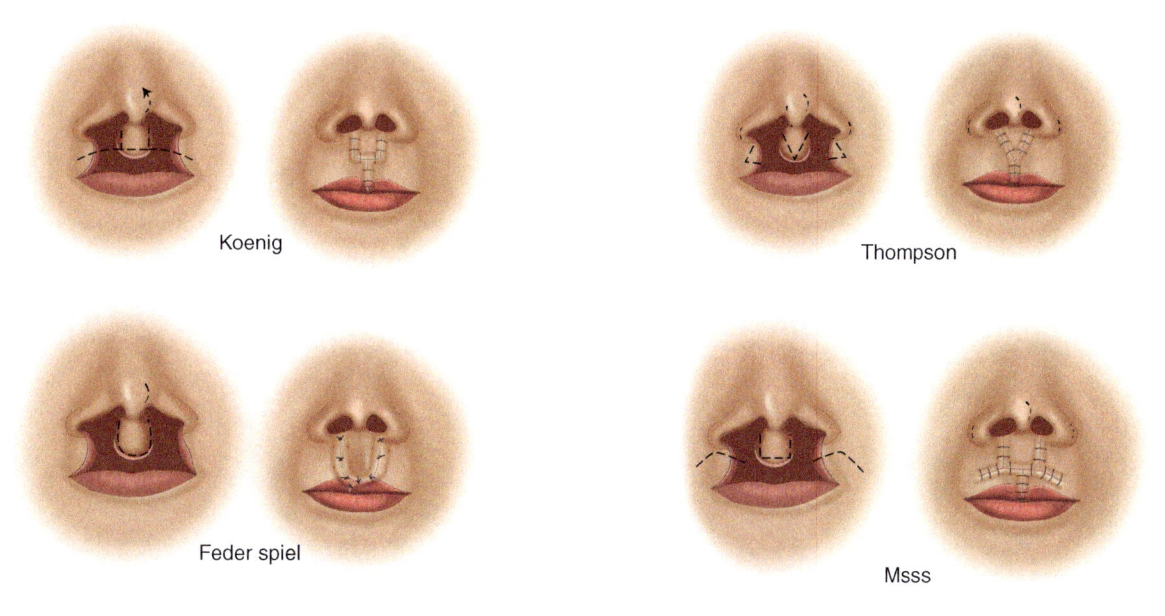

Koenig

Thompson

Feder spiel

Msss

The Best!

Illustrations by Dr. Millard Jr. *Cleft Craft* 1980

## 9.1 Lip Surgery in Complete Bilateral Cleft Lip and Palate

### 9.1.1 Mucosa and Muscle Joined Behind the Prolabium

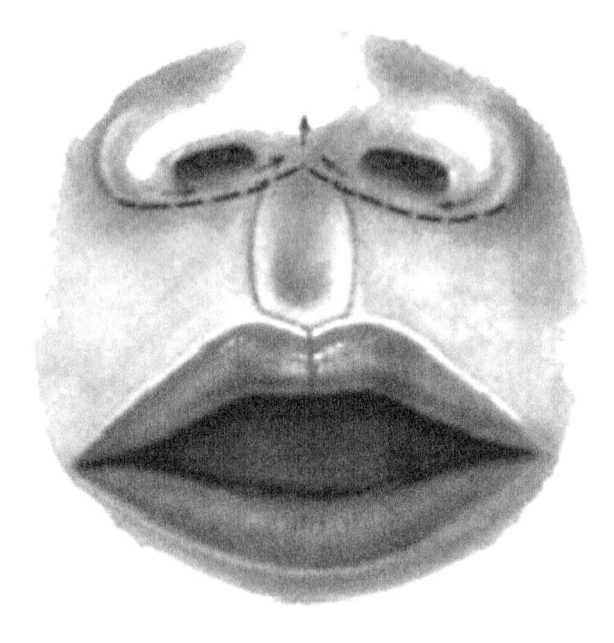

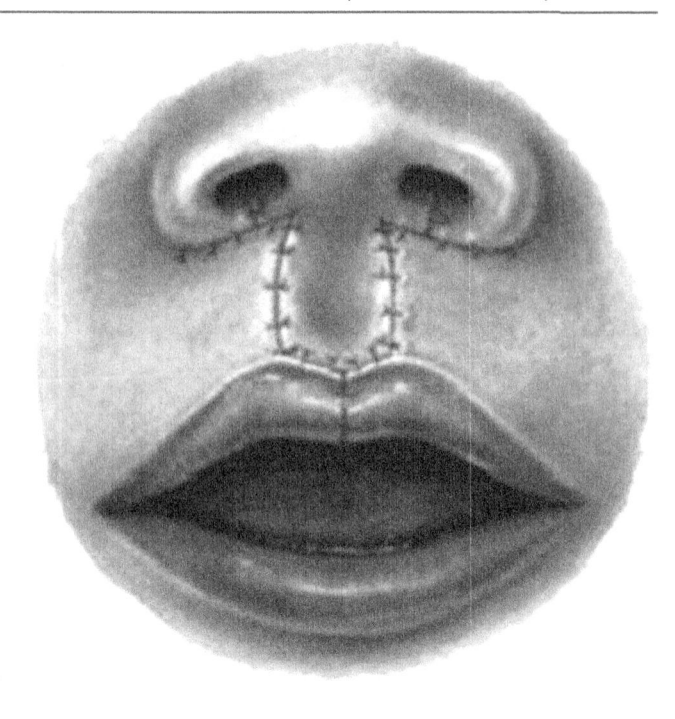

If columella slightly short keep wide floors for later advancement.

The suture closure after tying dimple stitch.

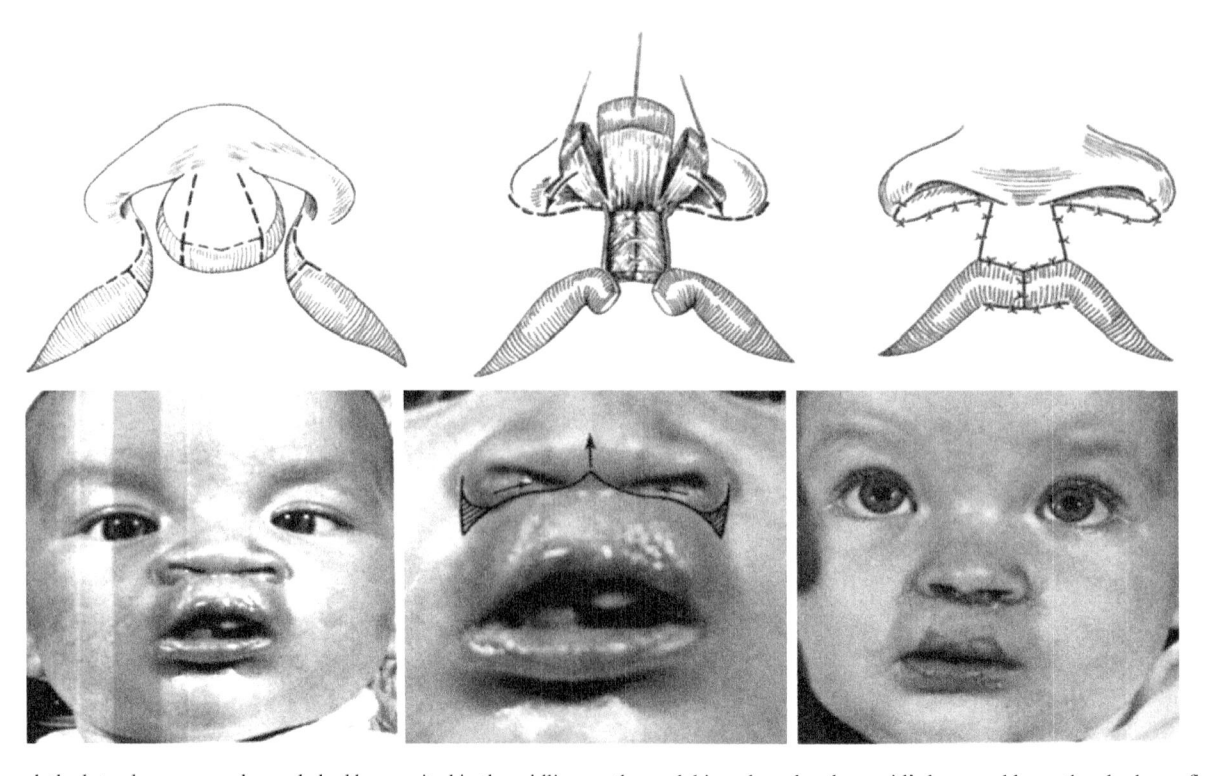

Although the lateral mucosa and muscle had been united in the midline, the upper muscle approximation had been timid and the alar bases had not been advanced medially in an attempt to leave a subalar gap in which to store the forks. This allowed subsequent lateral pull to spread the prolabium, broaden the cupid's bow, and leave the alar bases flared. Then, when it came time to shift the forked flap, advancement of the wide alar bases required. (Illustrations by Dr. Millard Jr. *Cleft Craft* 1980)

## 9.2 Variations of Palatal Segments to Each Other, and Premaxilla Size in Bilateral Cleft Lip and Palate

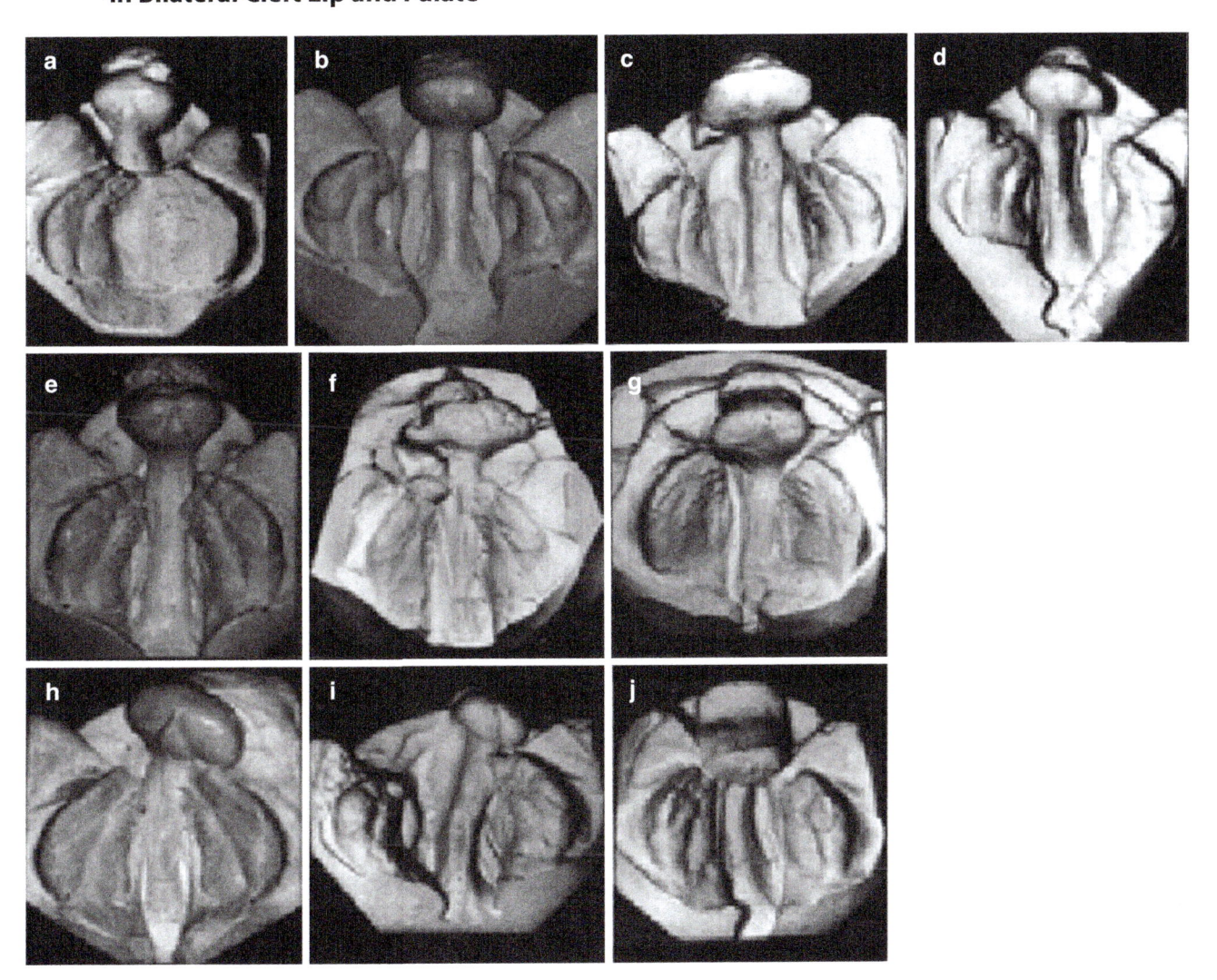

## 9.3 Protruding Premaxilla with Overexpanded Palatal Shelves

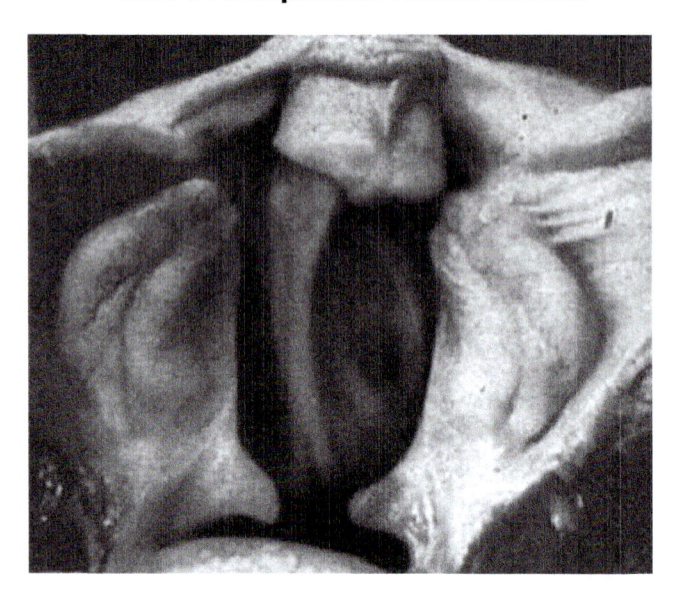

## 9.4 Growth of Premaxillary Vomerine Suture (PVS)

Growth occurs at PVS—increase of pellet distance on either side of PVS

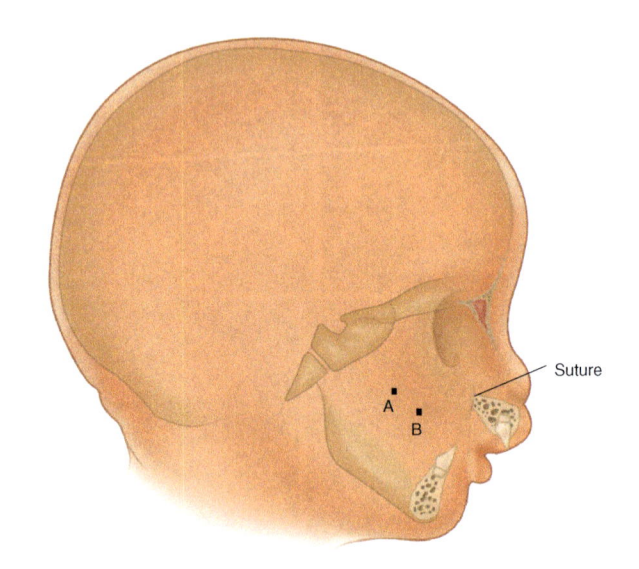

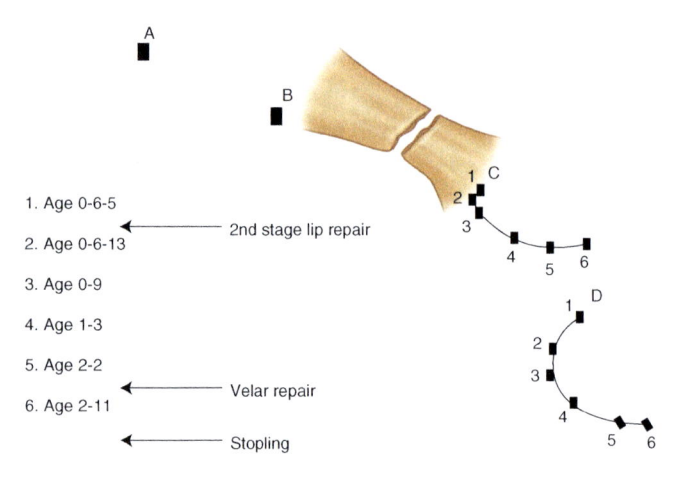

1. Age 0-6-5
2. Age 0-6-13 ← 2nd stage lip repair
3. Age 0-9
4. Age 1-3
5. Age 2-2
6. Age 2-11 ← Velar repair
   ← Stopling

## 9.5 Various Possible CBCLP Treatments

1. Lip repair only.
2. Excision of premaxilla.
3. Early setback of premaxilla.
4. Late setback of premaxilla.

## 9.6 Complete Bilateral Cleft Lip and Palate Conservative Treatment

The following cases were selected to demonstrate that staged treatment is necessary to achieve excellent facial aesthetics, good occlusion, and speech.

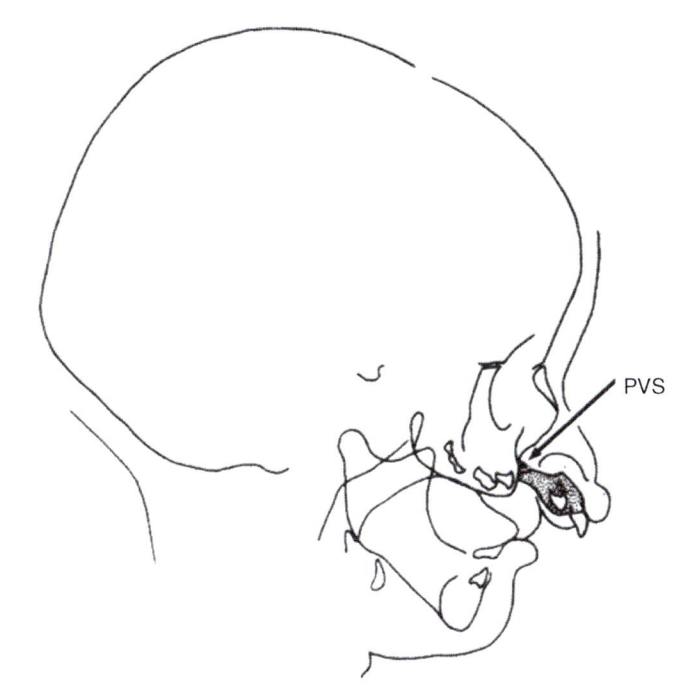

There are no surgical procedures that could be used at birth to permit these goals to be achieved by surgery alone.

Although the classification system designates similarity in cleft type, these cases demonstrate that the facial growth pattern, degree of osteogenic deficiency, and palatal growth are the variables which need to be taken into consideration.

One needs to focus on the premaxillary vomerine suture to better understand its importance in achieving good facial aesthetics. The premaxilla's forward growth is retarded by the repaired lip while the lateral palatal segments (the maxilla) grow forward closing the anterior cleft space in most cases.

## 9.6.1 Protruding Premaxilla Anterior and Posterior Cleft Spaces

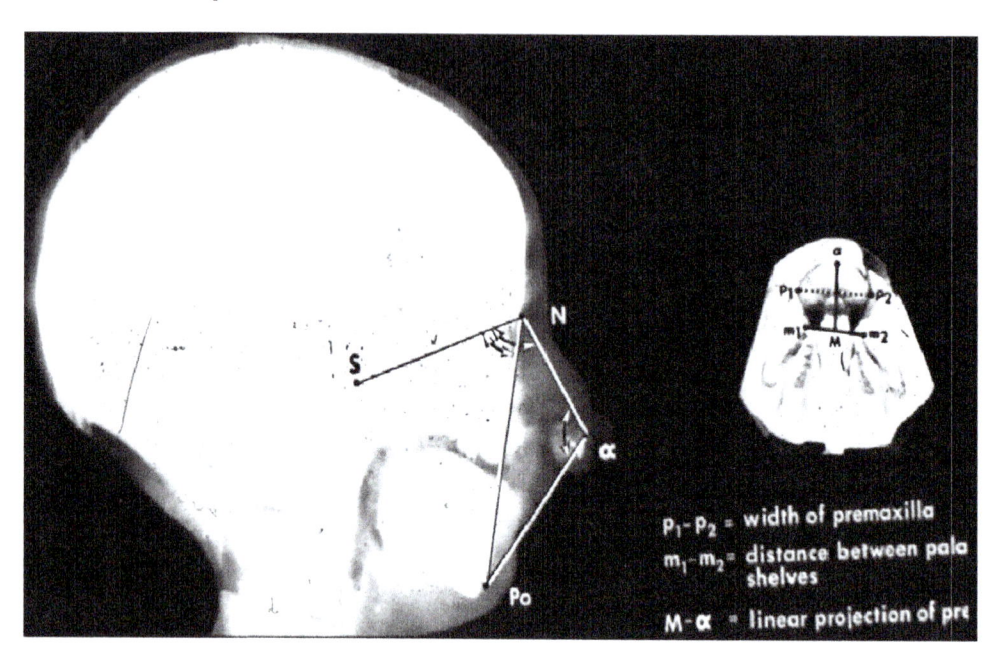

$p_1$-$p_2$ = width of premaxilla
$m_1$-$m_2$ = distance between pala shelves
M-$\alpha$ = linear projection of pre

## 9.7 Lateral Head X-Ray Shows The Kirschner Wire

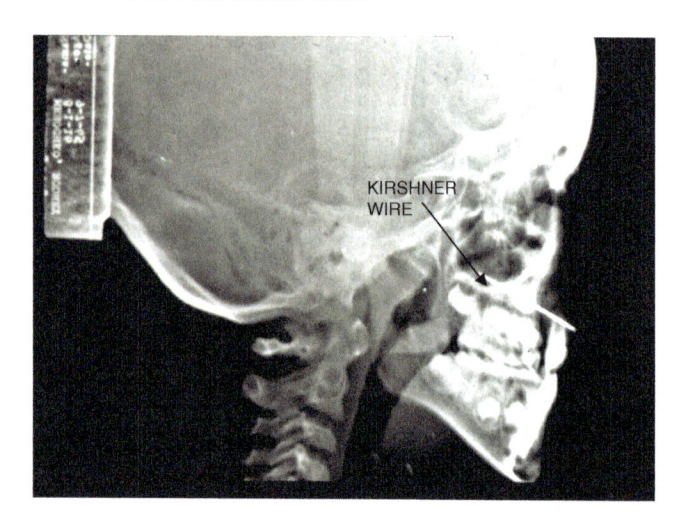

## 9.8 Premaxillary Surgical Setback

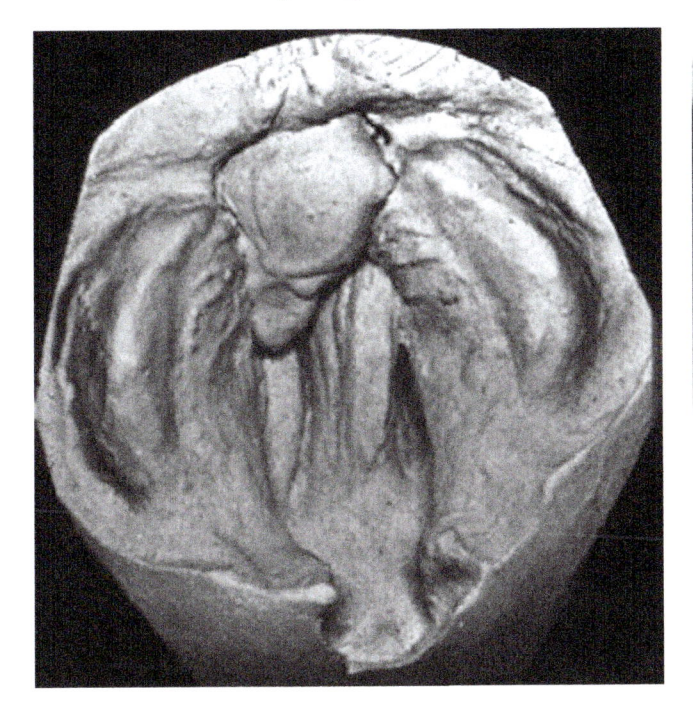

## 9.9 Kirschner Wire Placed in Premaxilla But Missing the Vomer

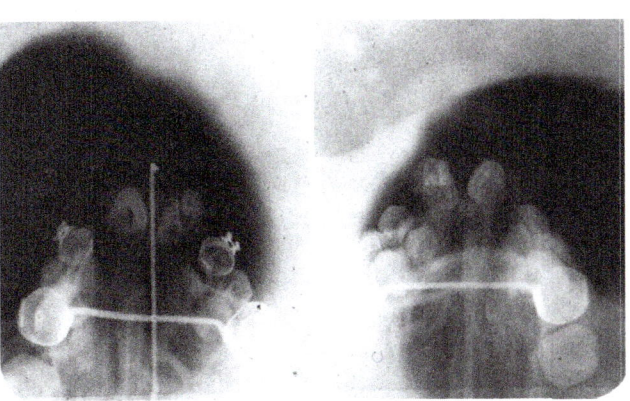

## 9.10 A Case Where Kirschner Wire Was Used, Hopefully to Stabilize Retropositional Premaxilla

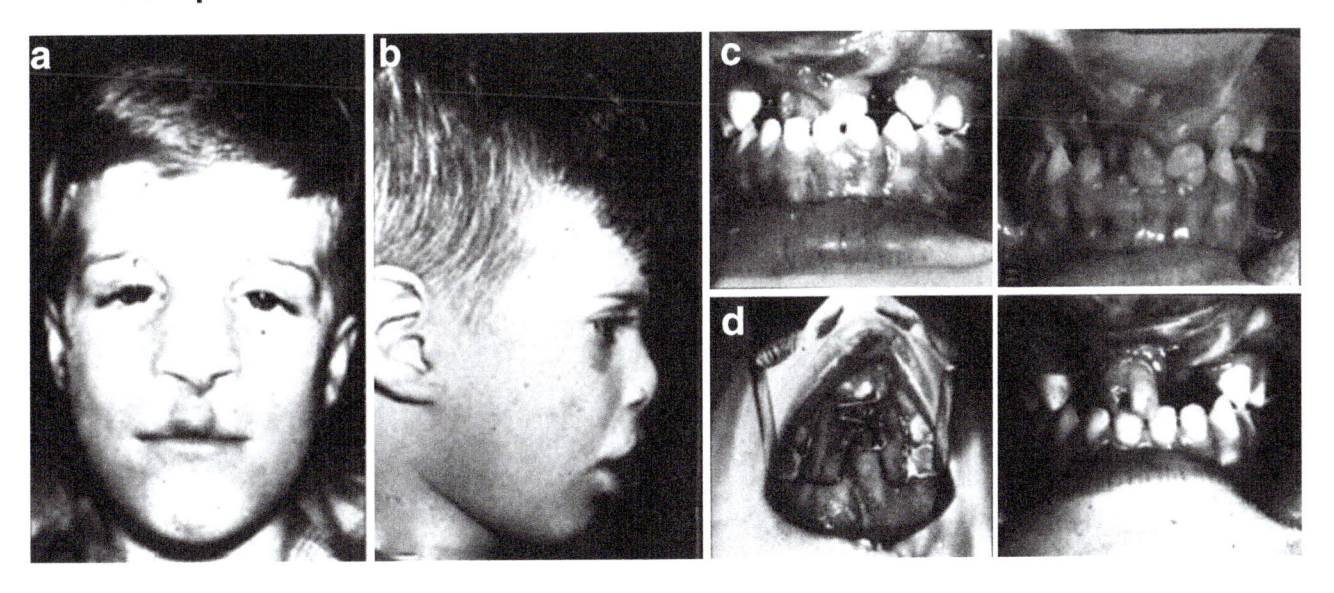

Most facial and palatal skeletal malformations in cleft patients are the result of surgical procedures that cause some growth retardation or there are osteogenic deficiencies that lead to maxillary hypoplasia. All maxillary discrepancies are 3 dimensional, and bone size relative to cleft size at the time of surgery is crucial.

Differences between surgeons, variance in the performance by the same surgeon from day to day, and during the course of several years, and differences in techniques that are difficult to identify and compare, complicate analysis. However, the research objectives to test the influence of presurgical orthopedic treatment and the relationship of cleft palate space to surgical outcome can be reached. It is possible to statistically test and covary for effects because of difference between and within surgeons.

## 9.11 The Value of Longitudinal Facial and Dental Cast Record in Clinical Research and Treatment Analysis

After 40 years of treating children with various types of clefts, the author has concluded that the success or failure of a surgical procedure depends on the degree of palatal cleft defect at the time of surgery and the resulting facial growth pattern as well as the surgical skills and the surgical procedure utilized. This conclusion will not be new to the experienced orthodontist who in all probability recognizes that the progress recorded in treatment depends for the most part on the skeletal and facial growth patterns inherent in the patient and the interaction of surgery with facial and palatal growth.

### 9.11.1 Serial Cephaloradiographs and Casts of the Maxillary and Mandibular Dentition and Occlusion

To properly assess the results of treatment, there is a fundamental need for serial casts, lateral cephalometric films, and photographs in individual case reports.

## 9.12 The Reasons for Success or Failure Are Multifactorial and Are Not Often Related to the Surgeon's Surgical Procedure

A child with palatal tissue deficiency will have a different set of problems than the cleft palate patient with adequate palatal tissue and a cleft caused by failure of proper shelf force or failure to fuse.

In assessing failure in facial and palatal growth most surgeons focus on the surgical skills and/or surgical protocols involved, this leaves other possible explanations still unexplored.

### 9.12.1 Good Jaw Relationships

Central incisor pontics replacing missing ones

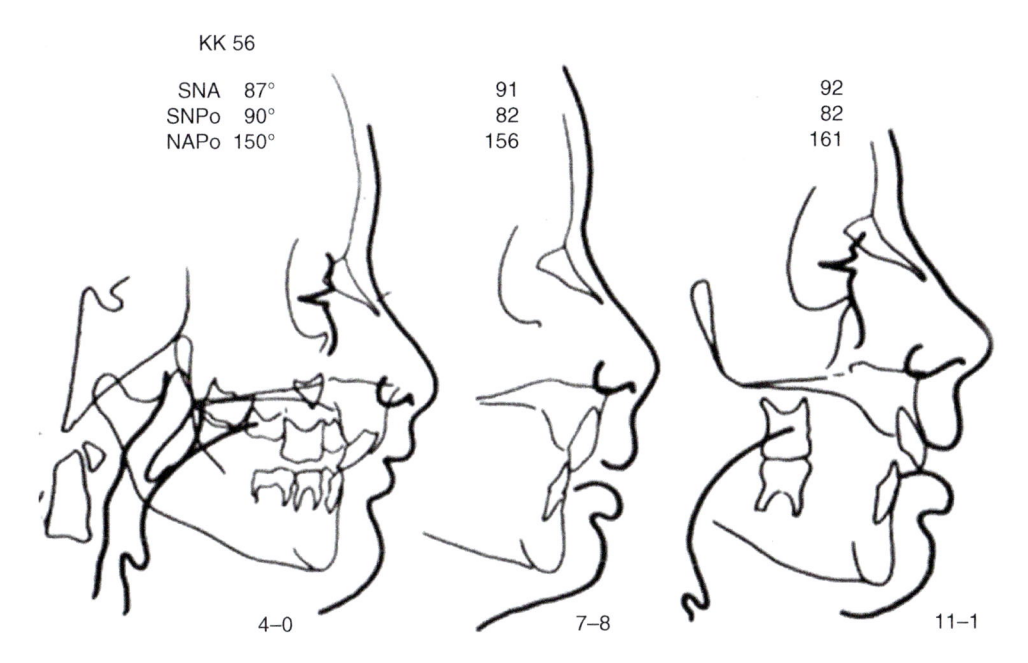

KK 56

| SNA 87° | 91 | 92 |
| SNPo 90° | 82 | 82 |
| NAPo 150° | 156 | 161 |

4–0   7–8   11–1

Central incisor pontics shown

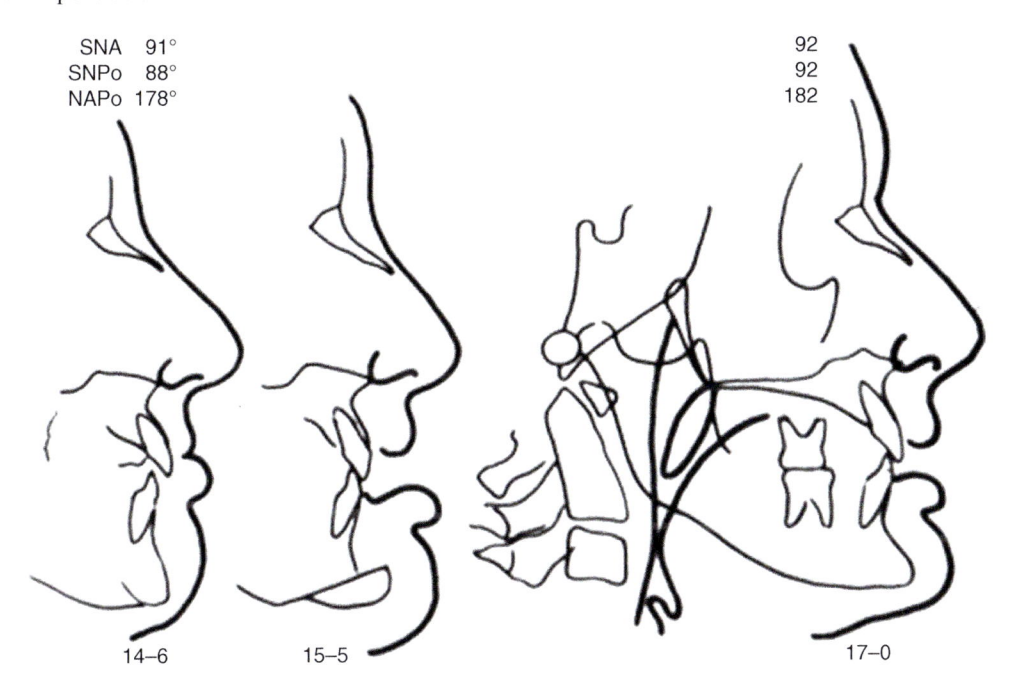

| SNA 91° | | 92 |
| SNPo 88° | | 92 |
| NAPo 178° | | 182 |

14–6   15–5   17–0

## 9.13 Variations in the Inclination of the Premaxilla at Similar Ages (Handelman)

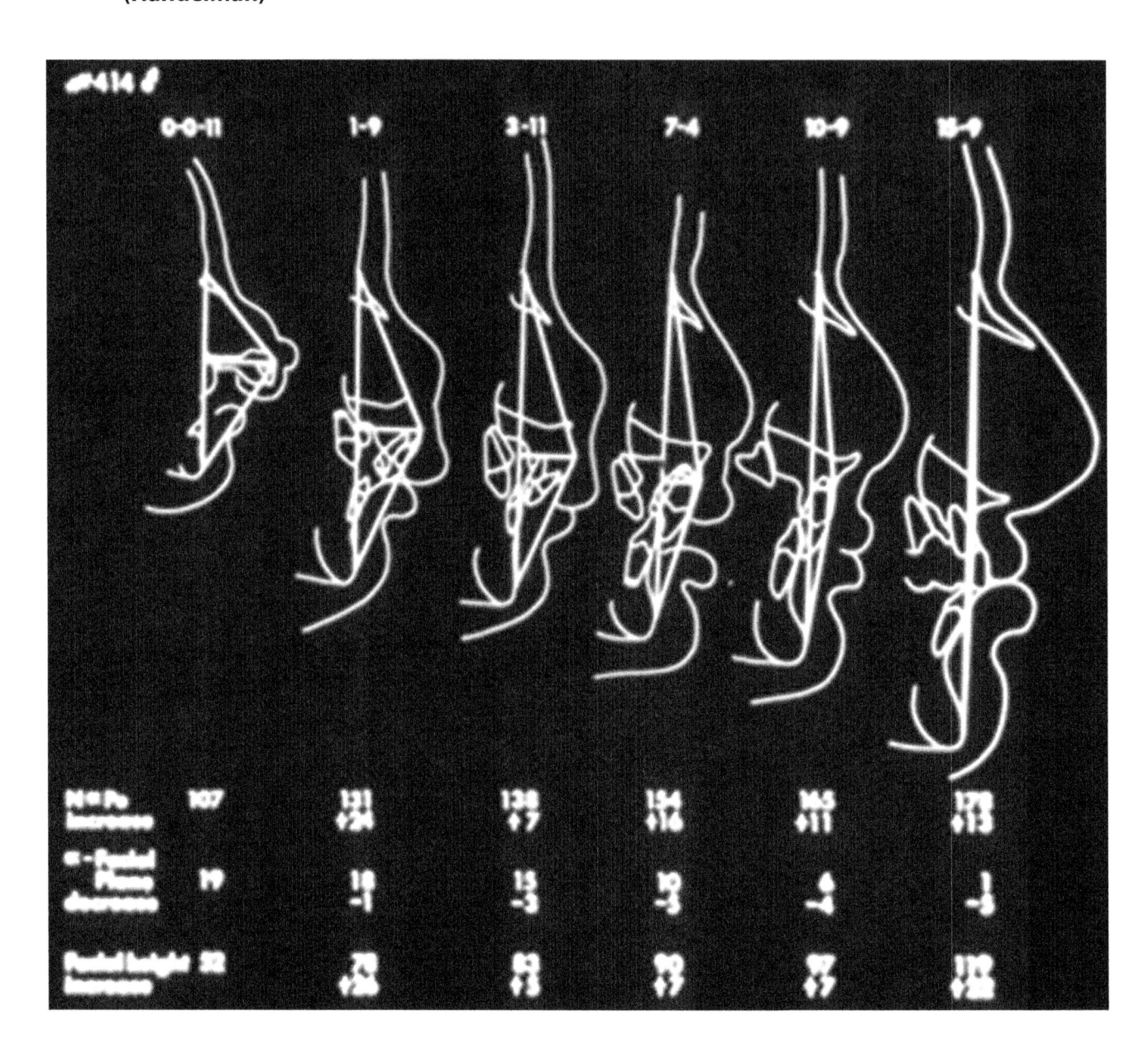

## 9.14 Gradual Flattening of the Facial Profile (Hans Friede)

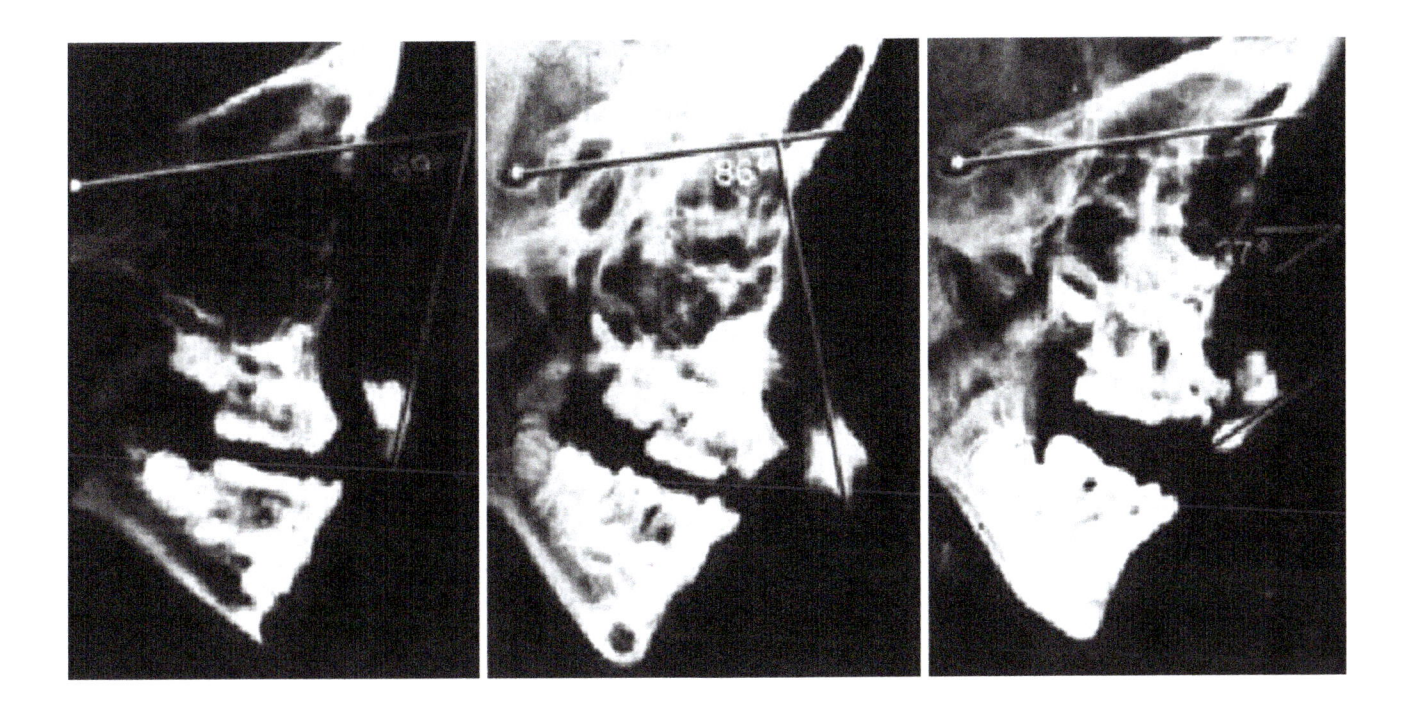

## 9.15 Two-Stage Lip

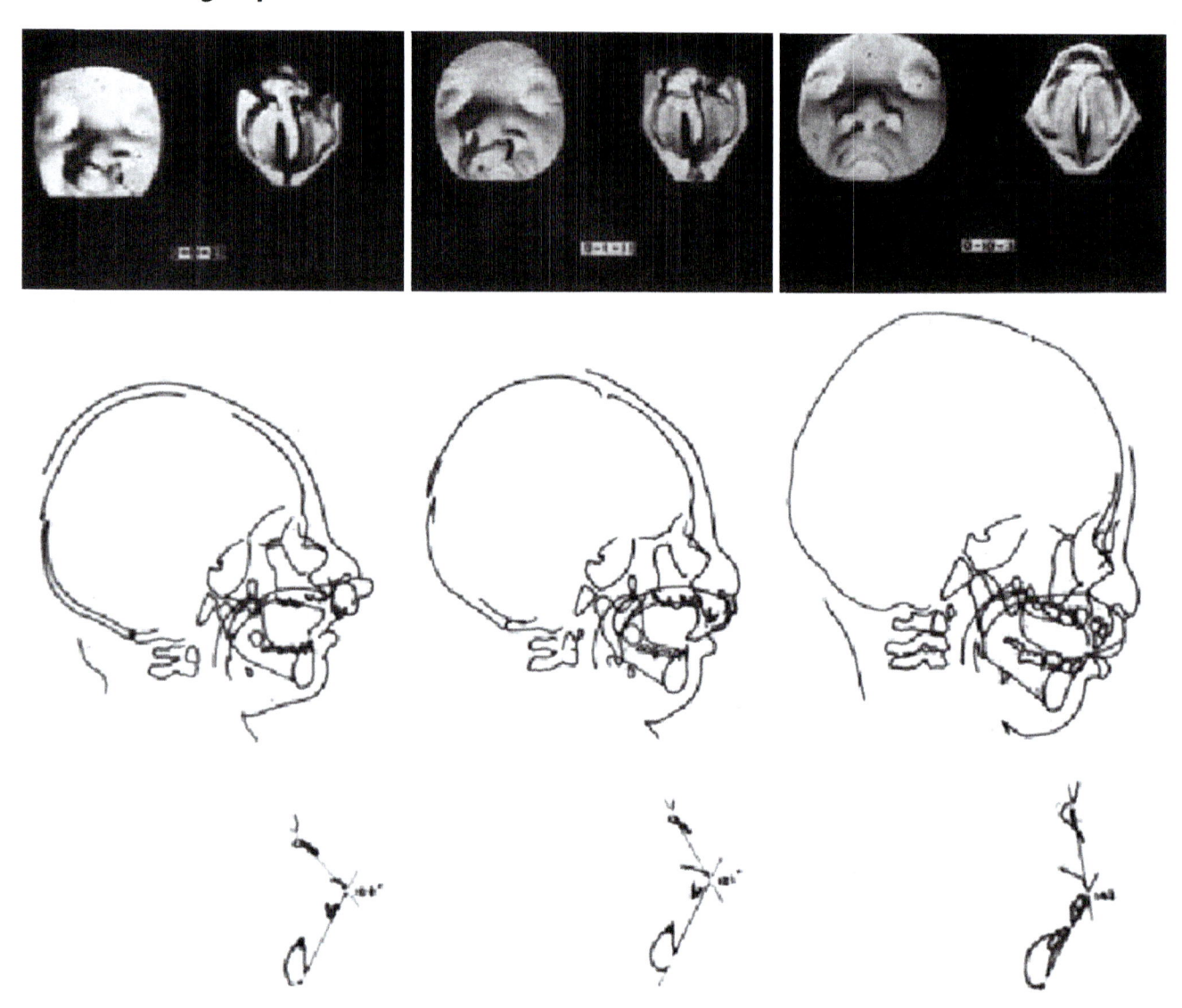

Changes in the angle of facial convexity over time

## 9.16 Various Analyses to Show Facial Growth Changes

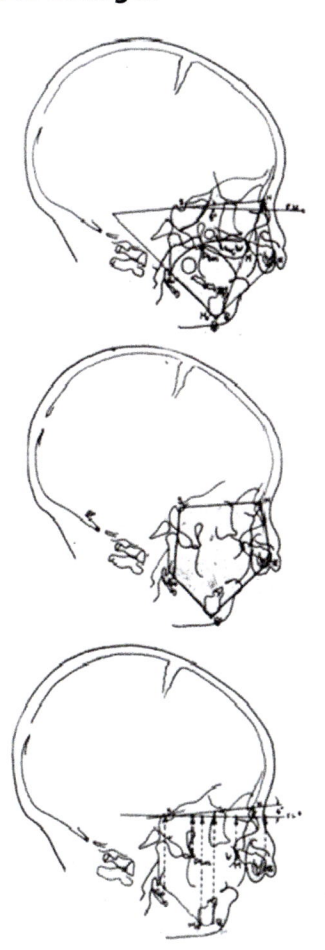

## 9.17 Bringing the Central Incisors Together to Allow for the Eruption of the Lateral Incisors

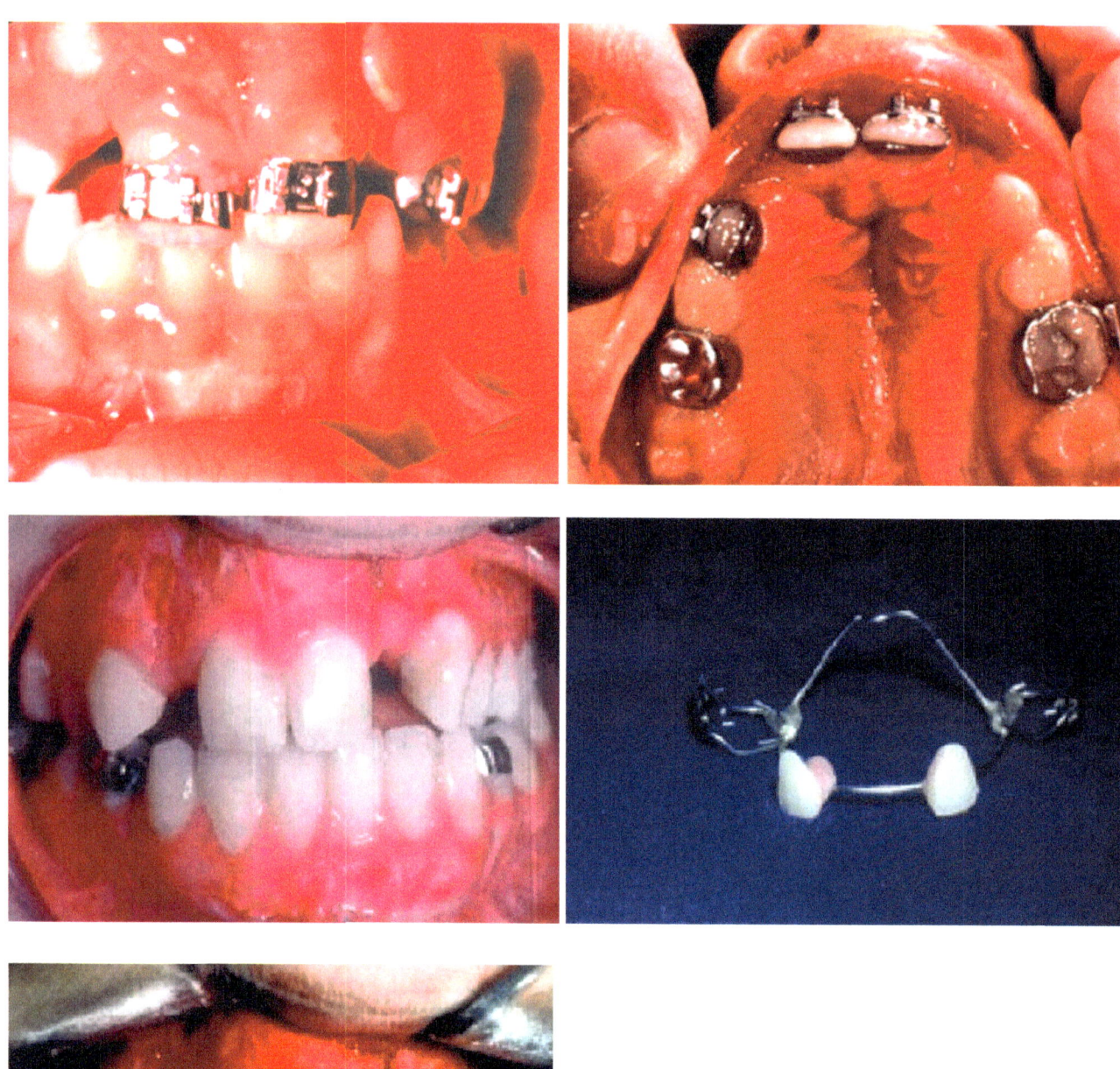

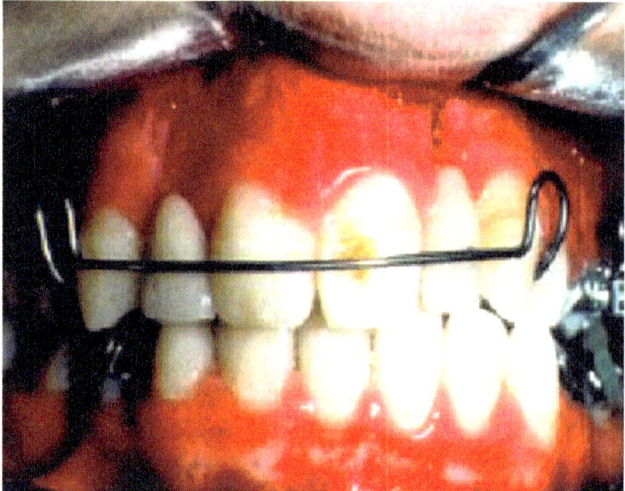

A temporary fixed retainer with lateral incisor pontics.

## 9.17 Bringing the Central Incisors Together to Allow for the Eruption of the Lateral Incisors

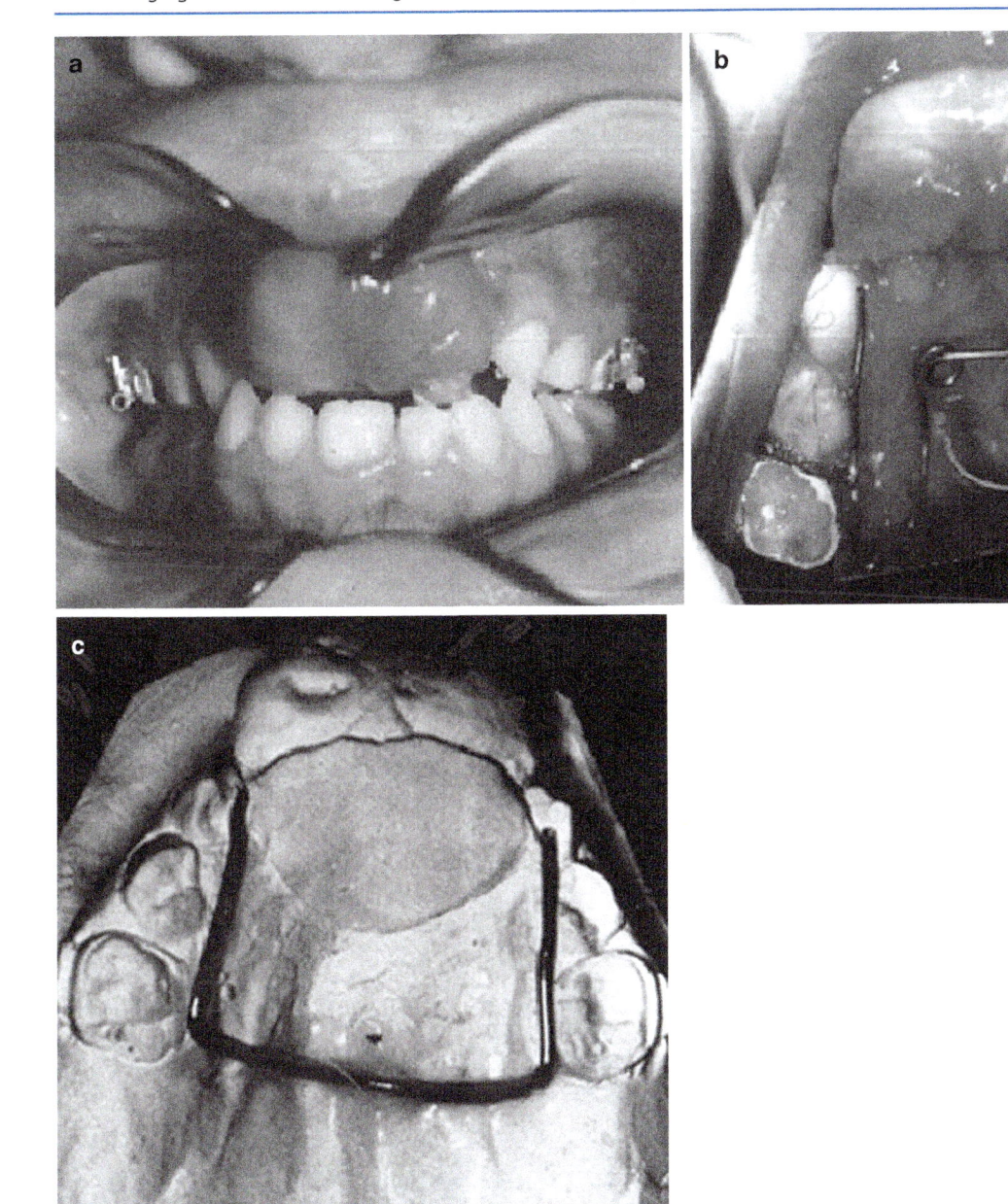

(**a–c**) The oversized premaxilla is due to the developing permanent maxillary incisors. The buccal crossbite had been corrected which allows for the premaxilla to be spontaneously aligned within the arch. The expansion was maintained with a fixed retainer.

## 9.18 Incomplete BLCLP

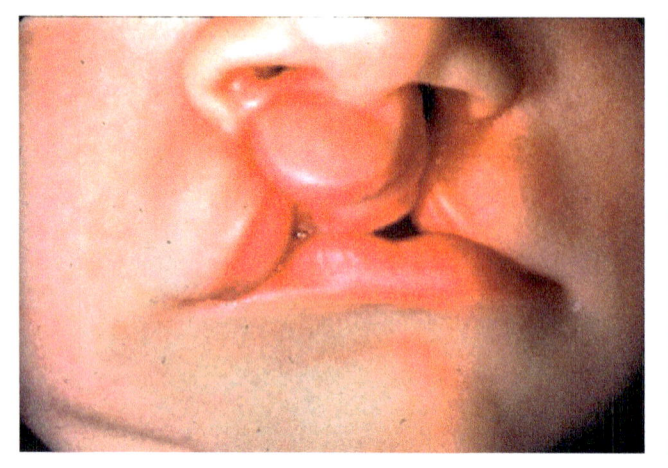

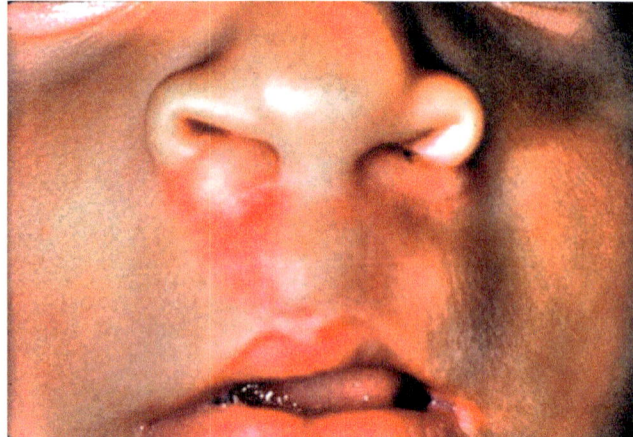

At birth

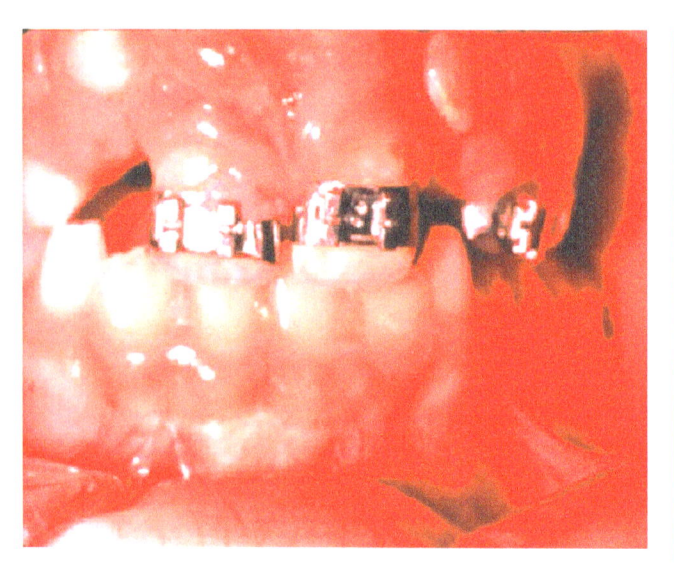

After banked fork flap

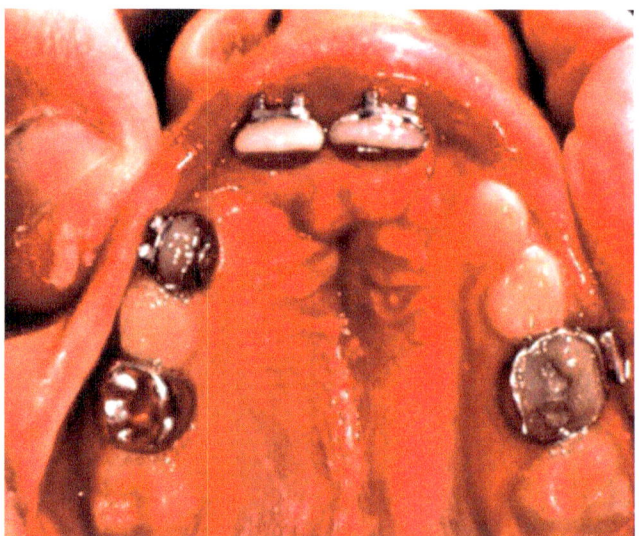

Bringing the central incisors together to allow for the eruption of the lateral incisors

## 9.19 Bilateral Cleft Lip and Palate

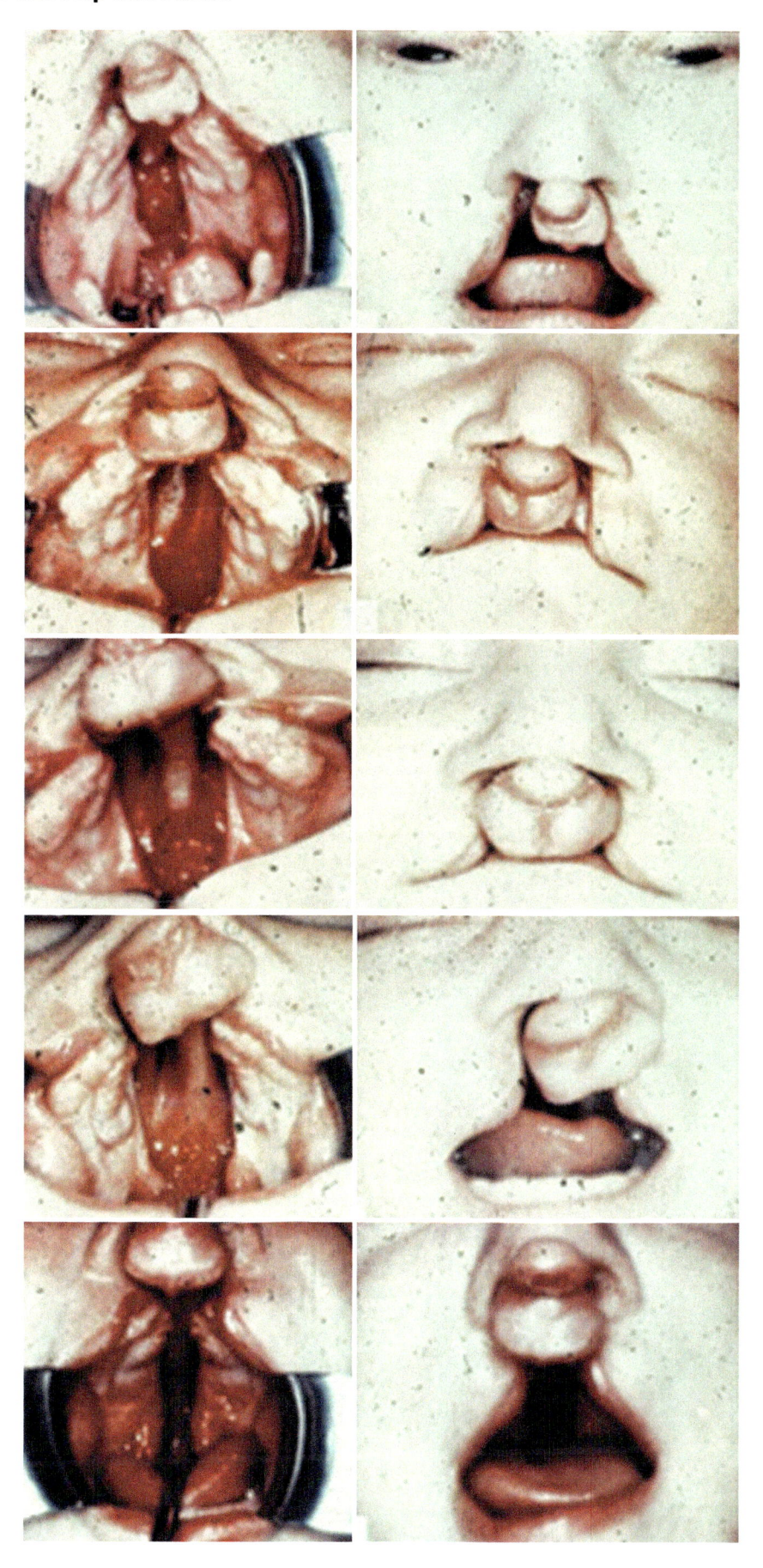

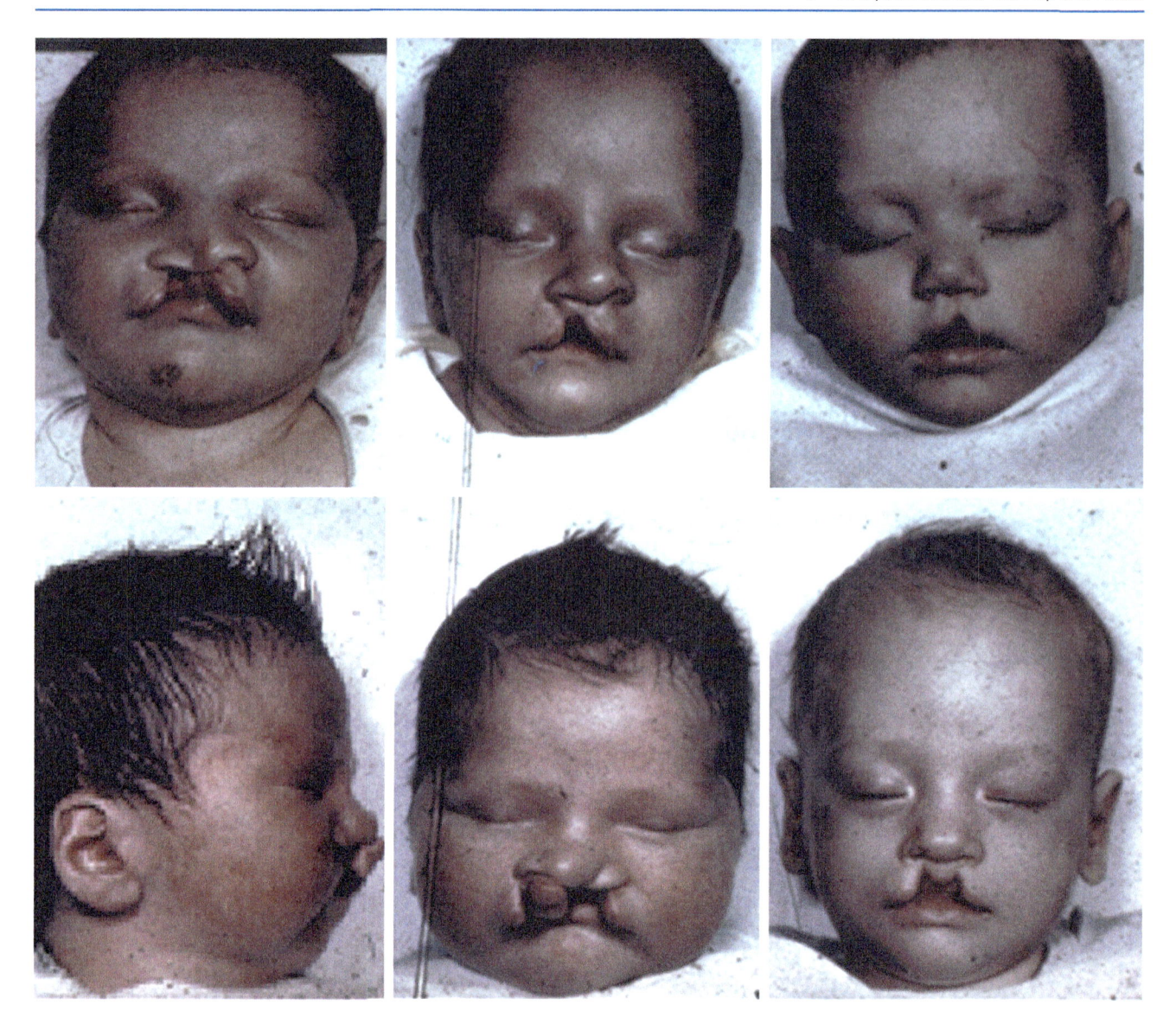

Should all these different children be treated the same way?

## 9.19 Bilateral Cleft Lip and Palate

Miami
Rapid narrowing of the cleft space.

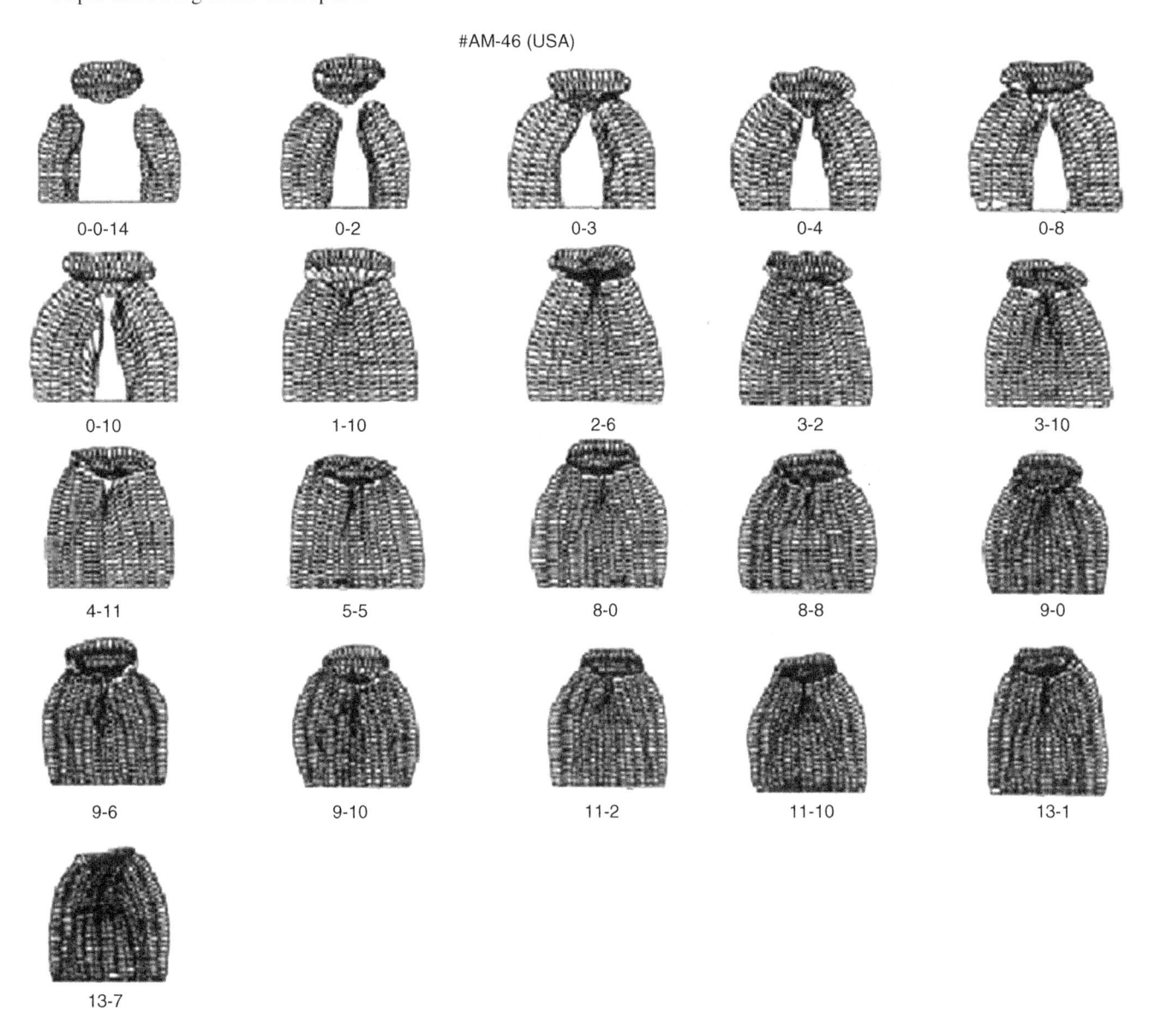

#AM-46 (USA)

0-0-14    0-2    0-3    0-4    0-8

0-10    1-10    2-6    3-2    3-10

4-11    5-5    8-0    8-8    9-0

9-6    9-10    11-2    11-10    13-1

13-7

Non-PSOT. Narrowing of the cleft space resulted in molding plus palatal growth.

Nijmegen

3471　　　　　　(ACTA)

0-0　　　　　　0-3

0-9　　　　　　1-6

PSOT prevents cleft space from narrowing. Appliance was removed at 1–4 years resulting in molding of palatal segments.

## 9.20 Serial Dental BCLP Casts

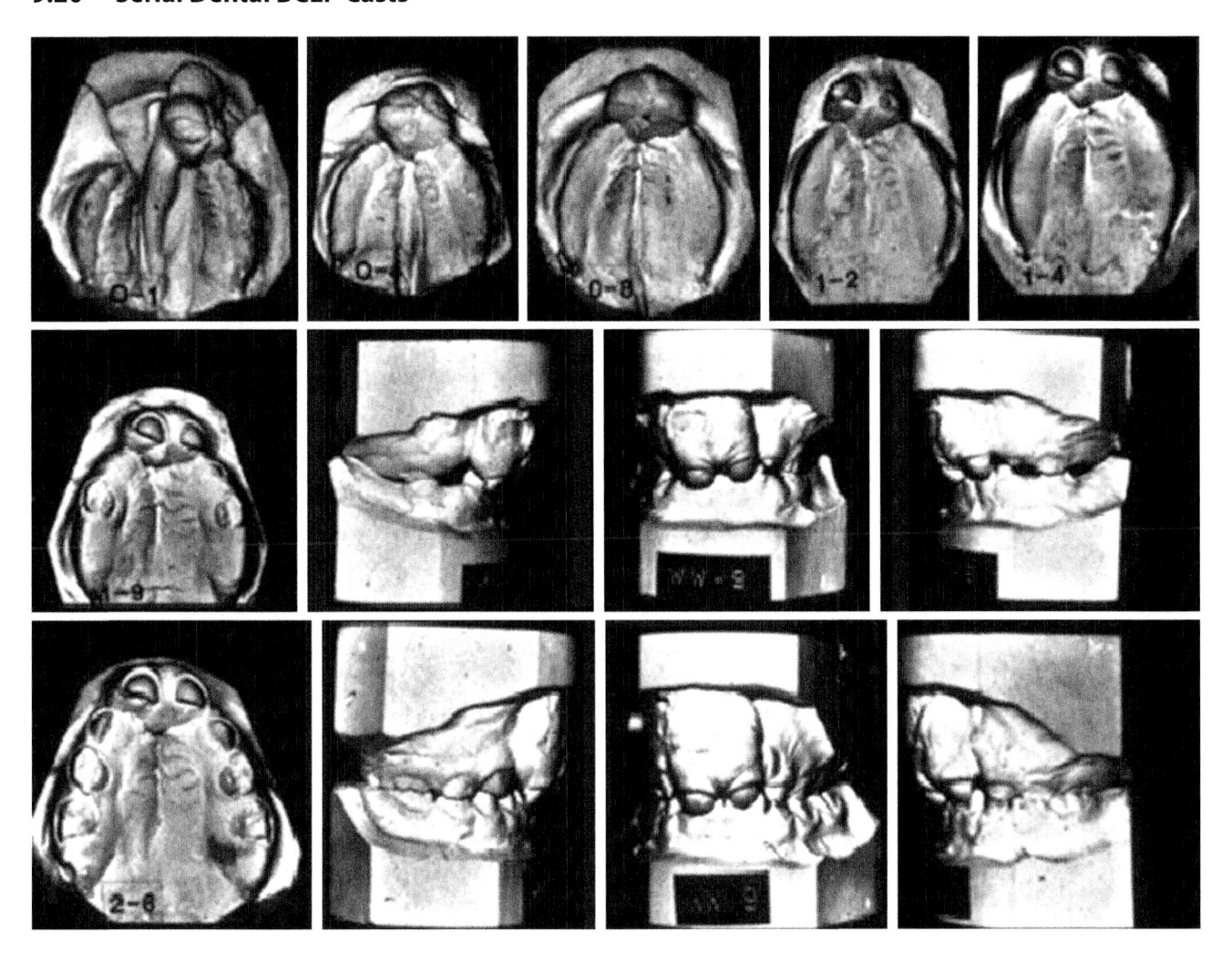

Note that the premaxilla is well forward of the lateral palatal segments soon after the lip is united.

The cleft space is greatly reduced with the molding action. It needs to be emphasized that the buccal segments have not been in crossbite at any time.

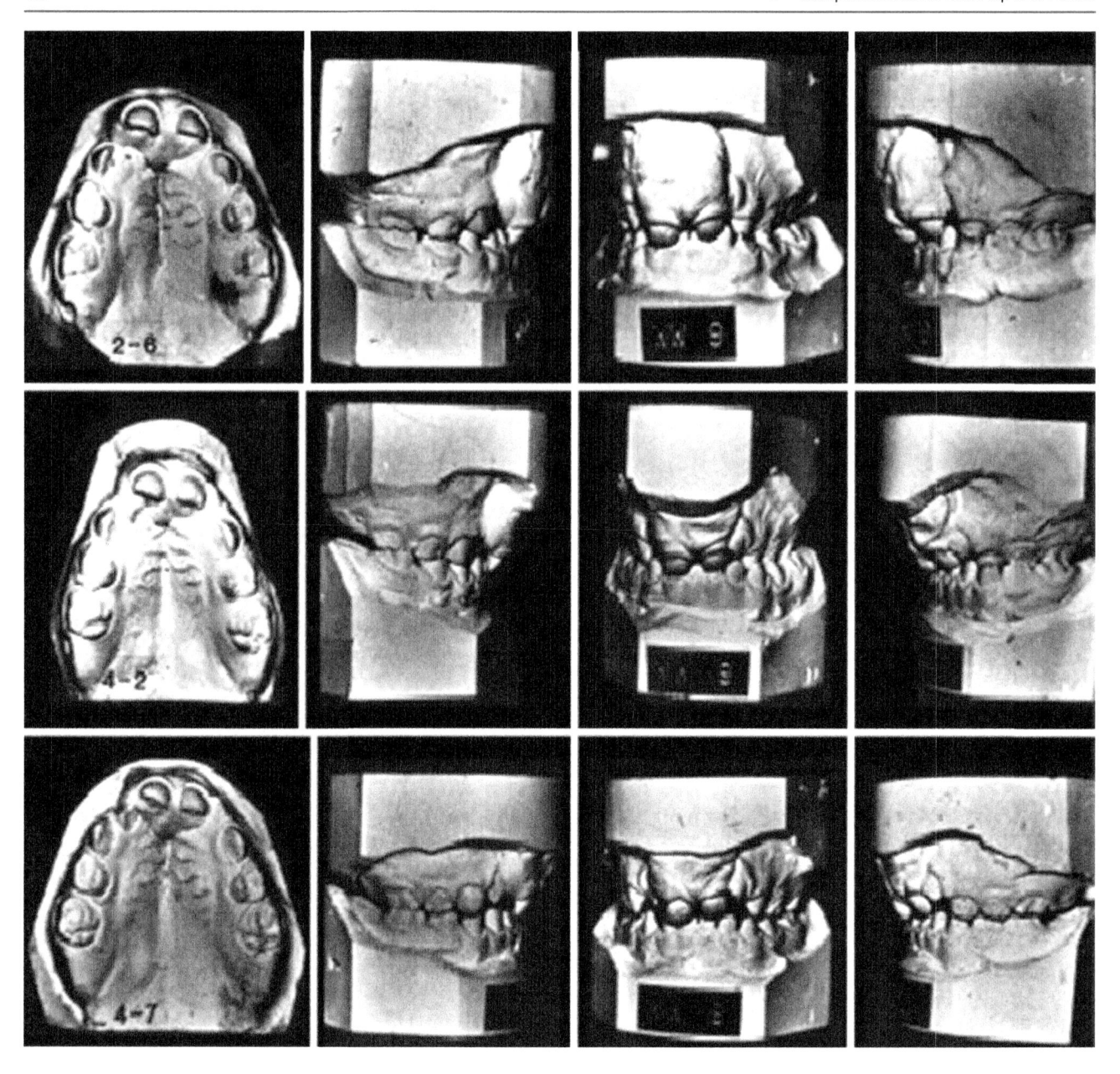

The premaxillary segment is in severe overbite and overjet early on but its protrusion is self-correcting with time.

9.20 Serial Dental BCLP Casts

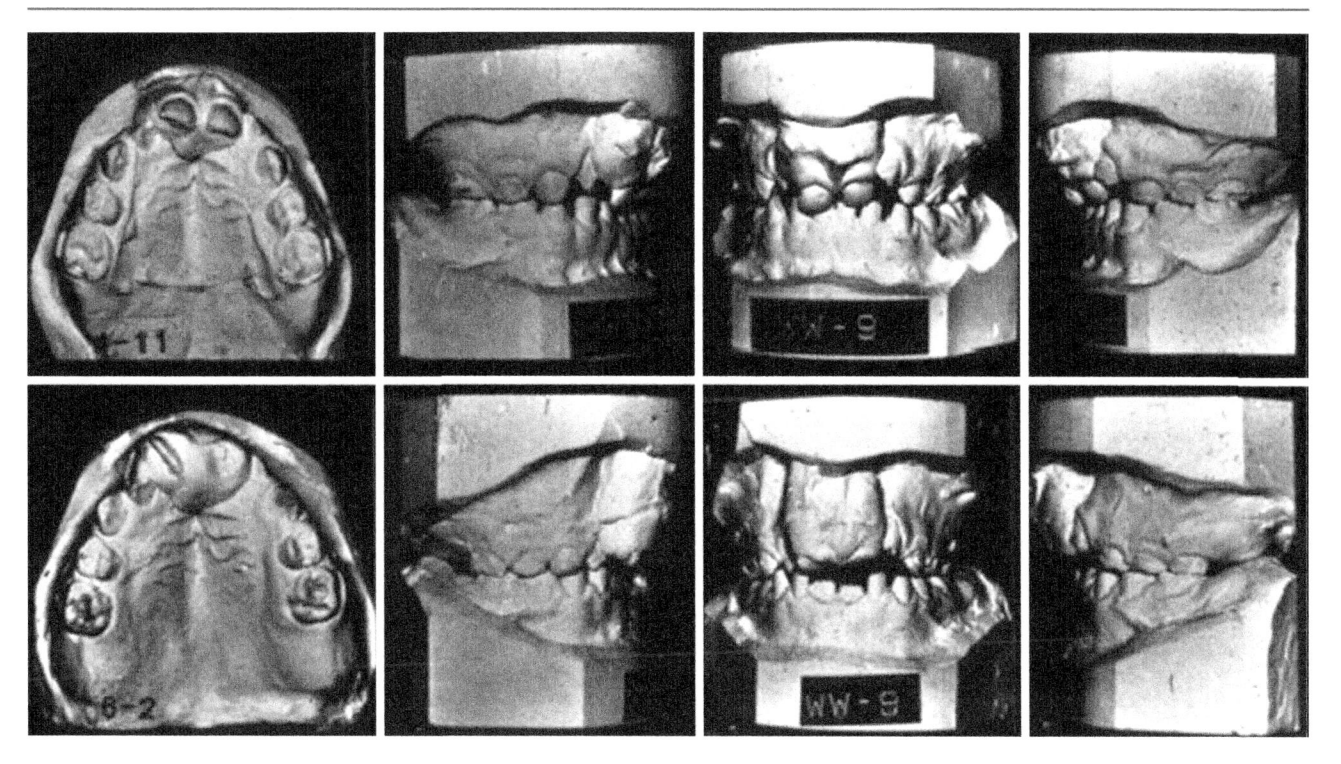

The upper anterior teeth are properly aligned prior to secondary alveolar bone grafting.
Usually performed between 8 and 10 years.

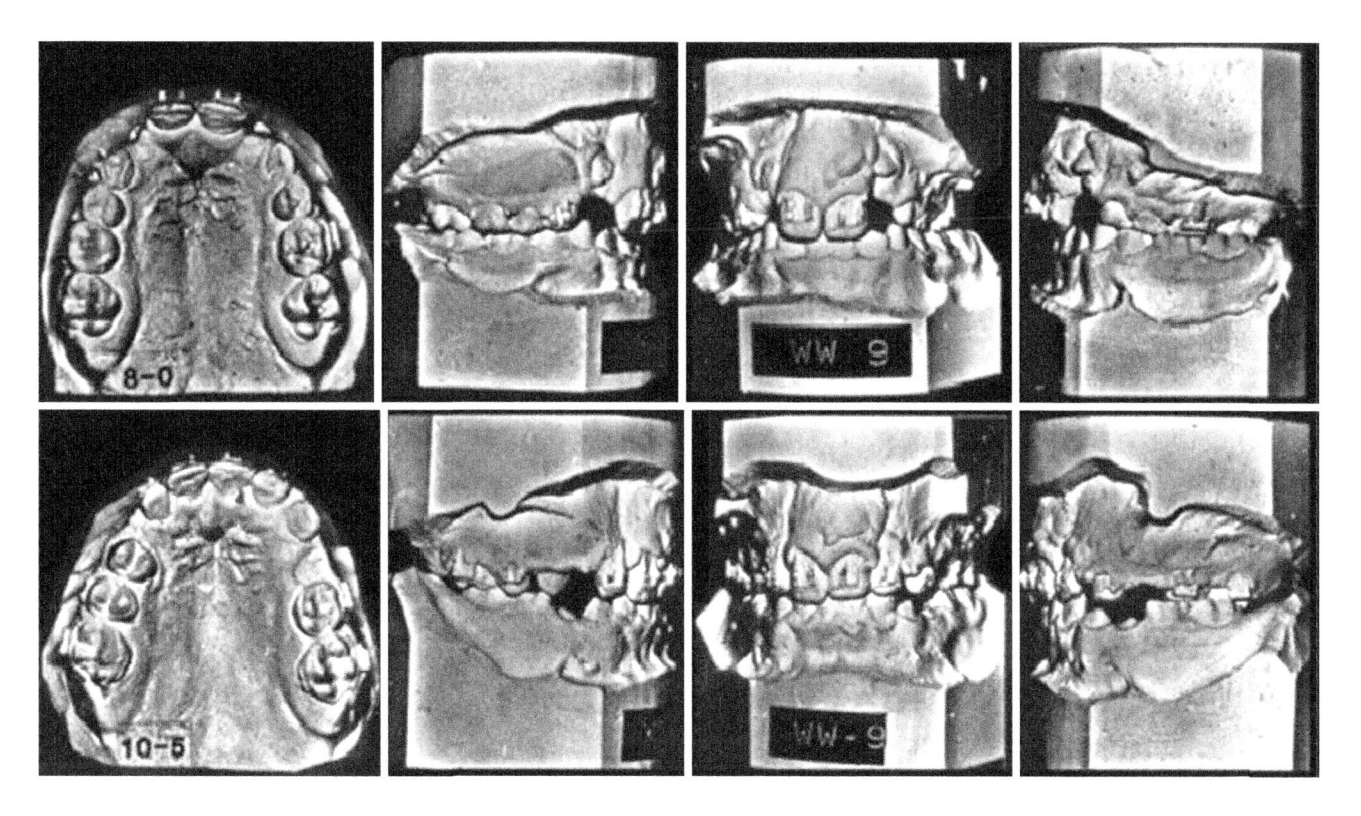

This allows the lateral incisors to erupt into position.
Conservative orthodontics follows, aligning all the teeth within the arches.

Case #TM. WW-9

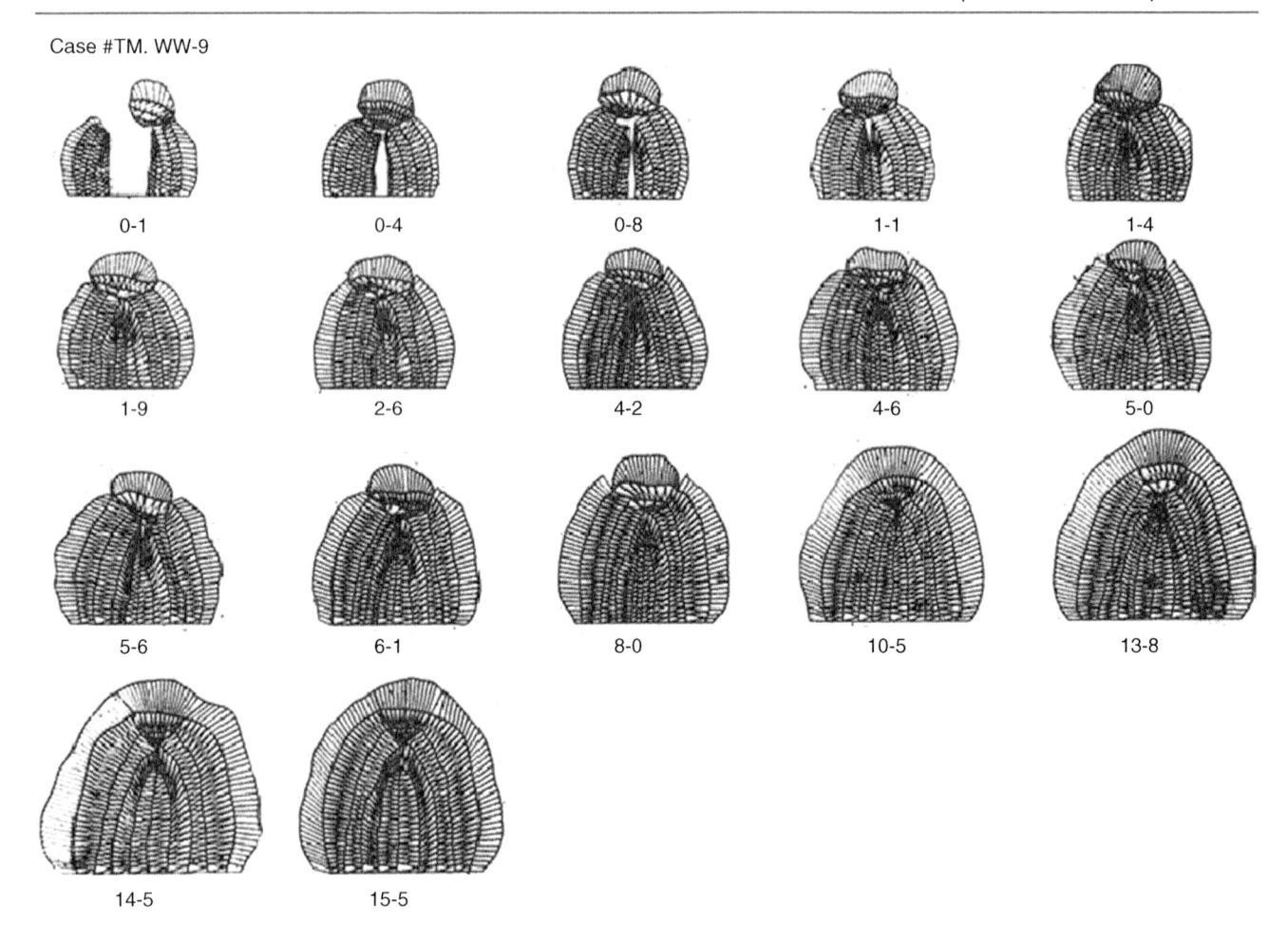

0-1   0-4   0-8   1-1   1-4

1-9   2-6   4-2   4-6   5-0

5-6   6-1   8-0   10-5   13-8

14-5   15-5

The forward positioned premaxilla relative to the lateral palatal segments is corrected spontaneously after palatal expansion at 3–6 months.

## 9.21 Excellent Facial Growth Pattern

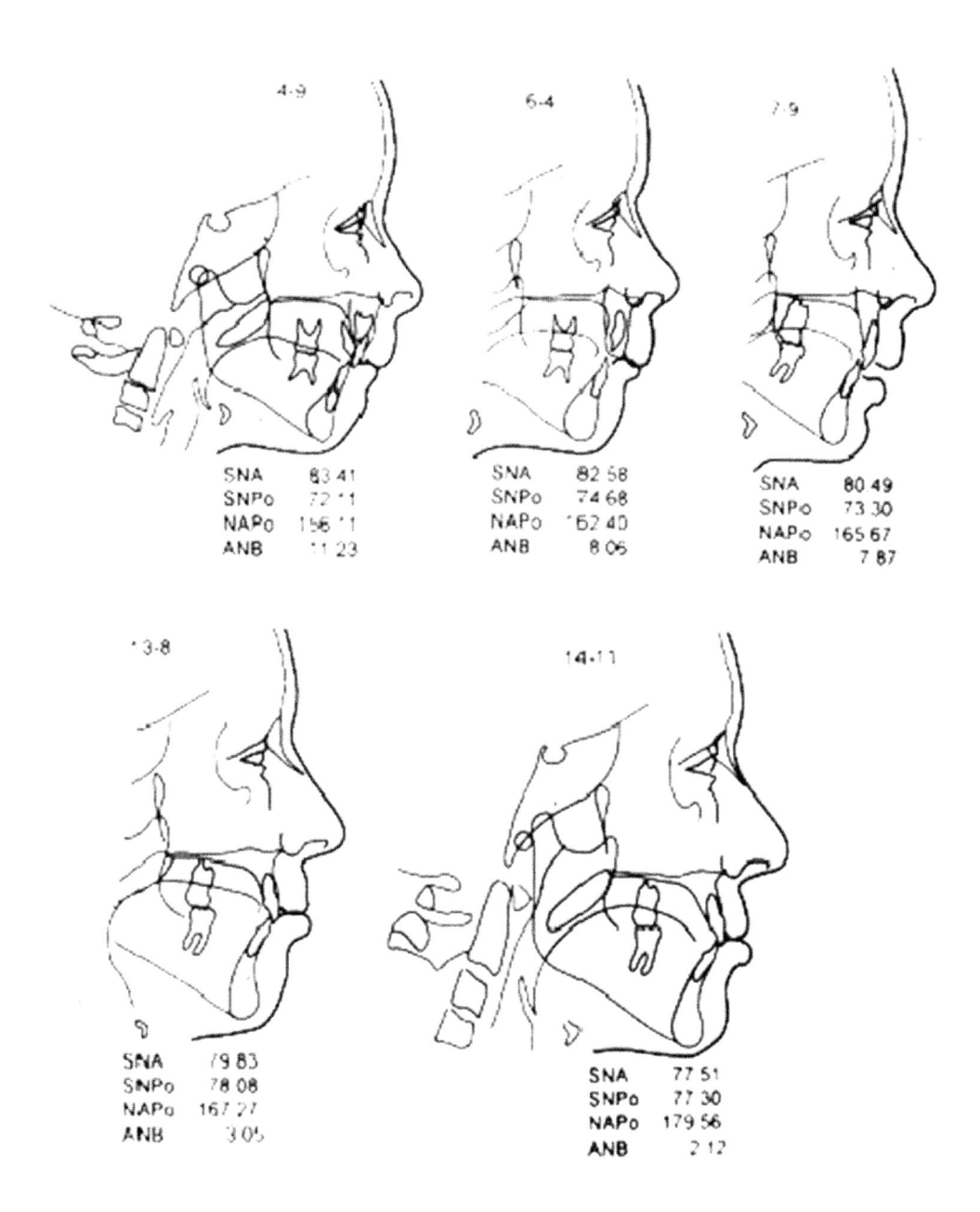

Case #TM WW-9

| Age | SNA | SNPo | NAPo | ANB |
|---|---|---|---|---|
| 4-9 | 83.41 | 72.11 | 156.11 | 11.23 |
| 6-4 | 82.58 | 74.68 | 162.40 | 8.05 |
| 7-9 | 80.49 | 73.30 | 165.67 | 7.87 |
| 13-8 | 79.83 | 78.08 | 167.27 | 3.05 |
| 14-11 | 77.51 | 77.30 | 179.56 | 2.12 |

Case #TM WW-9

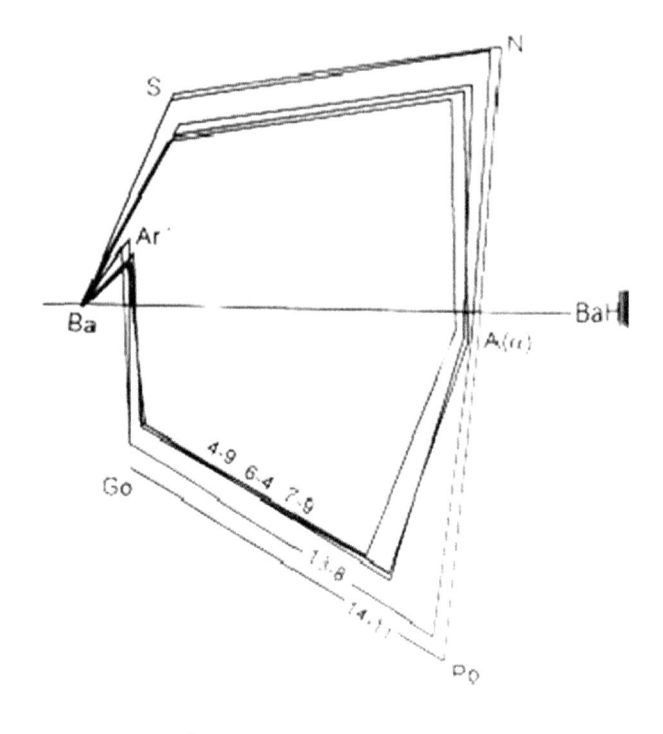

Case #MT WW-9

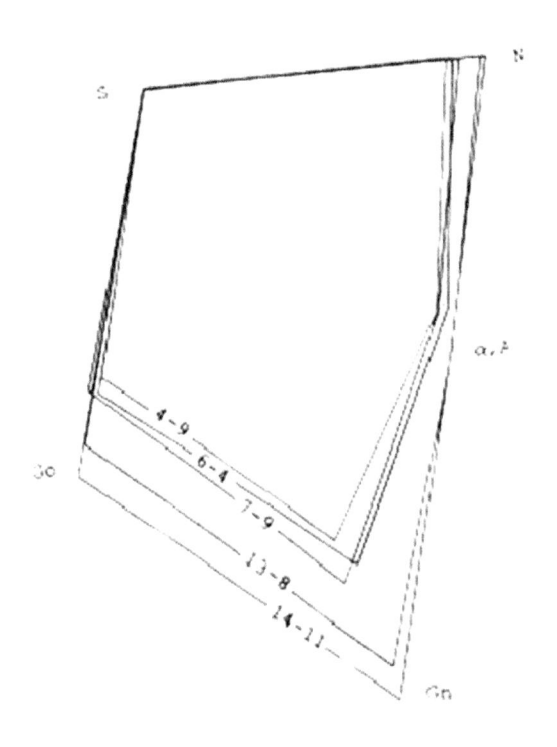

## 9.22 Excellent Facial Growth and Occlusion

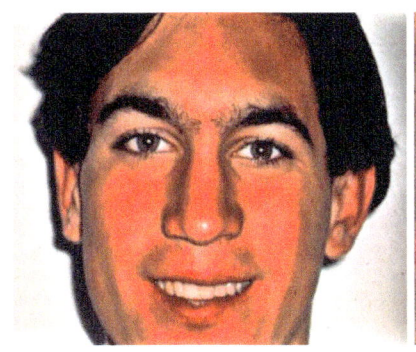

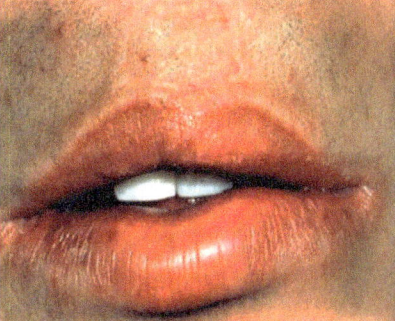

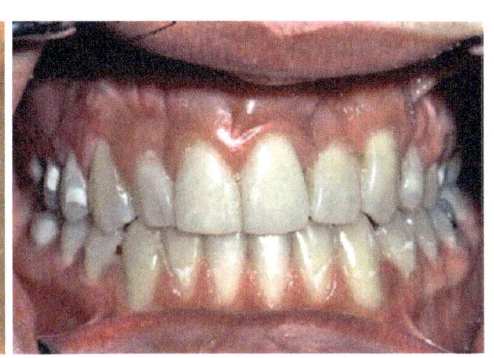

## 9.23 Incomplete Bilateral Cleft Lip and Palate: Both Lateral Incisors Are Missing—Excessive Symphysis Growth

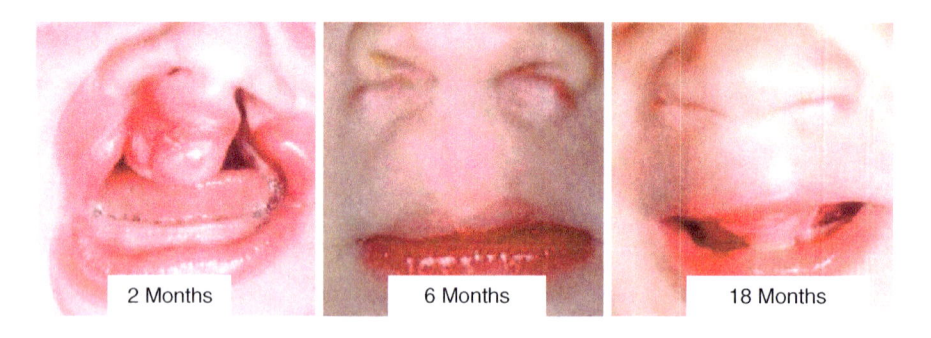

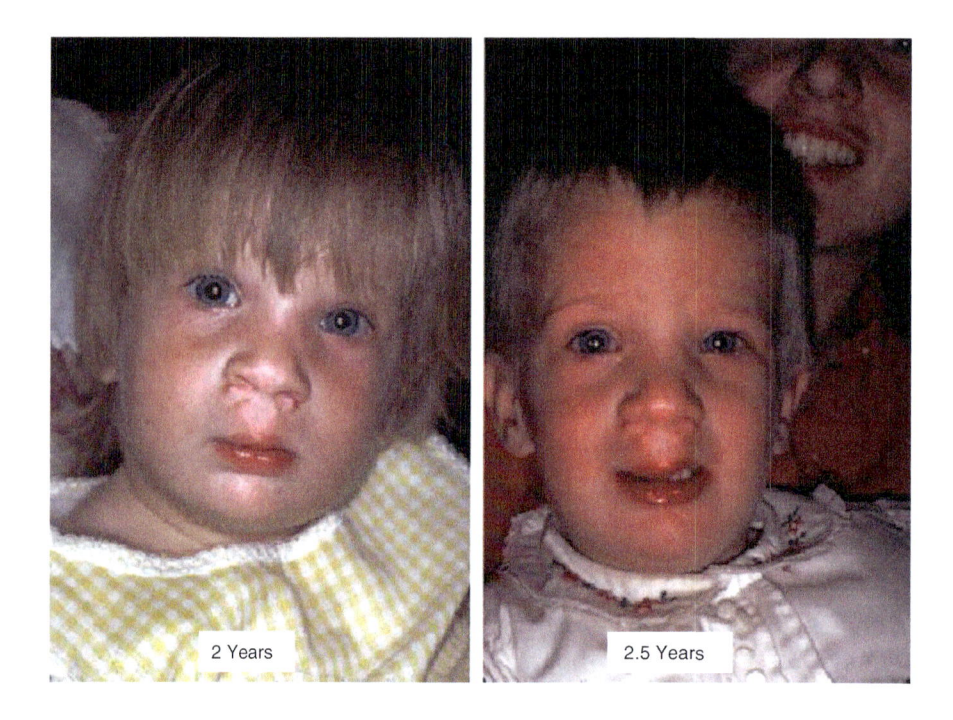

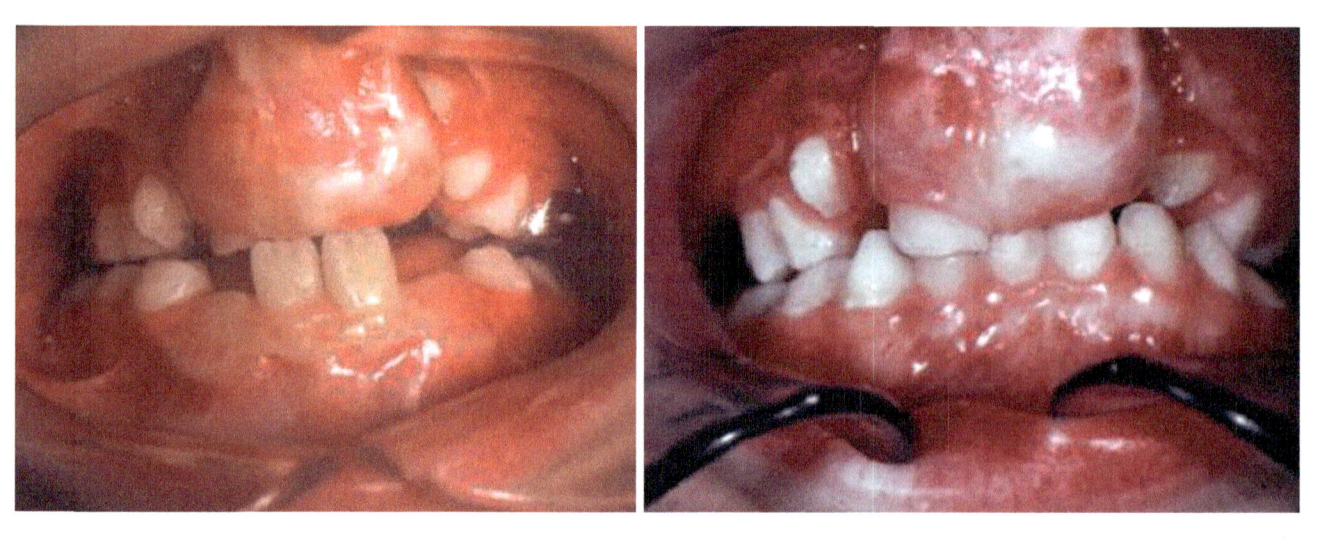

Forked flap to unite the lip after lip adhesion. The skin in the prolabium is used to increase the columella length

## 9.23 Incomplete Bilateral Cleft Lip and Palate: Both Lateral Incisors Are Missing—Excessive Symphysis Growth

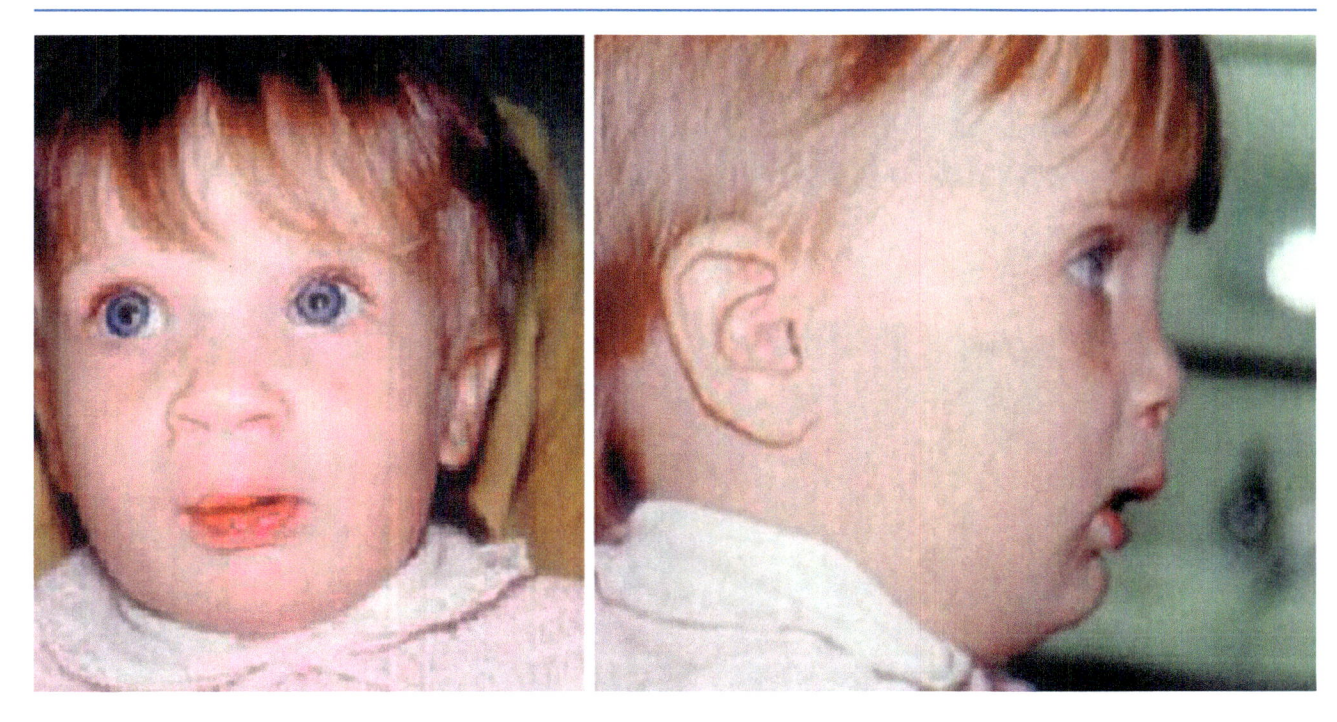

- **Forked flap**
- **Depressed nasal tip**

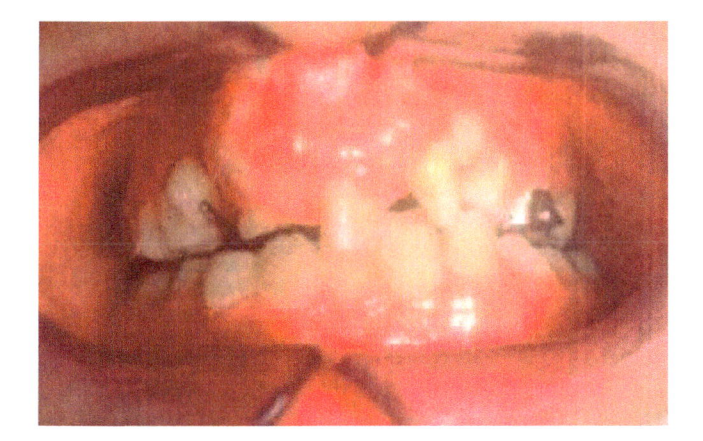

8 Years

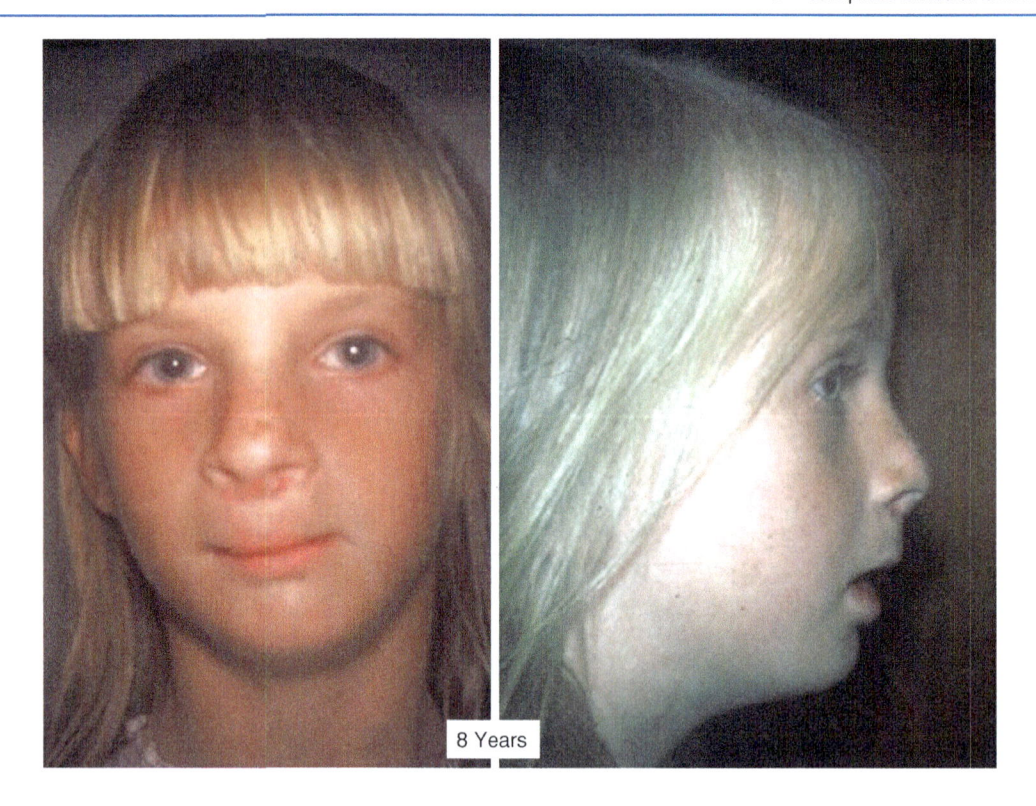

Palatal segments aligned and ready for secondary alveolar bone graft. Nasal tip was elevated with increased columella length.

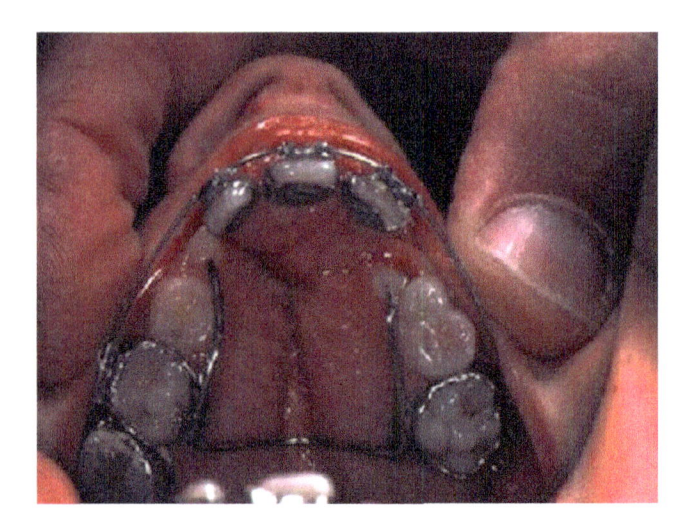

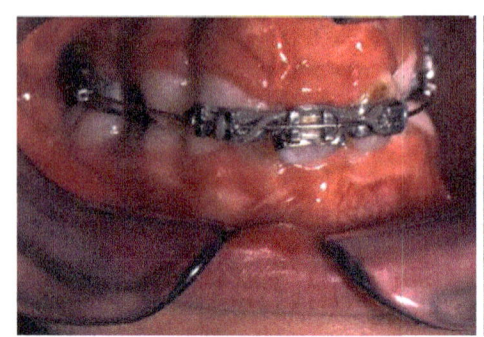

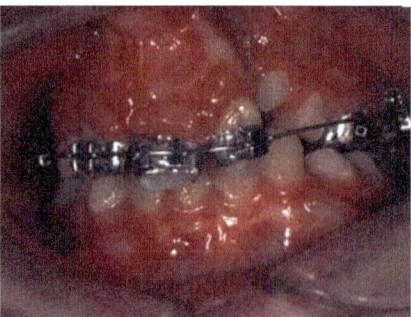

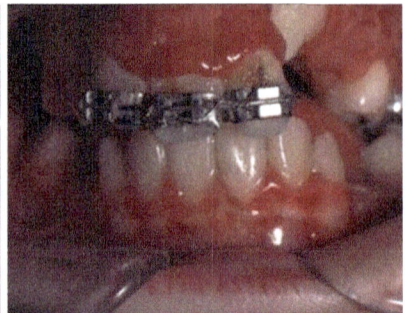

## 9.23 Incomplete Bilateral Cleft Lip and Palate: Both Lateral Incisors Are Missing—Excessive Symphysis Growth

14 Years

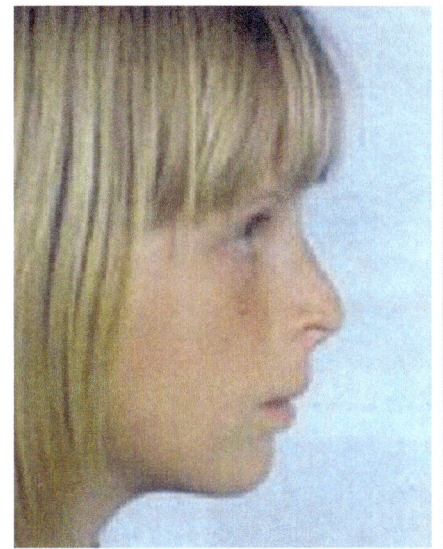

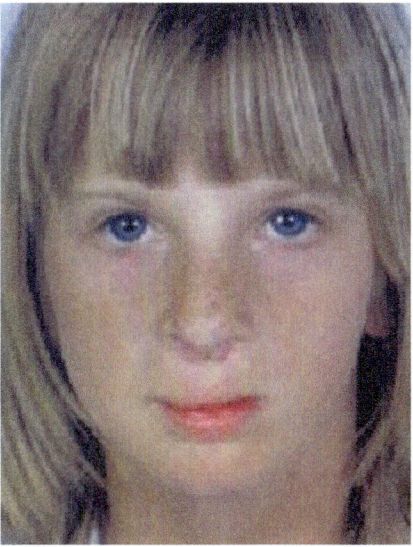

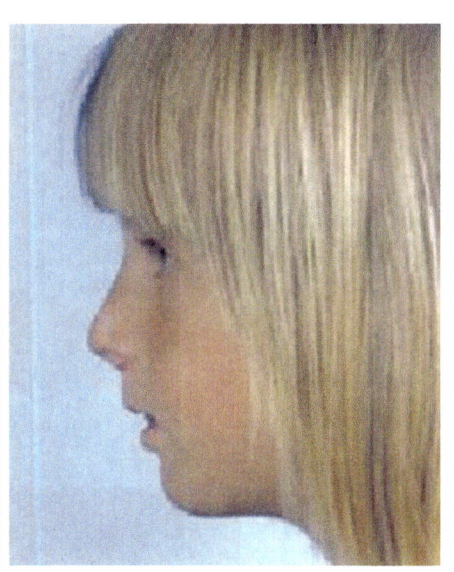

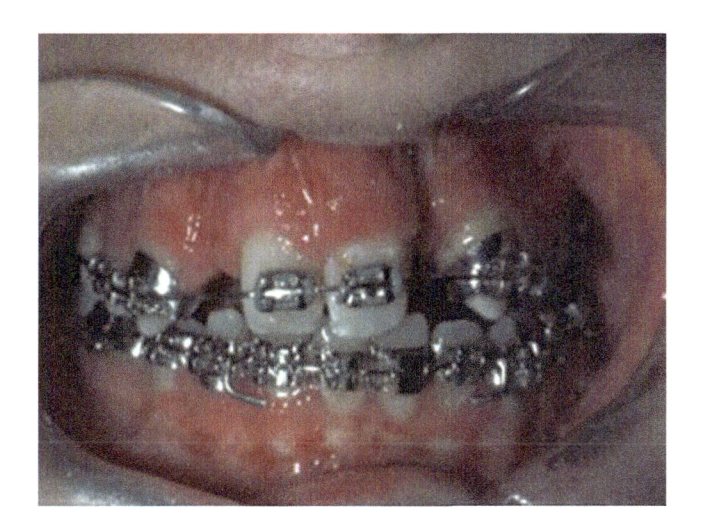

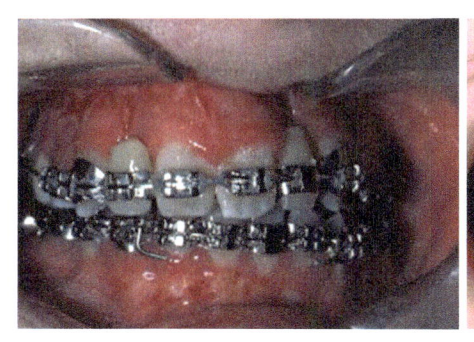

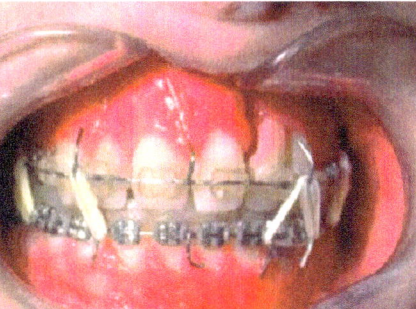

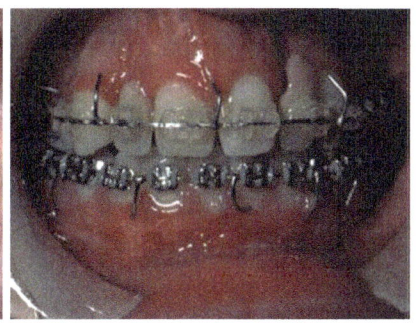

Lateral incisor pontics were attached to the arch wire.

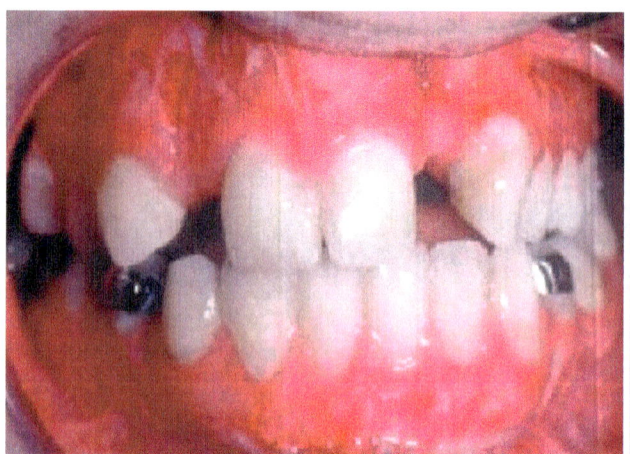

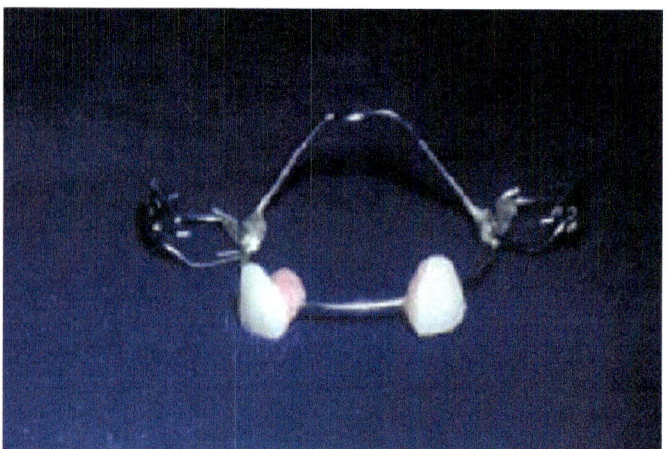

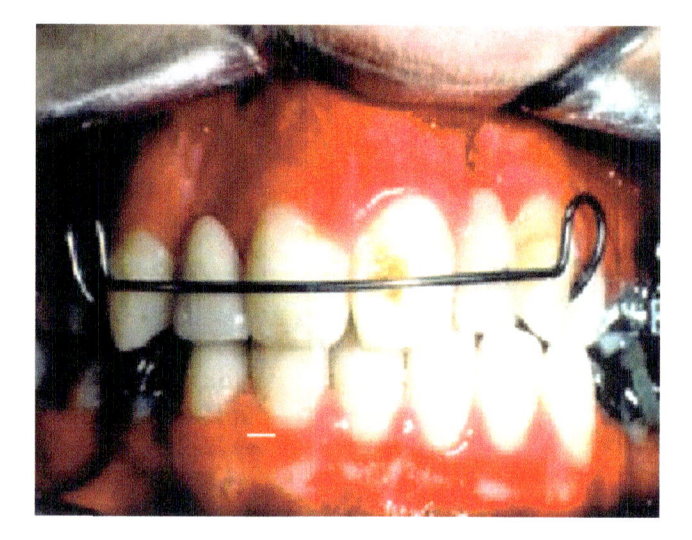

A temporary fixed retainer with lateral incisor pontics.

## 9.23 Incomplete Bilateral Cleft Lip and Palate: Both Lateral Incisors Are Missing—Excessive Symphysis Growth

16 Years: Fixed anterior bridge

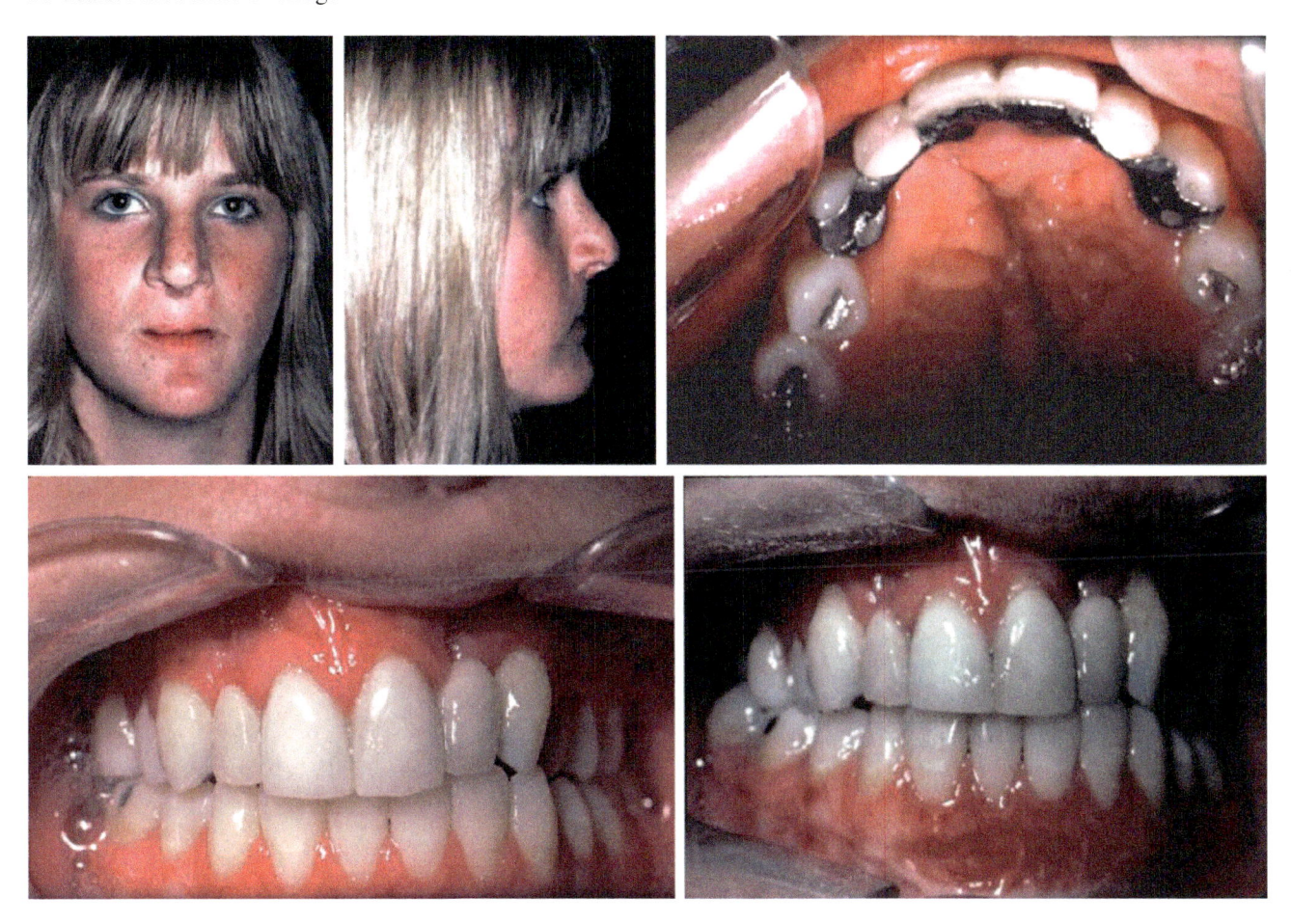

17 Years: Excellent aesthetics, occlusion, and speech

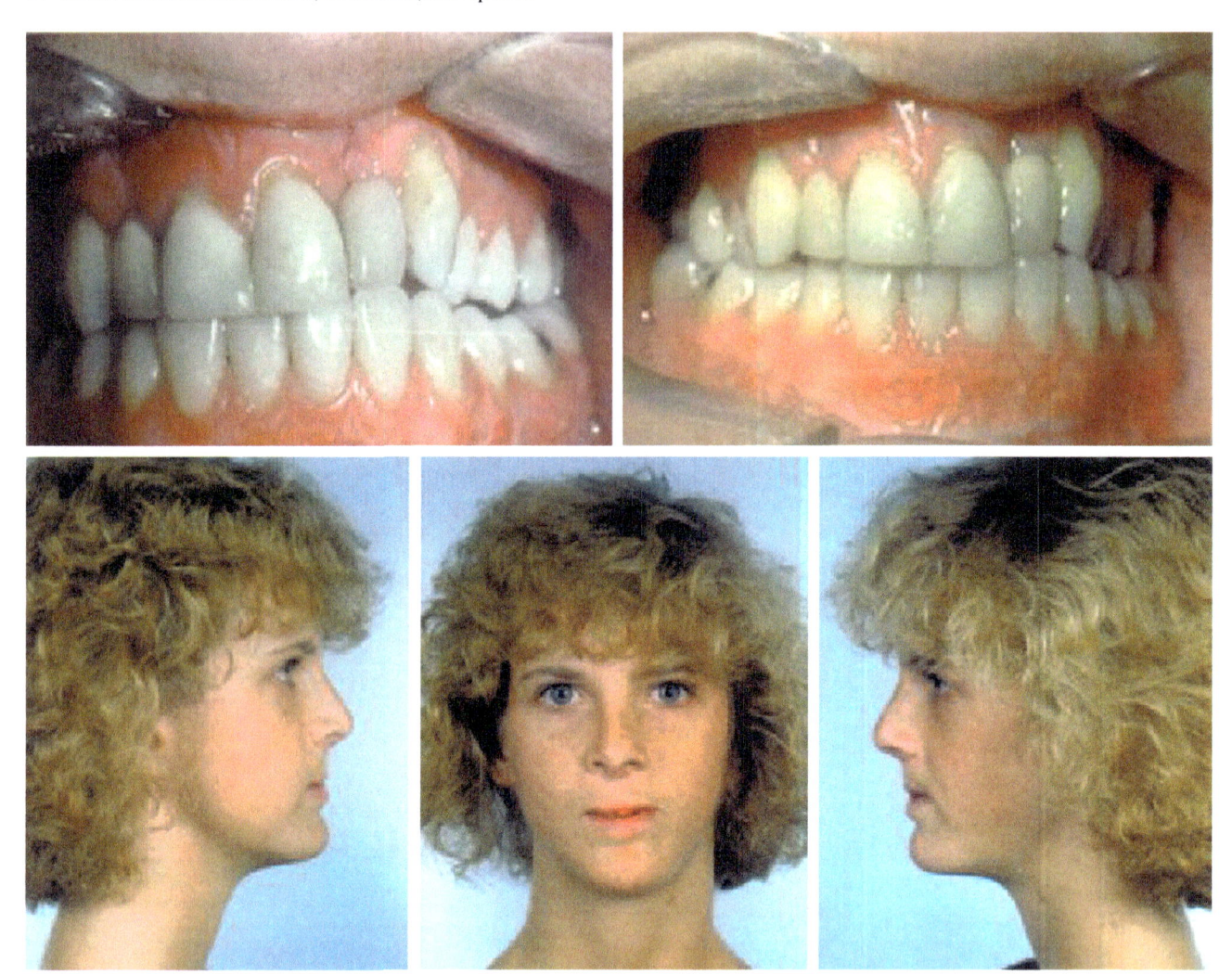

### 9.23 Incomplete Bilateral Cleft Lip and Palate: Both Lateral Incisors Are Missing—Excessive Symphysis Growth

Molding places the protruding premaxilla forward of both lateral palatal segments maintaining a protruding premaxilla with dental overjet.

The overjet is reduced spontaneously with facial palatal growth.

Note the alignment of the premaxilla within the arch without orthodontics creating a good overbite overjet incisor relationship.

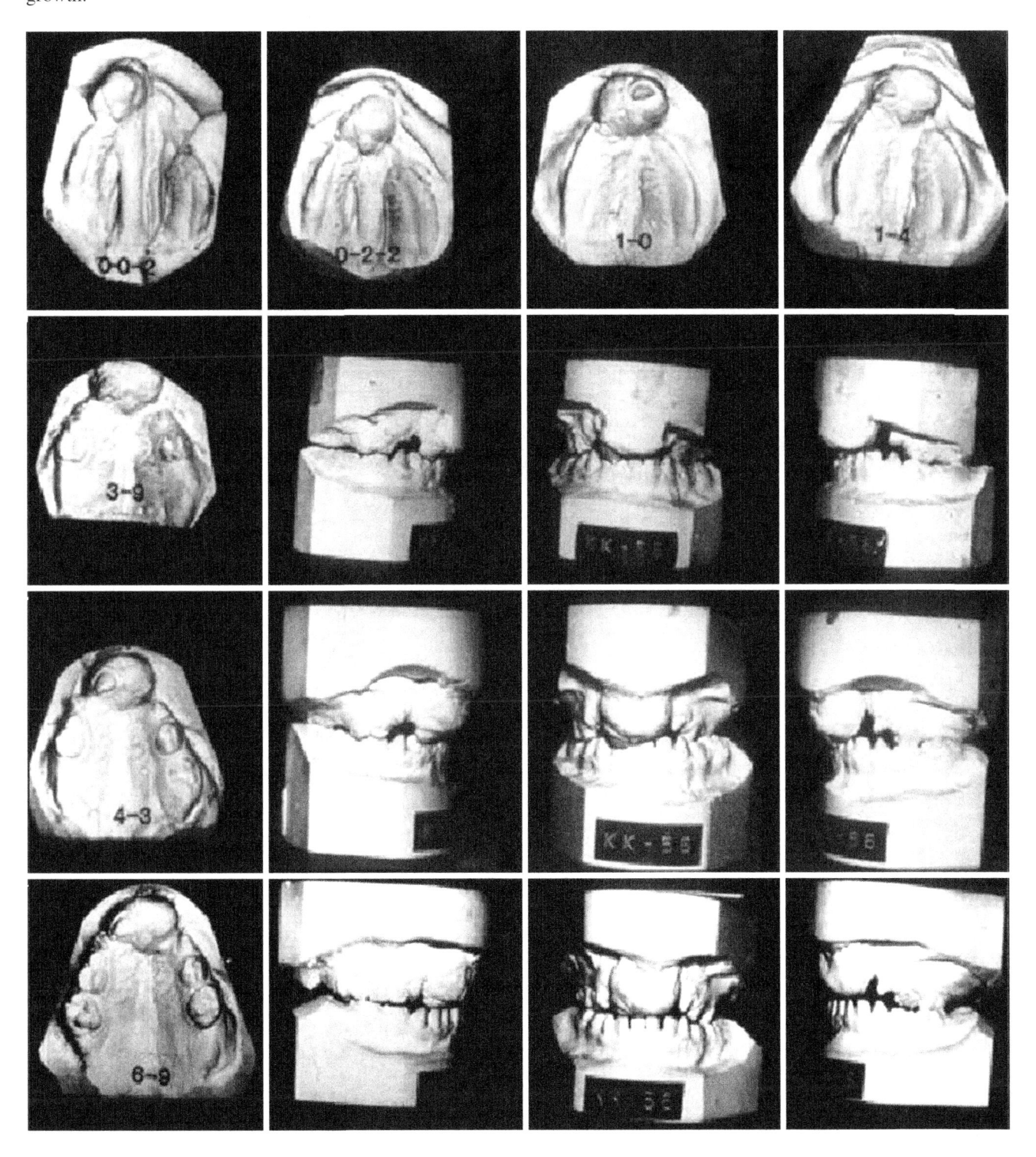

In order to maintain upper and lower anterior arch congruency, the lateral incisor space was left open to be replaced by lateral incisors or by pontics.

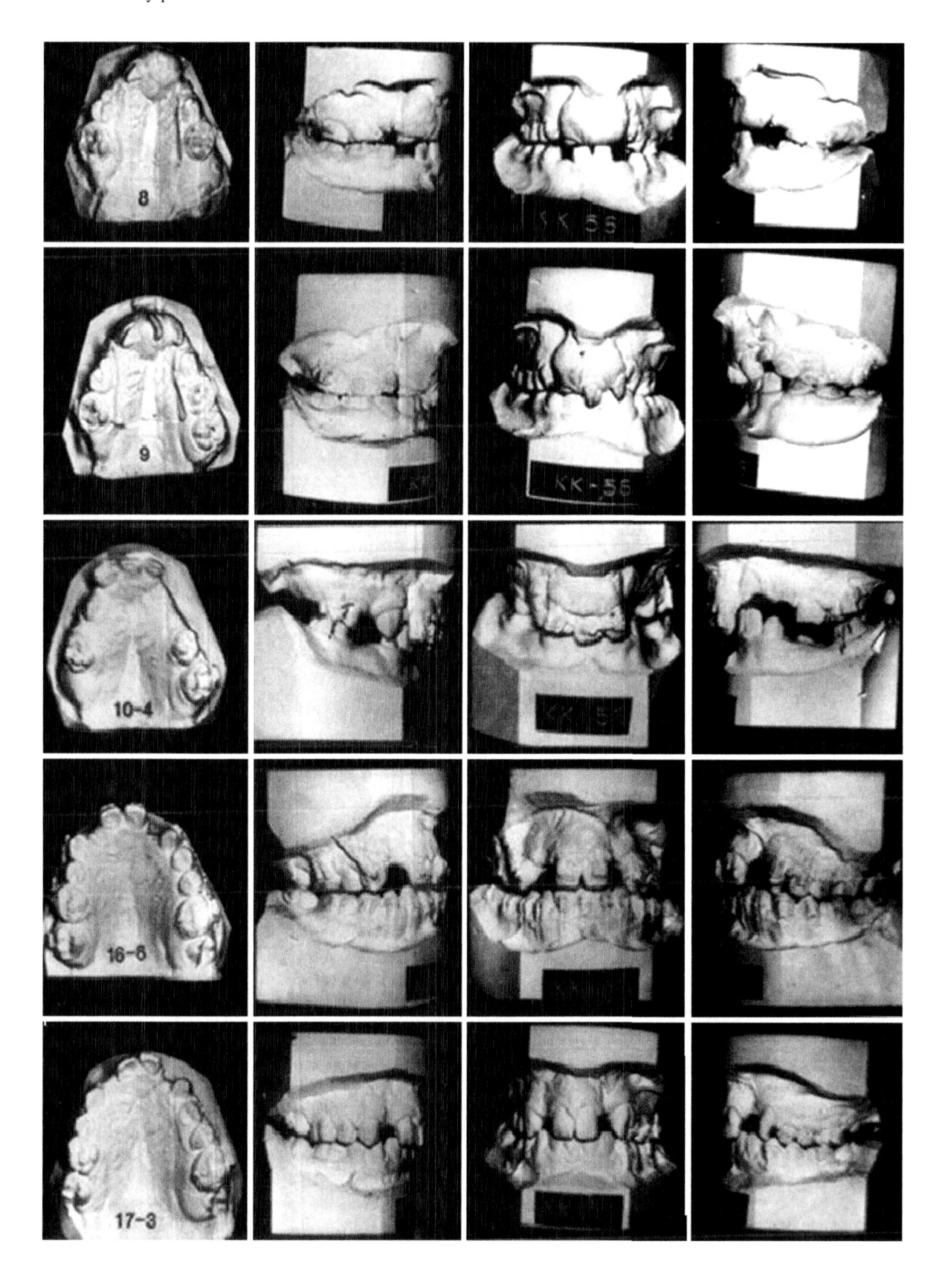

## 9.24 Exceptional Forward Mandibular Growth Flattening the Facial Profile

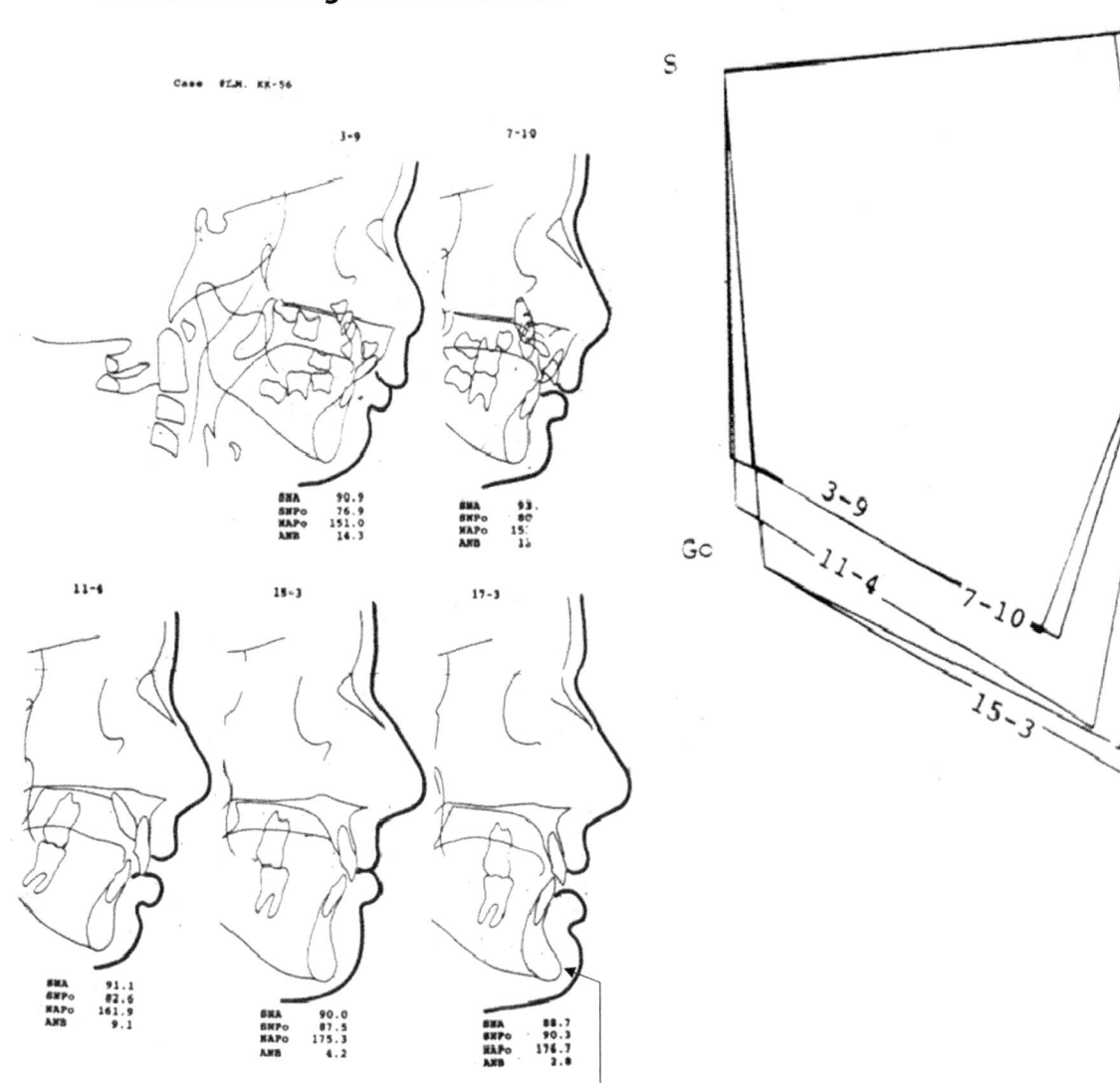

Exceptionally large symphysis.

144    9  Complete Bilateral Cleft Lip and Palate

## 9.25 CBCLP Demonstrating Facial Profile Going from Protrusion to Retrusion

**4 months**

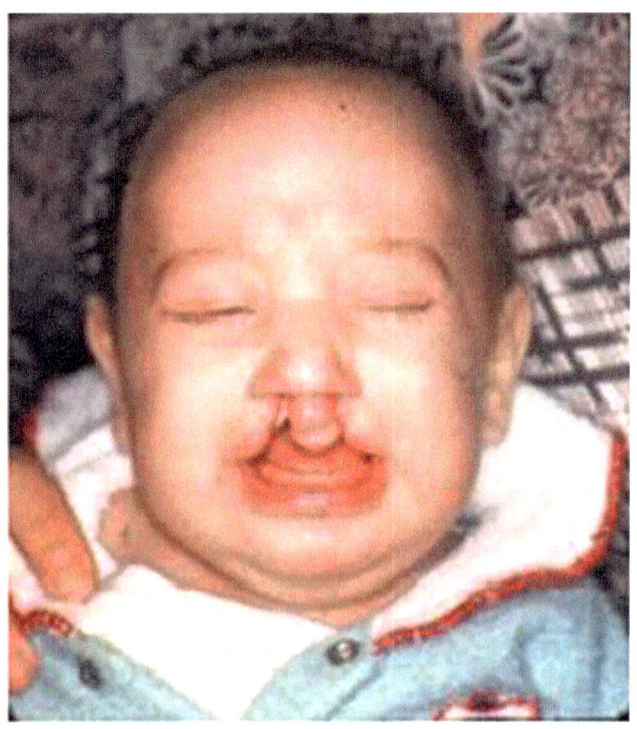

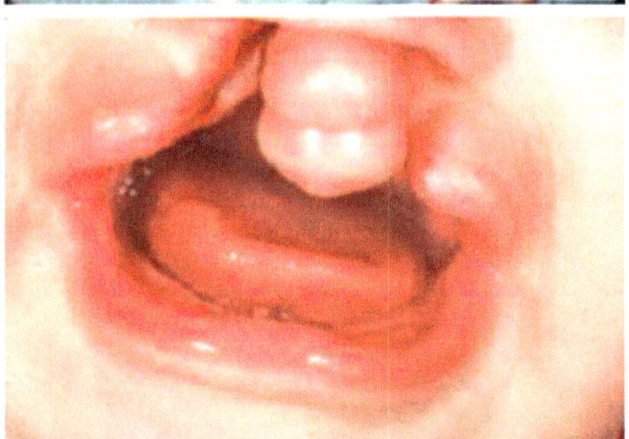

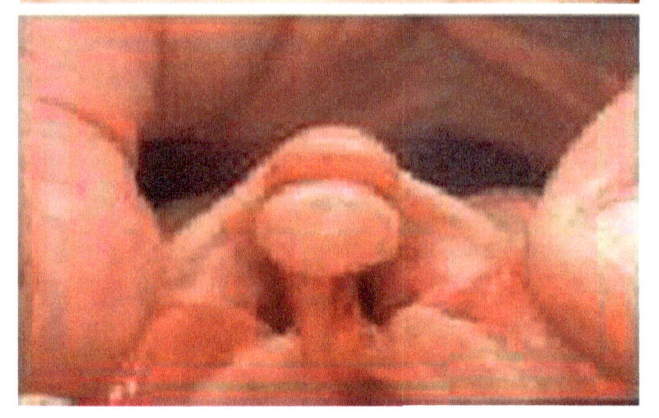

**6 months**

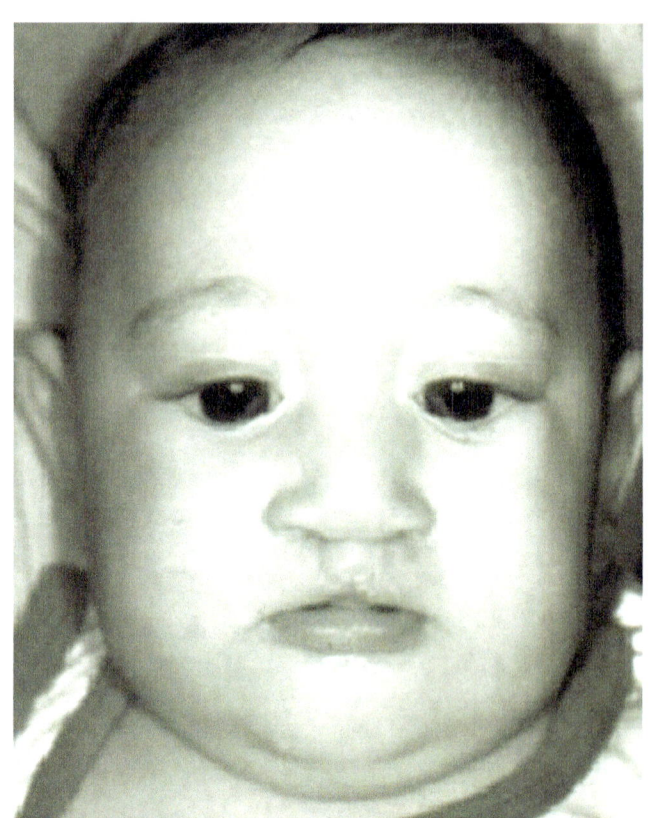

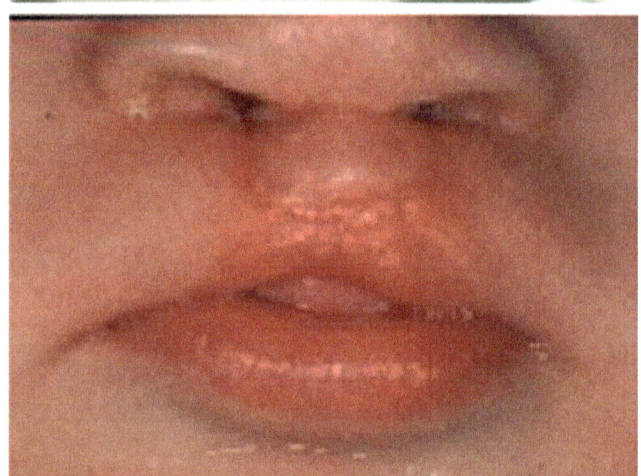

After lip adhesion (3 months) and definitive lips repairs (8 months). Prolabium used to create a philtrum.

Very small and extremely protrusive premaxilla.

9.25 CBCLP Demonstrating Facial Profile Going from Protrusion to Retrusion

**1 year 2 months**

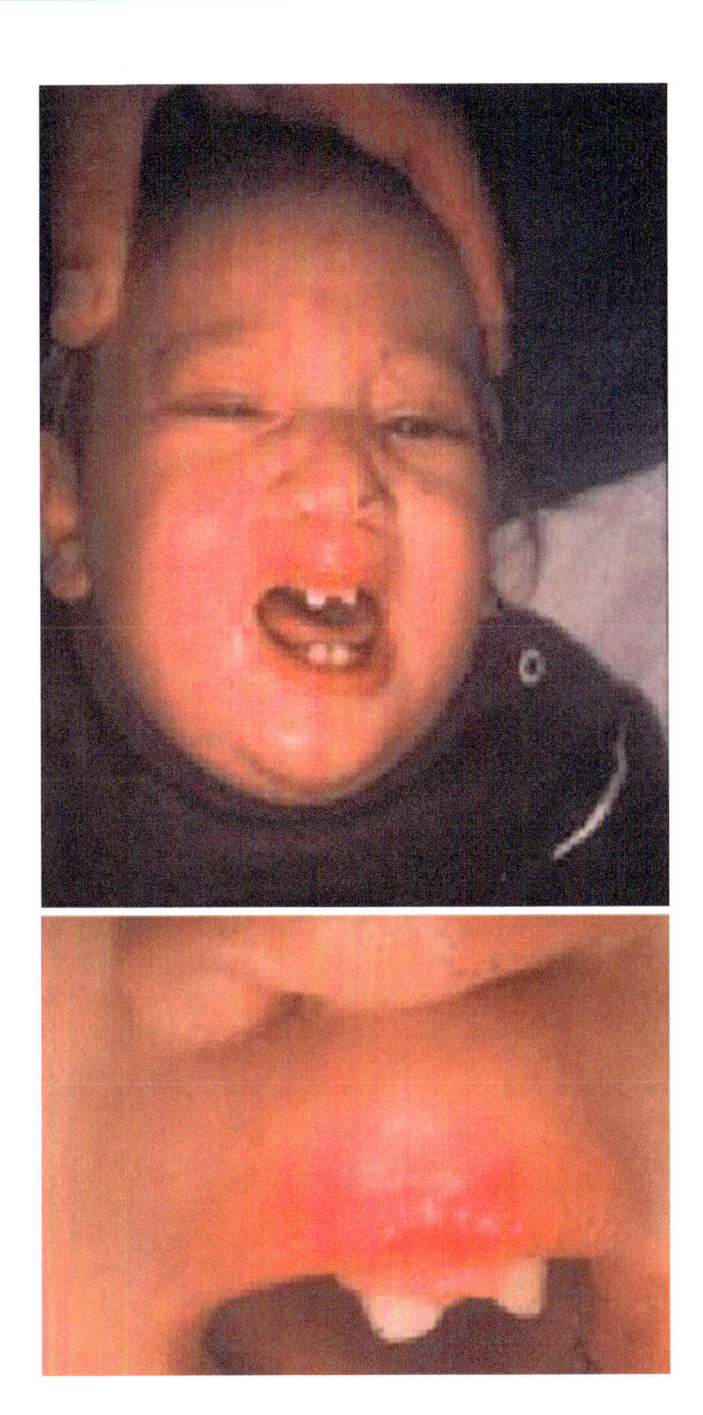

Nasal tip depressed.

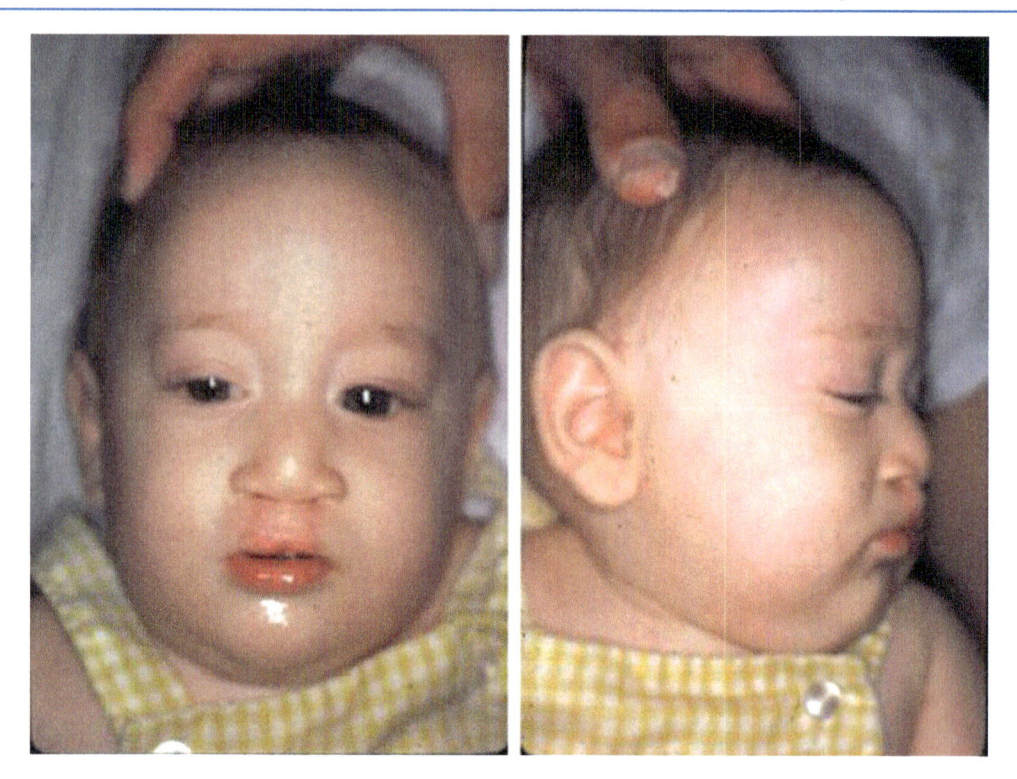

**1 year**
Good upper lip length—Slightly protrusive.

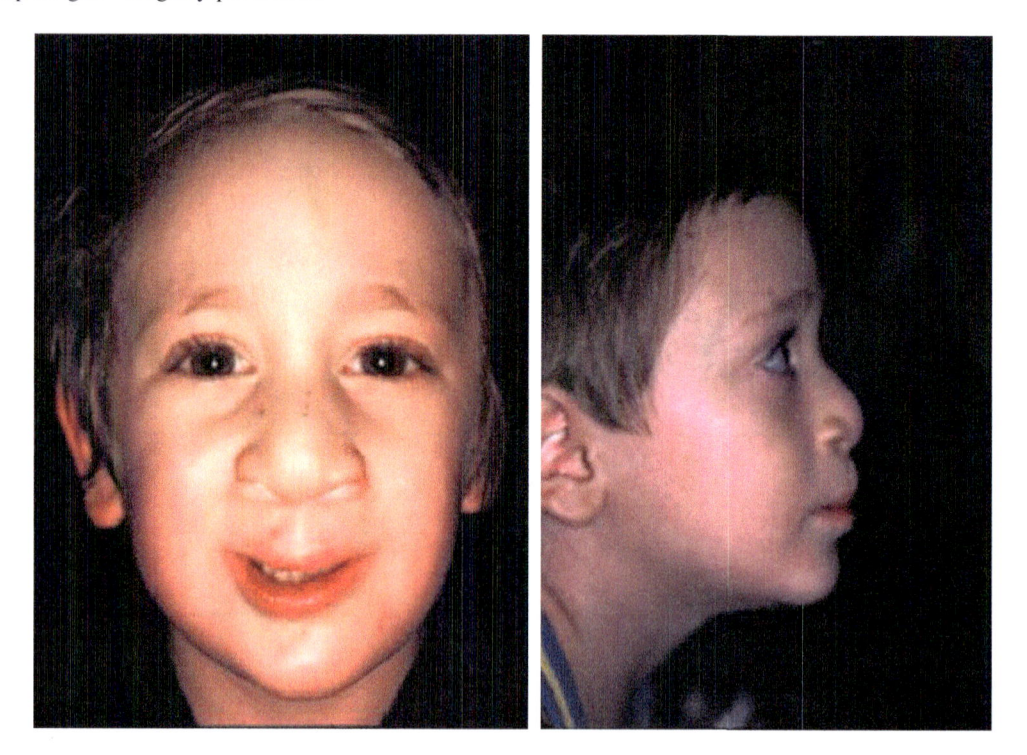

**4 years**
The premaxilla is only slightly protrusive.

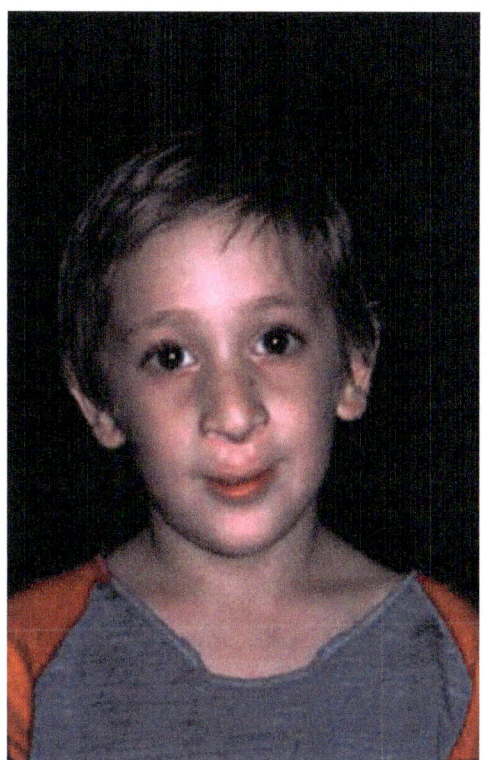

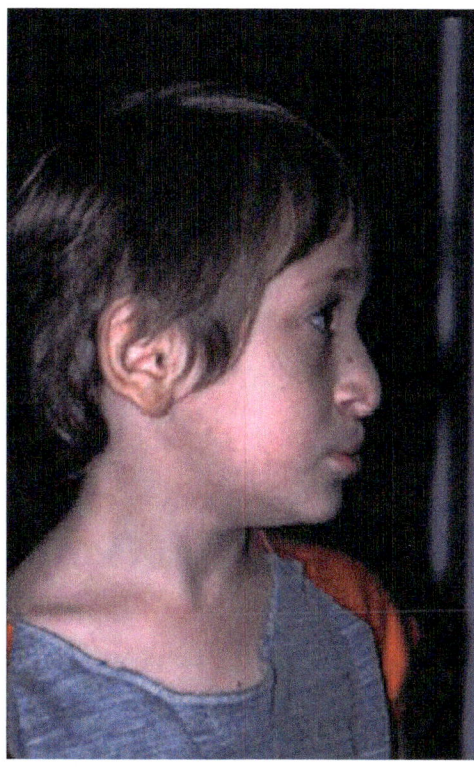

9.25 CBCLP Demonstrating Facial Profile Going from Protrusion to Retrusion

**6 years**

At 3 years:
Von Langenbeck with modified vomer palatal flap closure leaving the anterior cleft open for future secondary alveolar bone grafts.

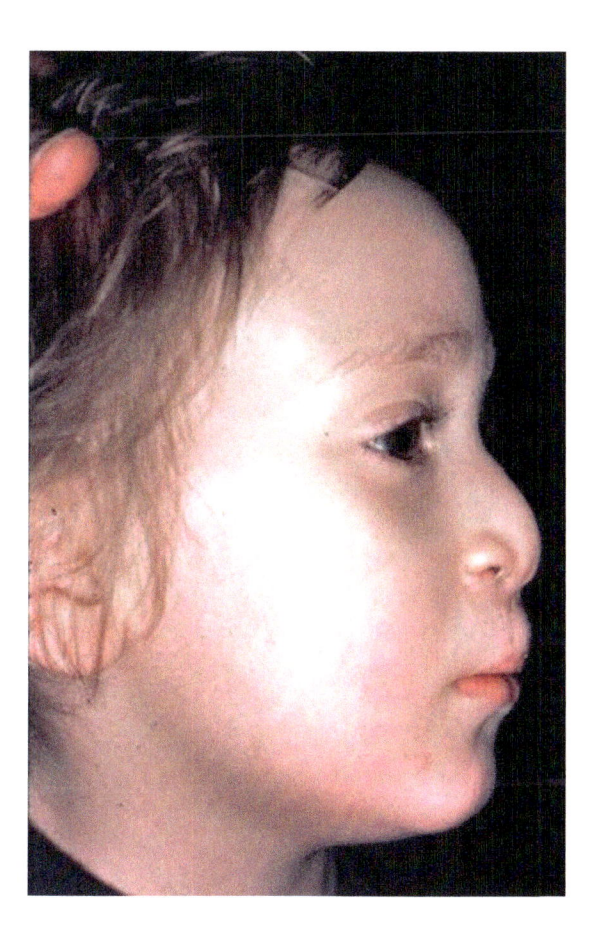

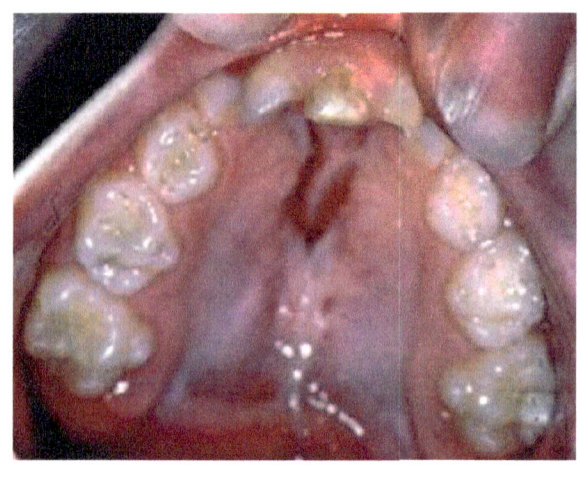

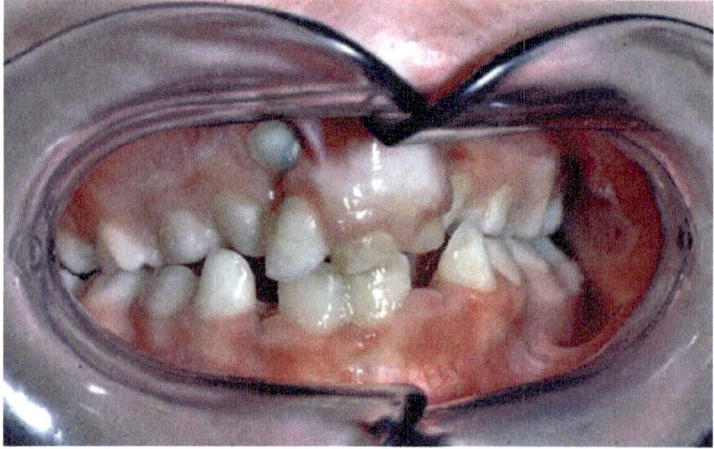

**At 7 years:**

Note the relative flatness of the profile with the reduction of premaxillary protrusion. Good buccal occlusion. The anterior cleft was purposely left open. It will be closed with a secondary alveolar bone graft.

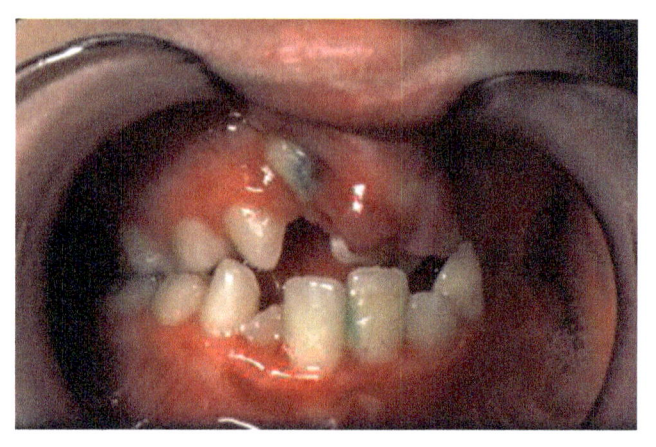

**Age: 7–11**
Anterior and buccal crossbite

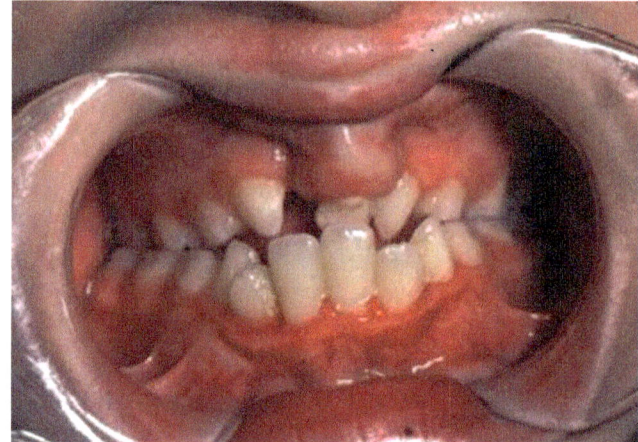

**Age: 8–11**
Dental crossbite still remains, with slight narrowing across the maxillary cuspids. Protruding and crowded lower anterior teeth.

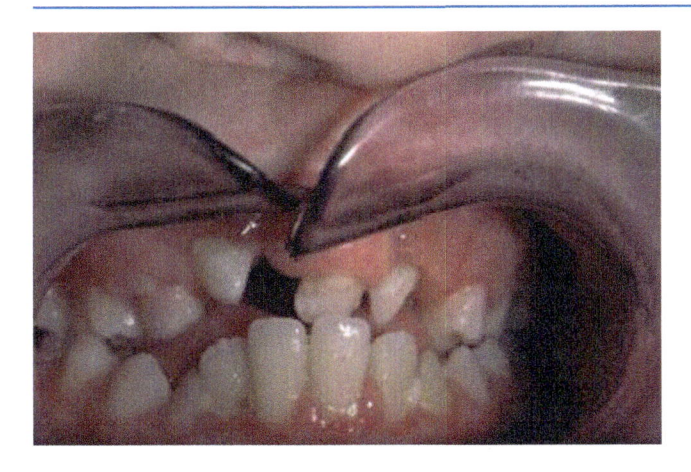

### 9.25 CBCLP Demonstrating Facial Profile Going from Protrusion to Retrusion

**Age: 10–5**
No change in occlusion.

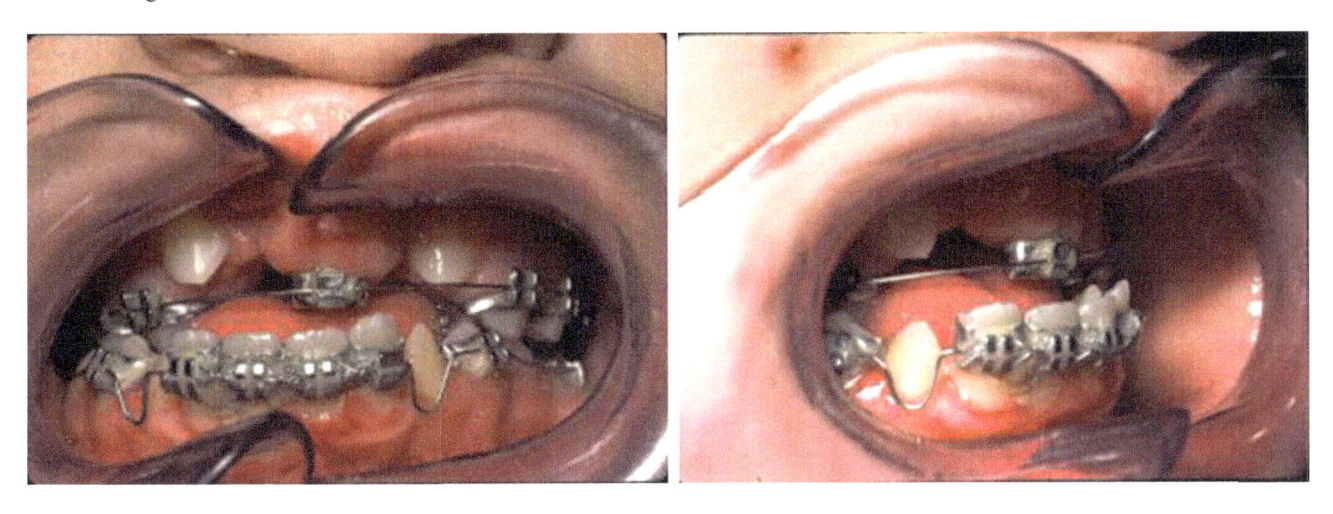

**Age: 11–5**
Advanced crowded lower incisors created a more severe anterior crossbite.

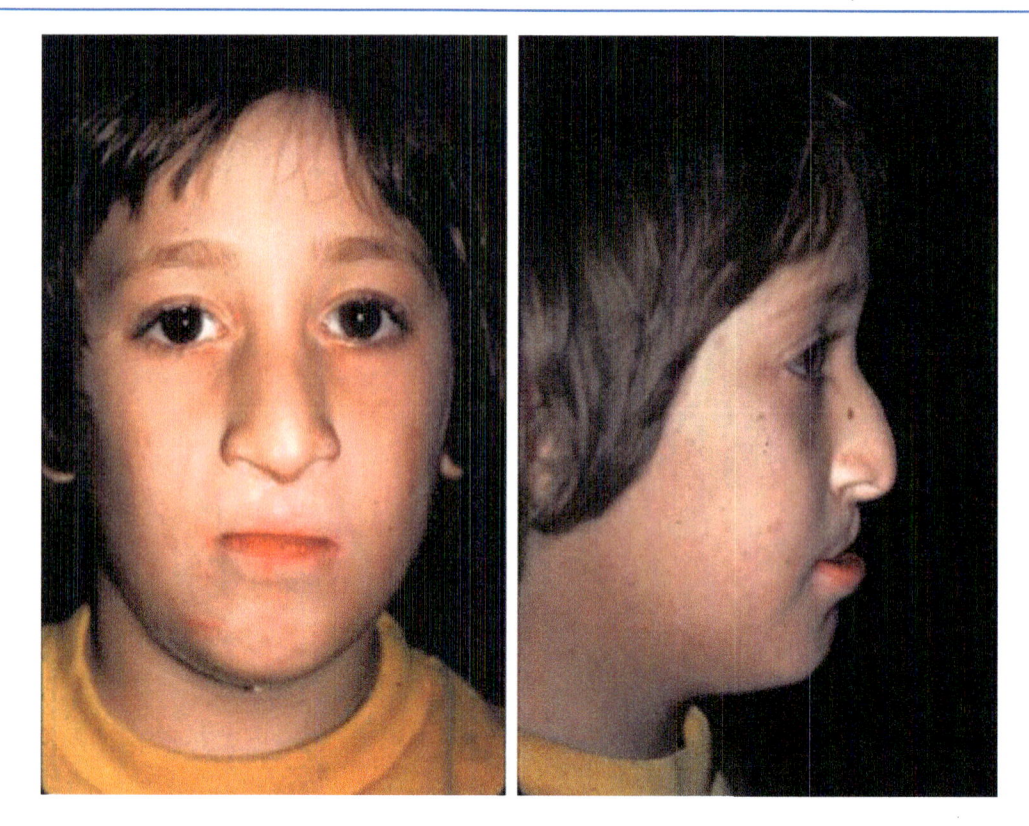

**9 years**
   Nasal tip was elevated.

## 9.26 Concave Facial Profile

**11.5 years**

No permanent incisor teeth were present in the premaxilla. One deciduous tooth remained. Lip pressure against the premaxilla to the nasal septum coupled with mandibular growth was responsible for the recessive midface. The crowed lower incisors were advanced creating flaring incisors with an anterior crossbite. NO GOOD!

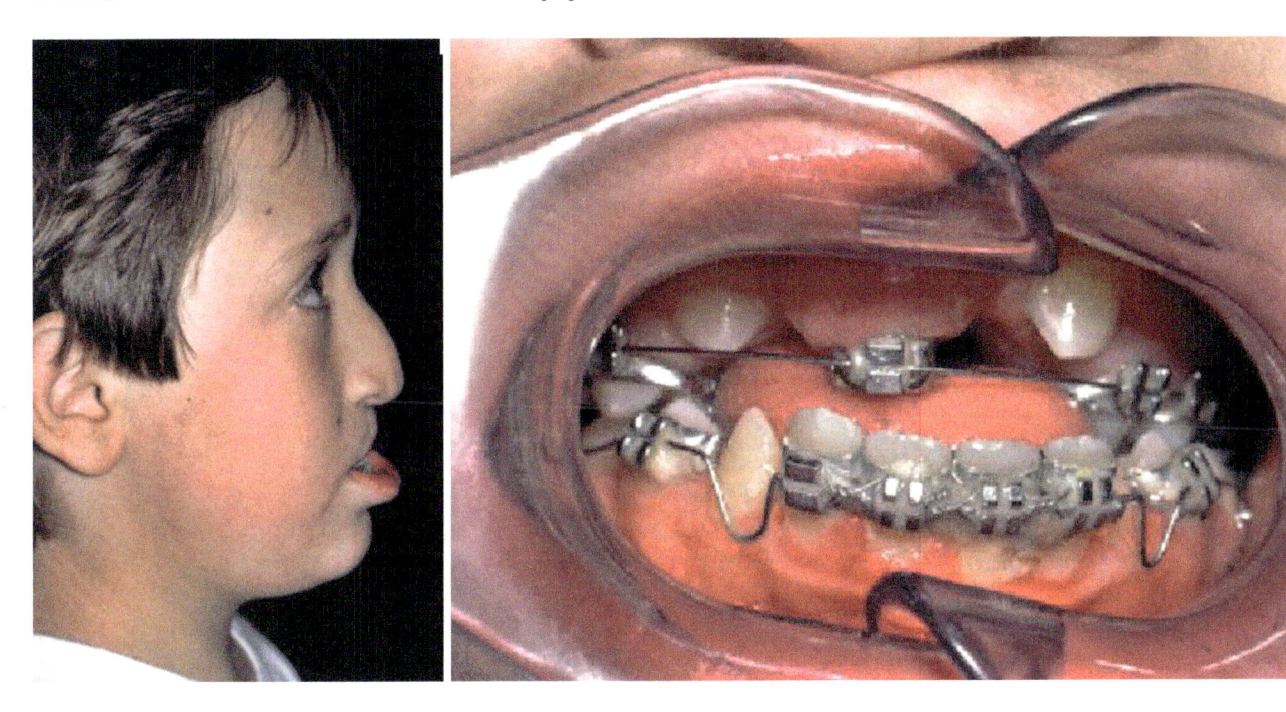

**12 years**

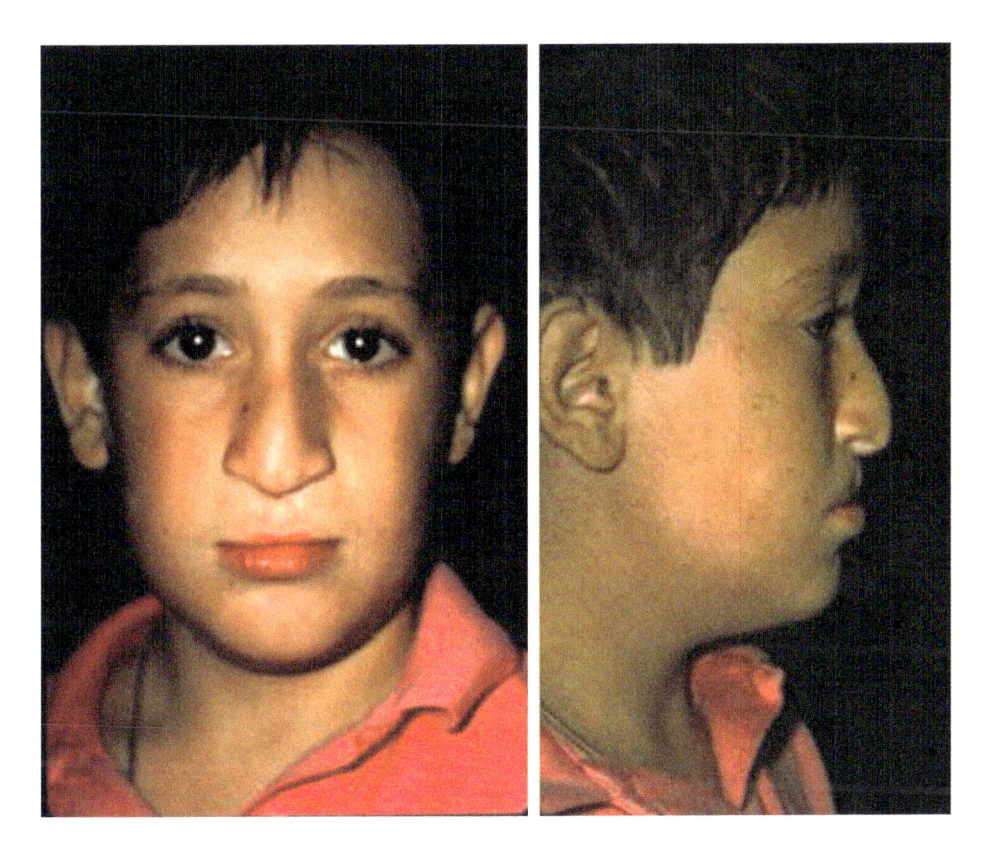

Midface is now very recessive.

**13 years**

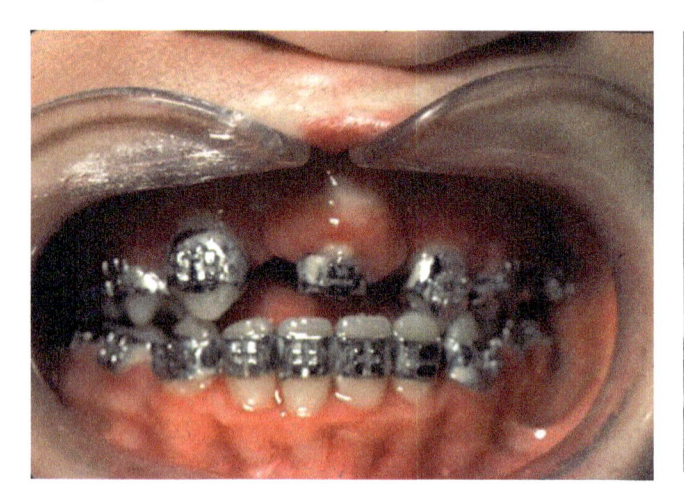

**15 years**

The lower first bicuspids were extracted and the lower incisors retracted creating proper axial teeth inclinations.

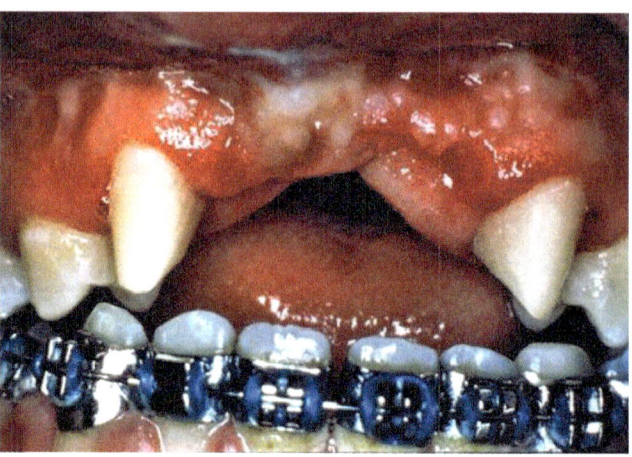

No permanent incisors were present, therefore the remaining deciduous tooth was removed and replaced by a fixed anterior bridge.

## 9.26 Concave Facial Profile

**17 years** Final face

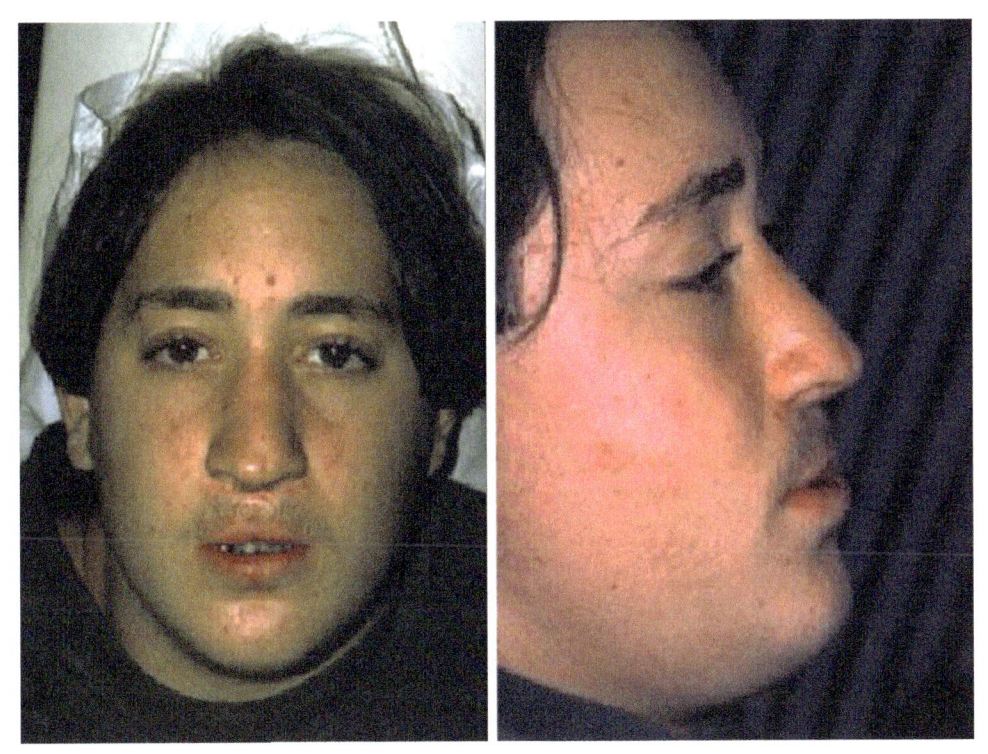

Good lip balance with fixed anterior bridge replacing all missing incisors

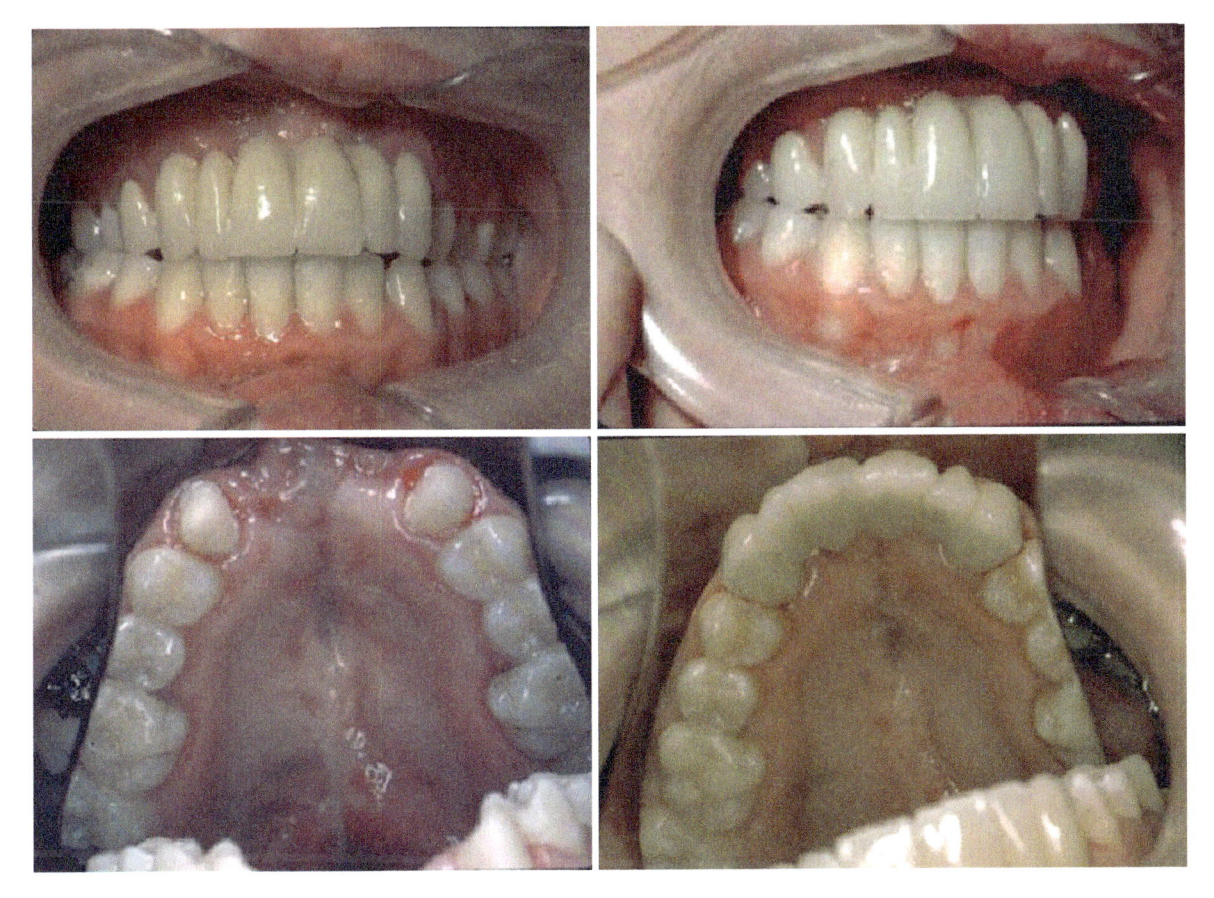

Anterior fixed bridge replaces missing maxillary central and lateral incisors, palatal fistula closed. Notice a normal palatal vault space.

Rapid reduction in the degree of premaxillary protrusion and closure of the anterior cleft space.

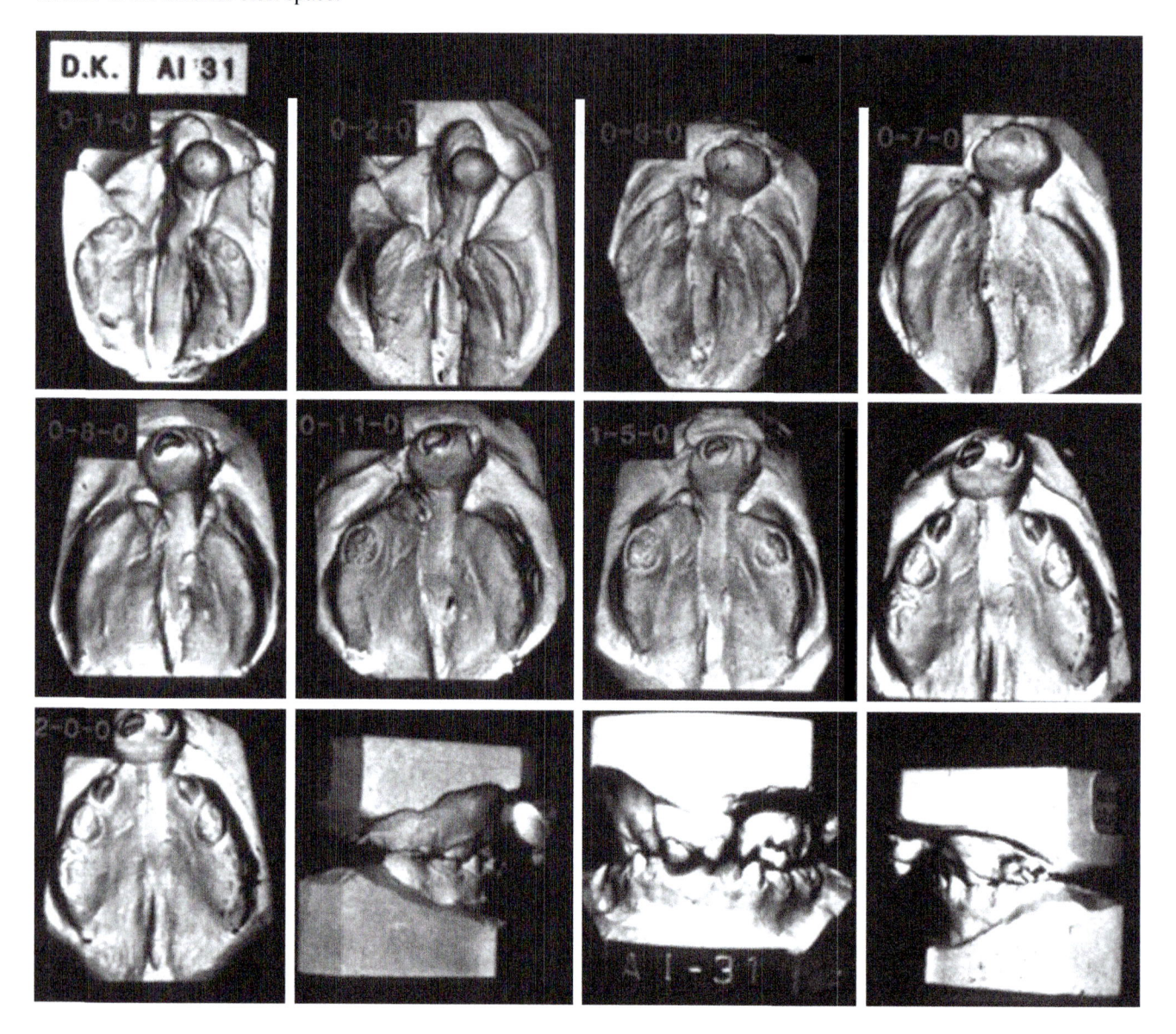

9.26 Concave Facial Profile

Good anterior overbite overjet relationship

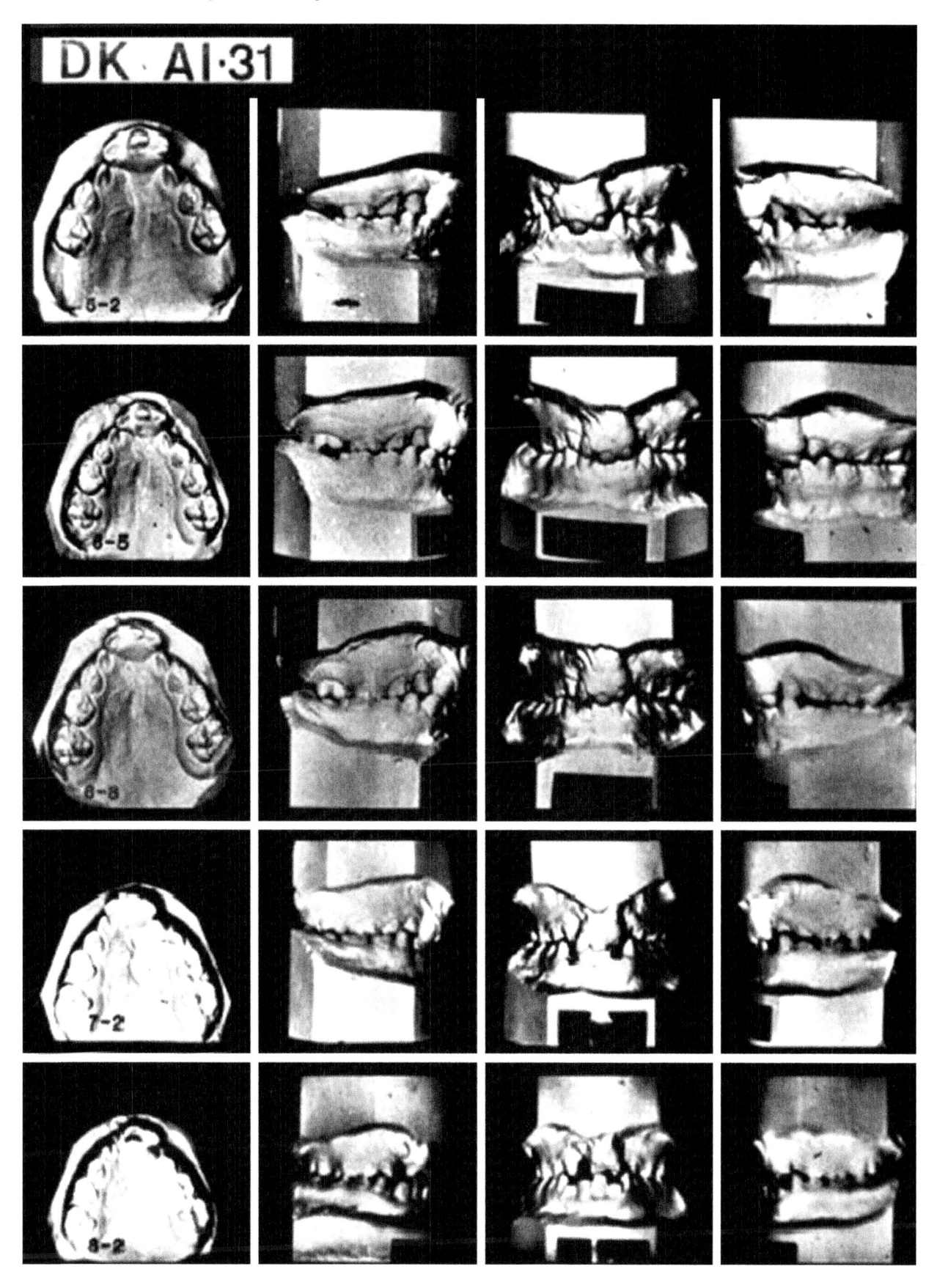

Lower anterior teeth advanced to uncrowd the lower incisors. This created severe axial flaring with a retruded midface. Lower first bicuspids were extracted and the incisors retracted.

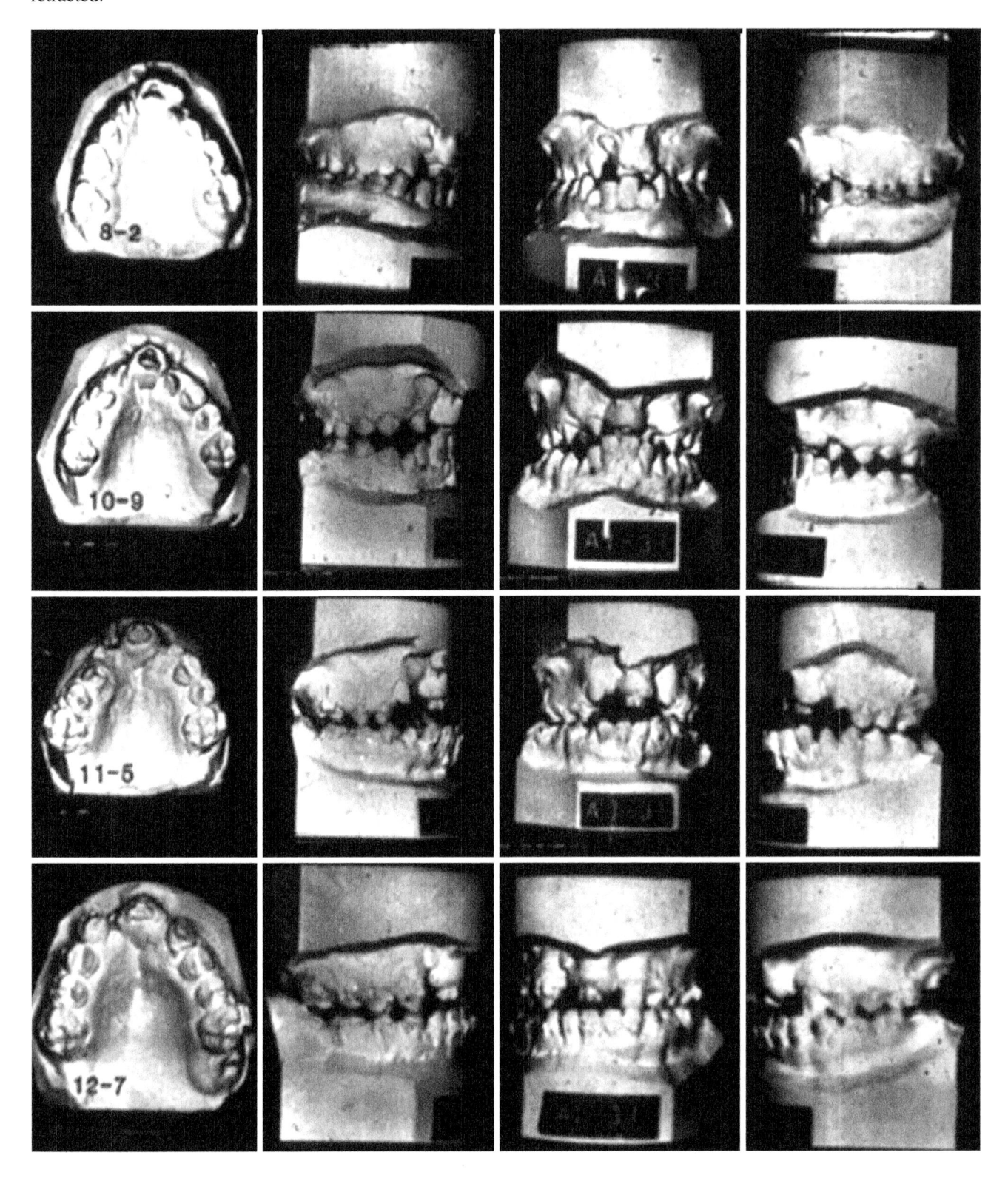

9.26 Concave Facial Profile

Replacement anterior maxillary bridge and final anterior and posterior occlusion.

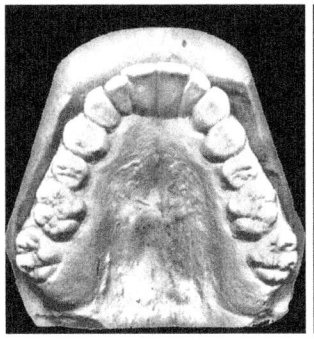

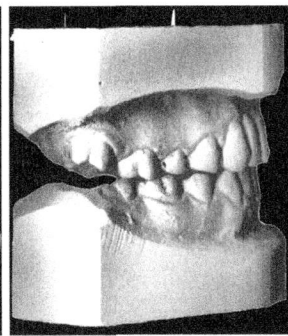

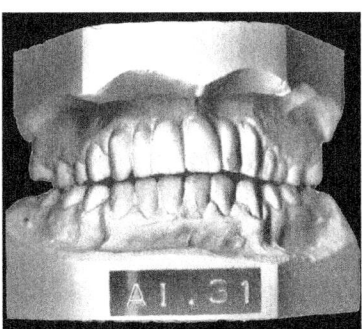

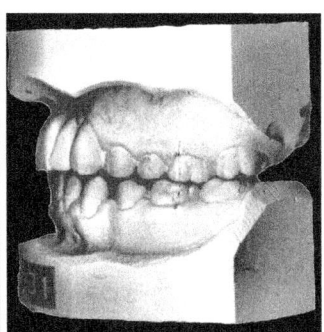

## 9.27 Gradual Reduction in the Anterior and Posterior Cleft Spaces as Seen in Computerized Serial Palatal Cast (Casts Are Not Drawn to Scale Relative To Size)

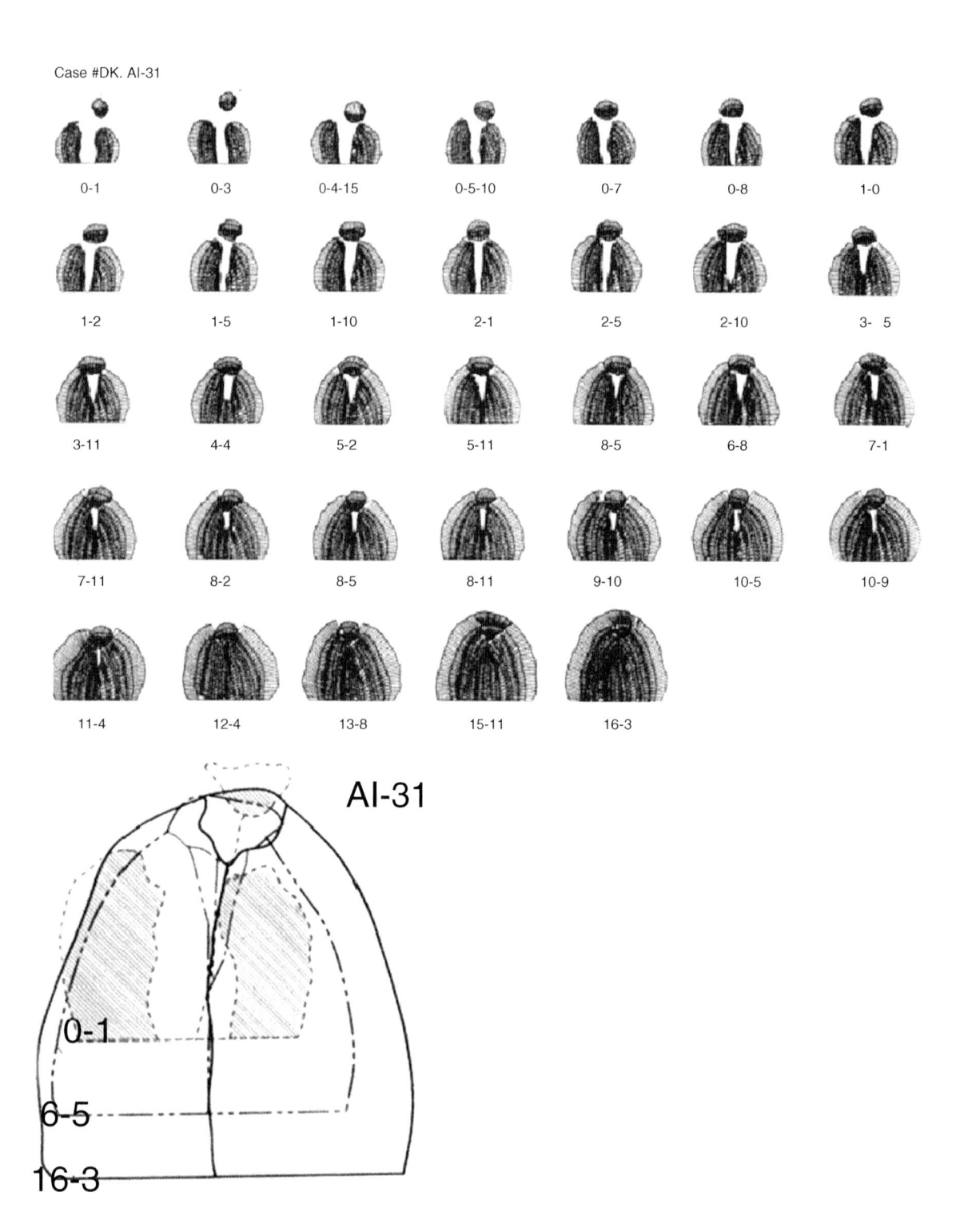

Case #DK. AI-31

| 0-1 | 0-3 | 0-4-15 | 0-5-10 | 0-7 | 0-8 | 1-0 |
| 1-2 | 1-5 | 1-10 | 2-1 | 2-5 | 2-10 | 3-5 |
| 3-11 | 4-4 | 5-2 | 5-11 | 8-5 | 6-8 | 7-1 |
| 7-11 | 8-2 | 8-5 | 8-11 | 9-10 | 10-5 | 10-9 |
| 11-4 | 12-4 | 13-8 | 15-11 | 16-3 | | |

AI-31

0-1
6-5
16-3

Superimposed serial palatal casts from birth to 16 years of age. Superimposed on rugae and registered on the Vomer (highest point of the vault)

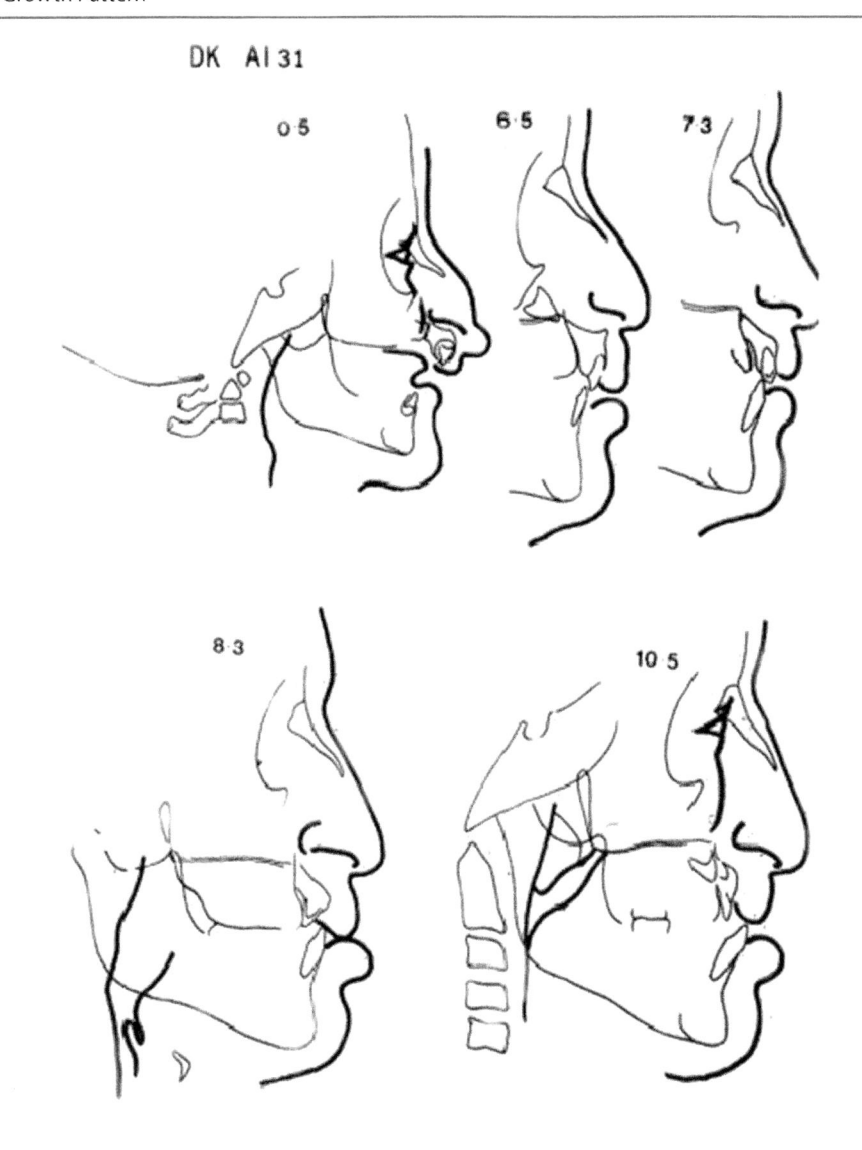

## 9.28 Excellent Facial Growth Pattern

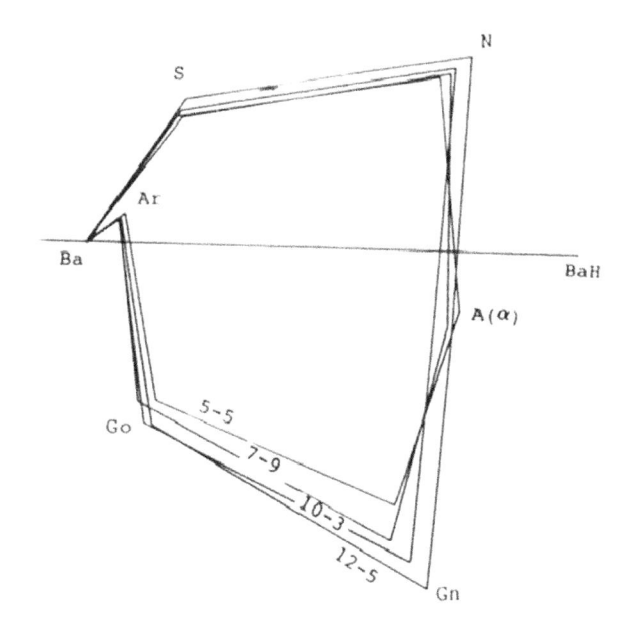

Spontaneous flattening of the midface.

## 9.29 Final Photographs

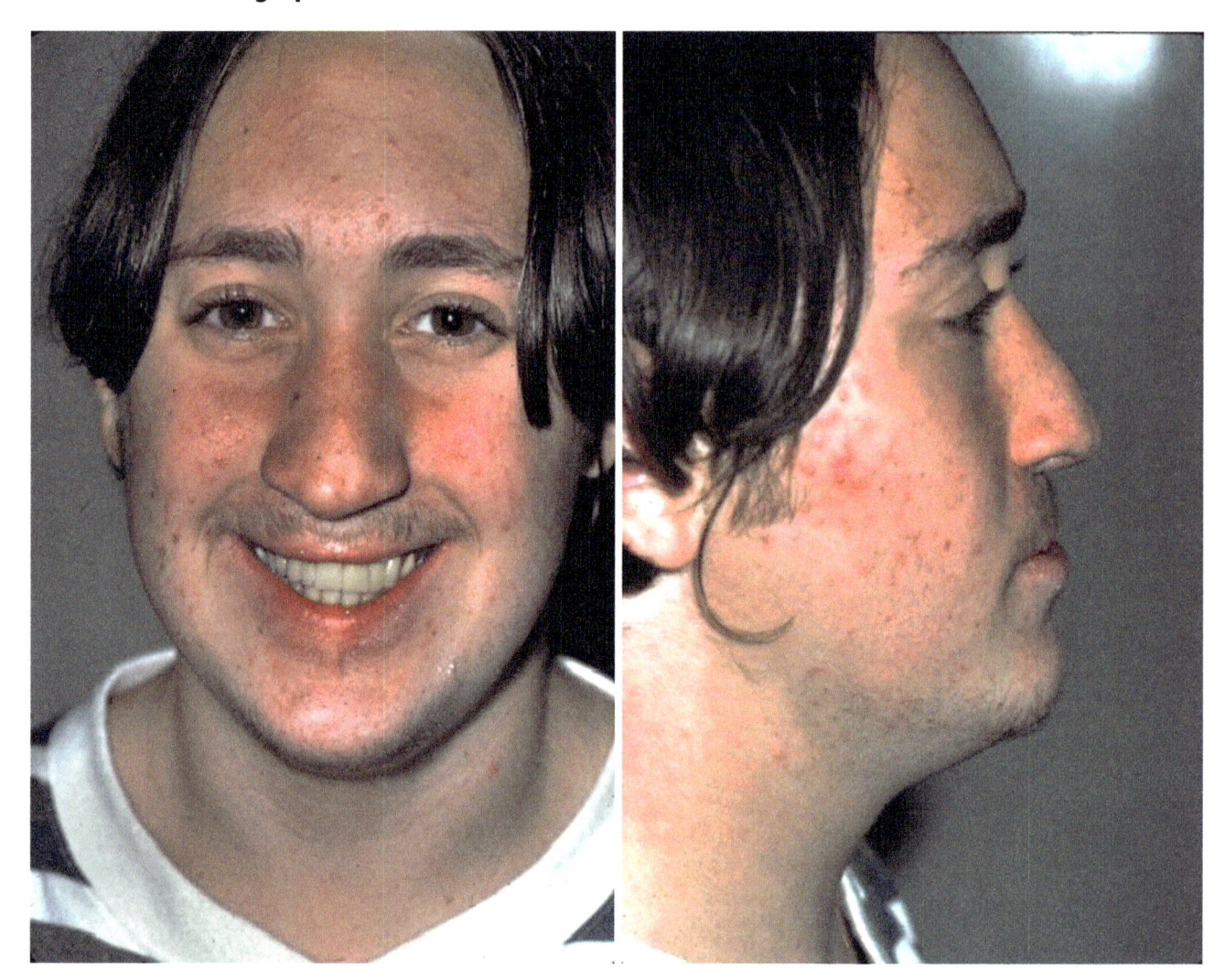

9.30 CBCLP: Ideal Treatment Results

## 9.30 CBCLP: Ideal Treatment Results

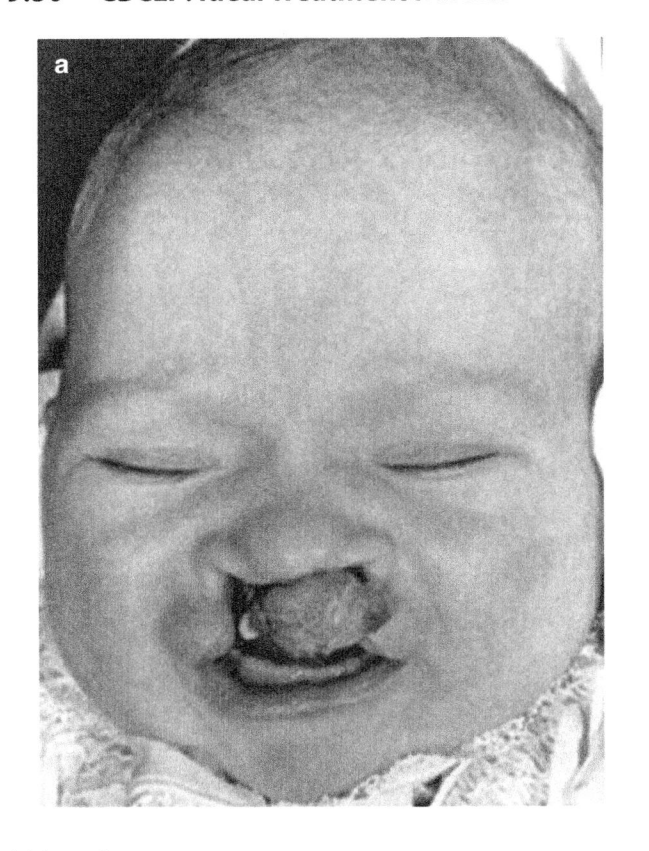

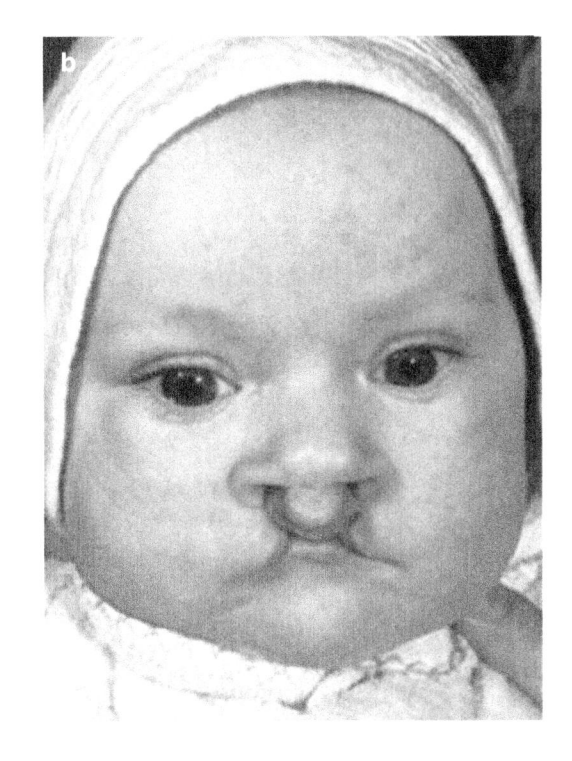

(**a**) 1 month

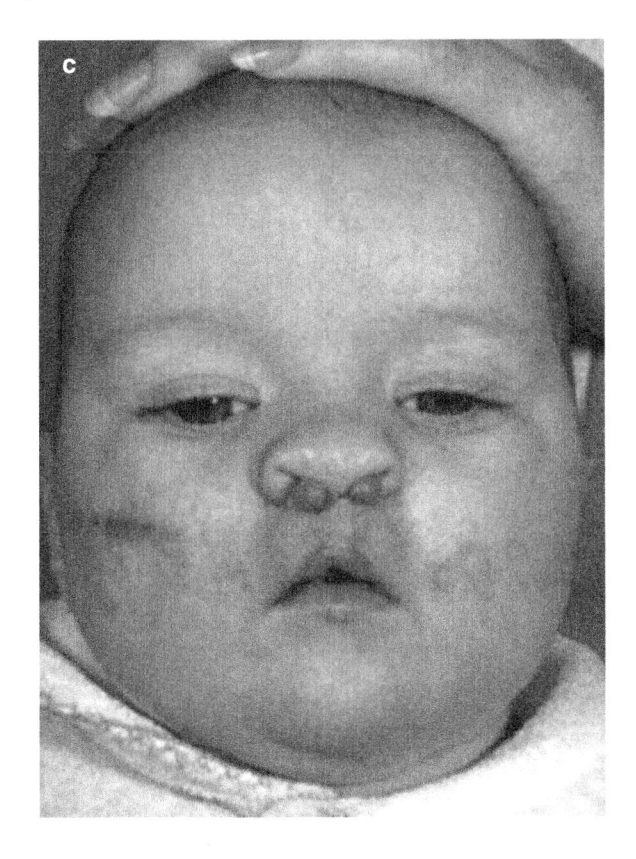

(**b**) 2 months after head bonnet and strap

(**c**) 6 months

(**d**) 1 month

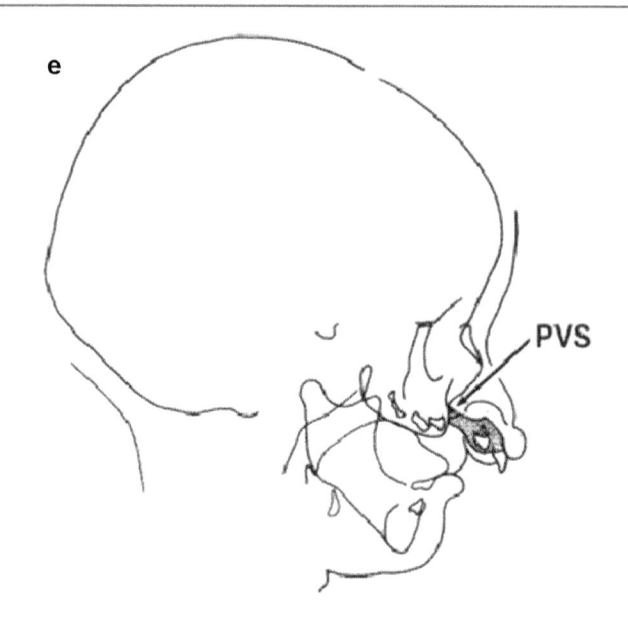

Lip united with banked forked flap.

a, b, d, e: Protruding premaxilla due to excessive growth at the premaxillary vomerine suture (PVS).

**This case was selected to show: (1) spontaneous narrowing of the palatal cleft. (2) The protruding premaxilla which is forward for the lateral palatal segments. (3) The protrusive midface reduces with growth and muscle restraint. (4) No presurgical orthopedics.**

(e) Example

7 months Ventroflexed premaxilla

1 year 11 months

2 years 1 month

### 9.30.1 Columella Lengthened, Nasal Tip Elevated

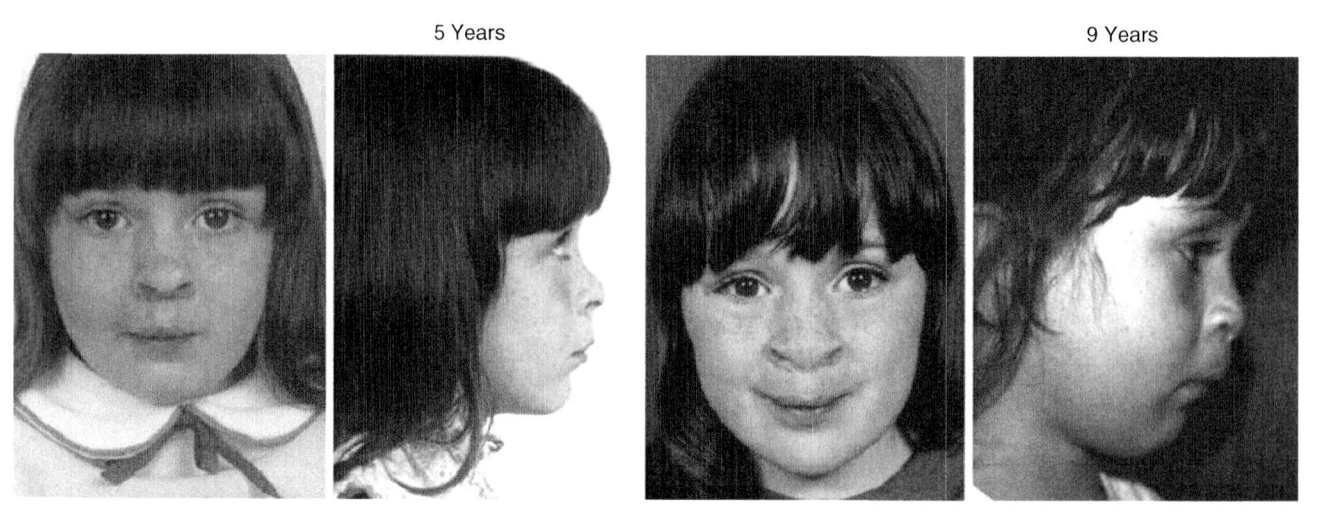

5 Years

9 Years

The midface is more protrusive after the eruption of the permanent maxillary anterior incisors.

9.30 CBCLP: Ideal Treatment Results

## 9.30.2 Profile Flattened Lip/Nose Revisions

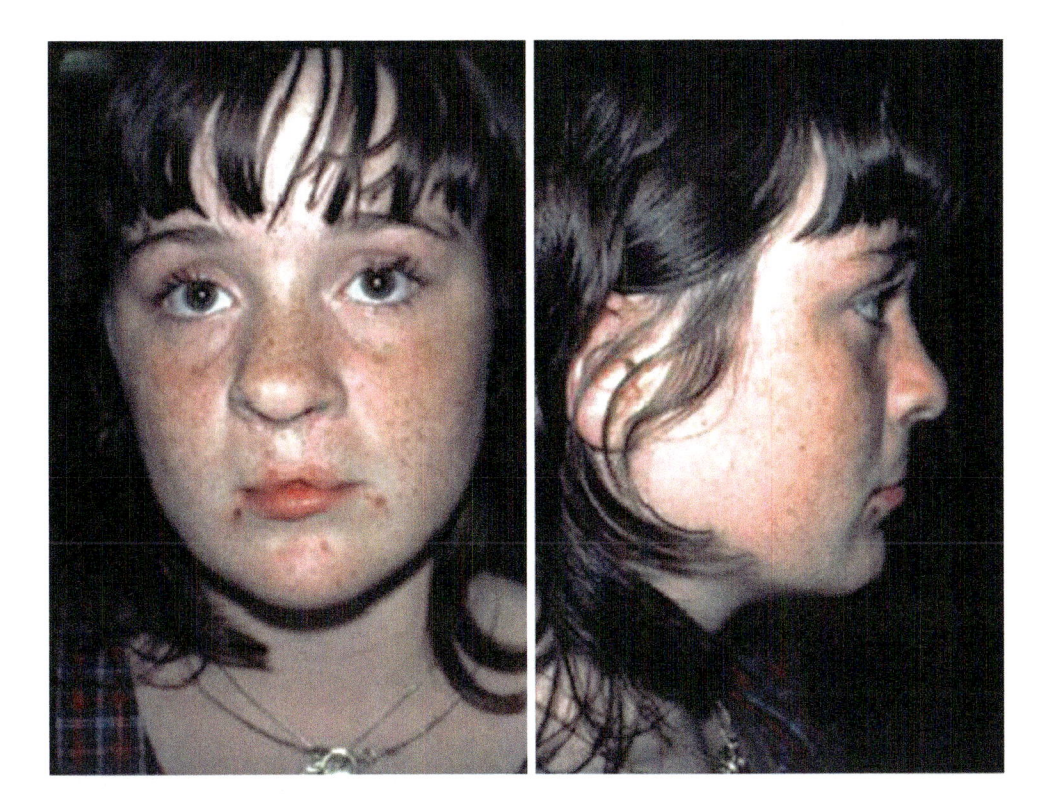

**11 years**

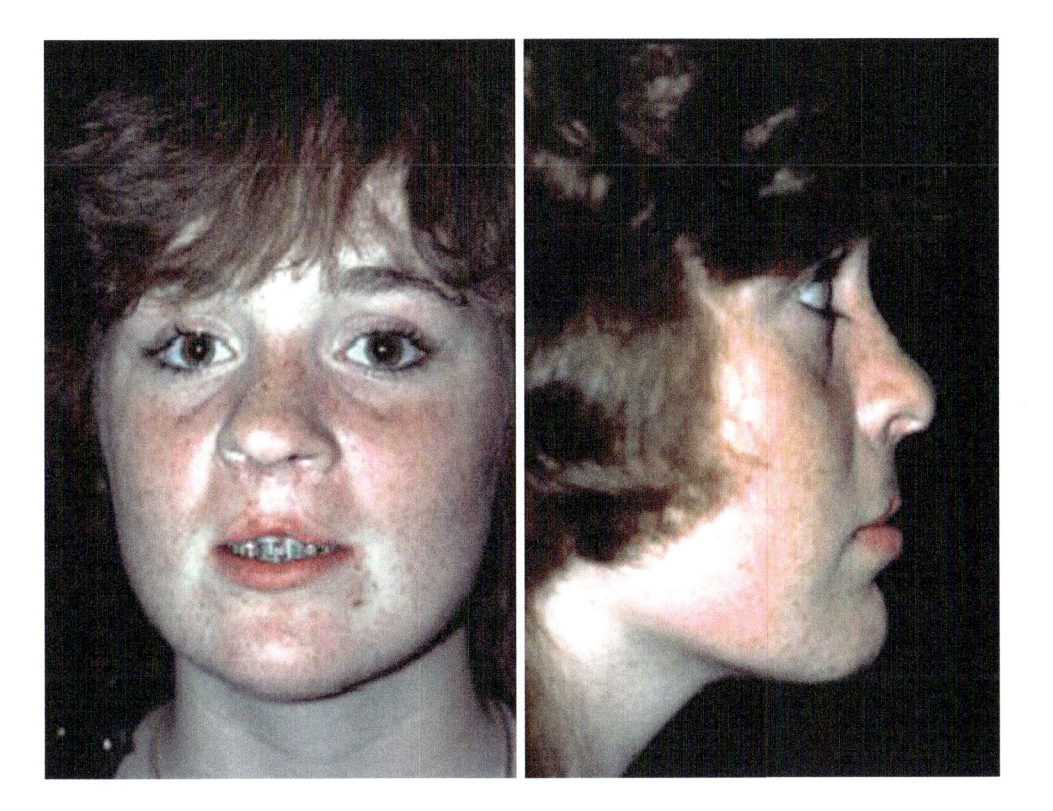

**12 years**

## 9.30.3 Nasal and Lip Revisions

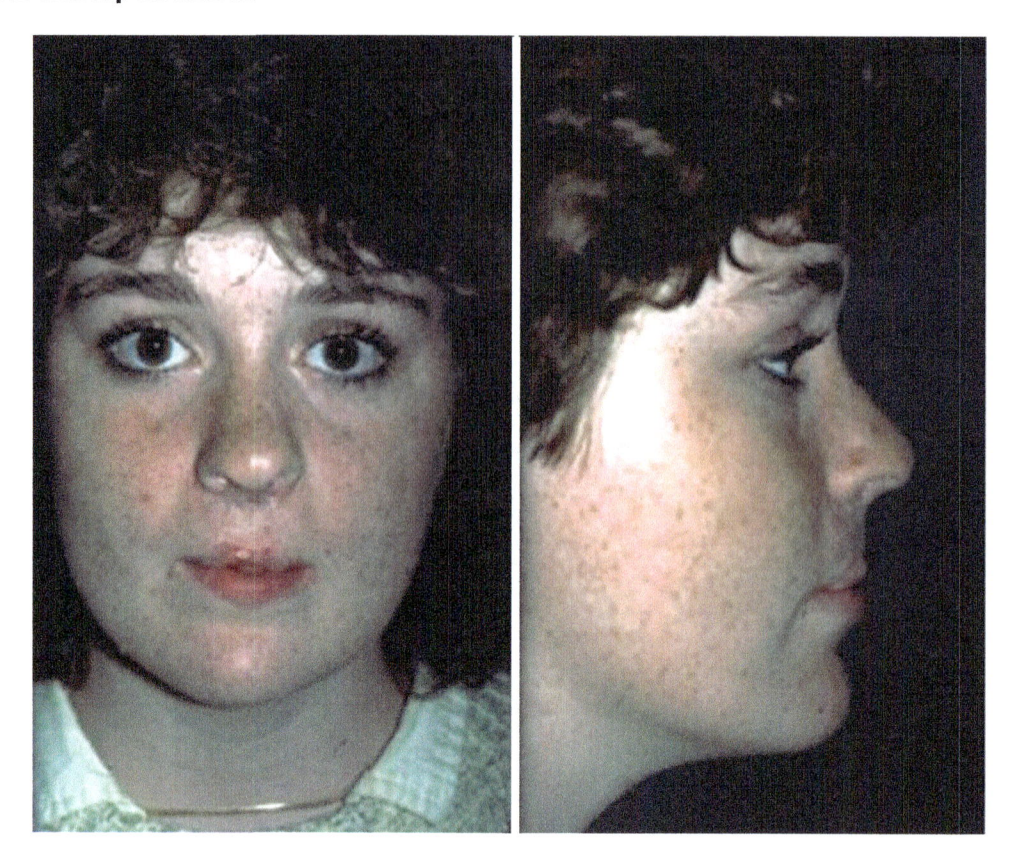

**14 years 10 months**

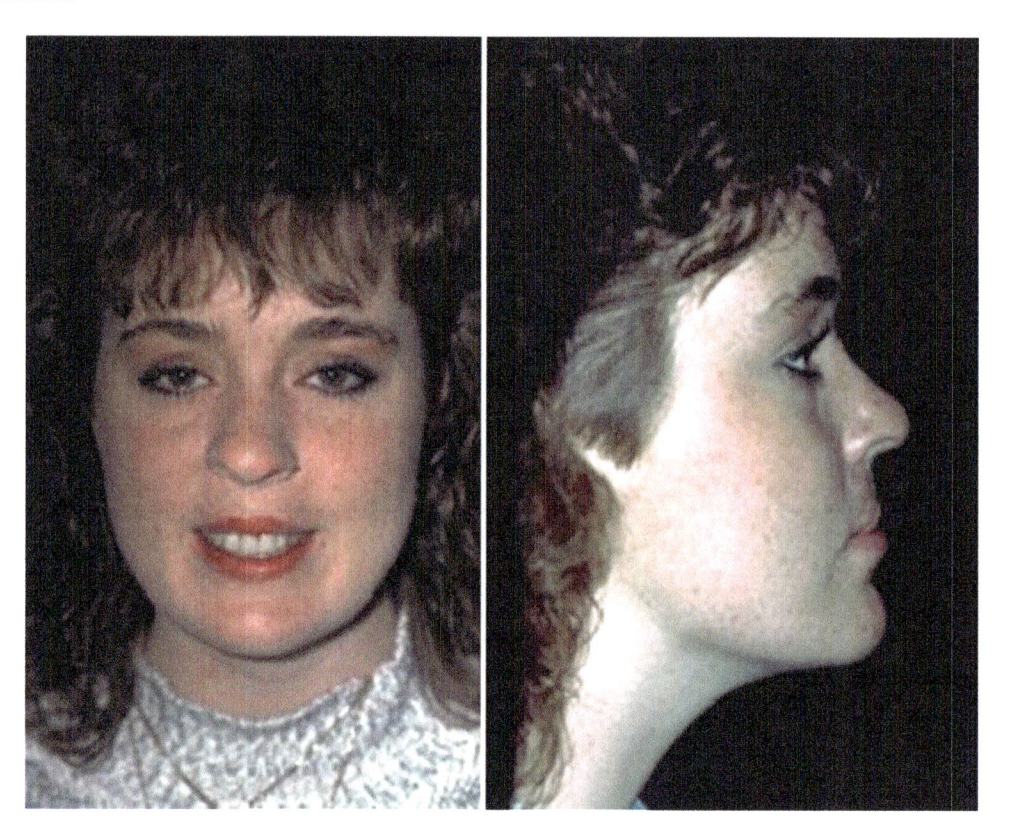

**20 years (Final)**

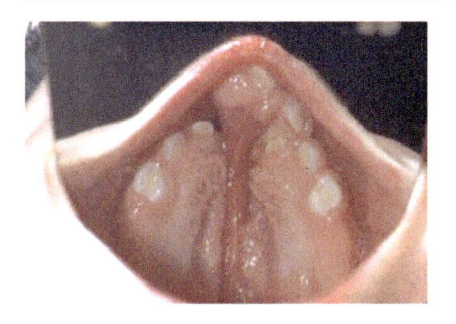

## 9.30 CBCLP: Ideal Treatment Results

**1 year 11 months**
Open palate and bilateral alveolar cleft **No anterior cleft**

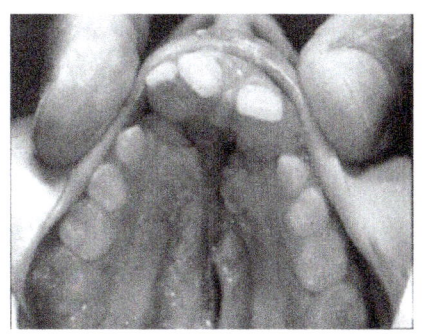

**7 years**
Anterior slight overbite and overjet Good buccal occlusion

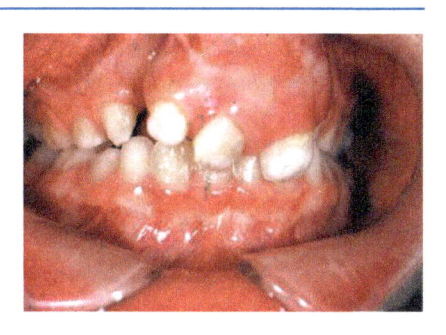

**7 years**

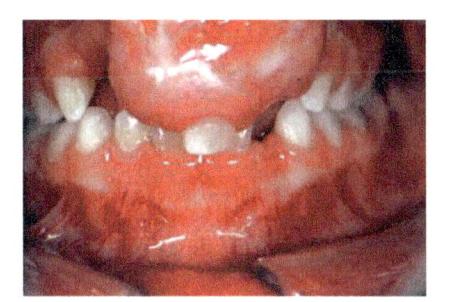

**7 years**
Anterior overjet and overbite. Good buccal occlusion. No orthodontics.

### 9.30.3.1 Final occlusion stabilized after orthodontics and secondary alveolar bone grafts

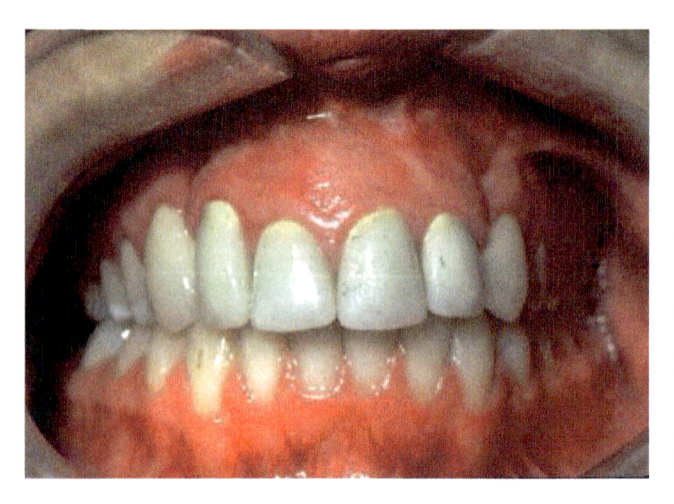

**18 years**

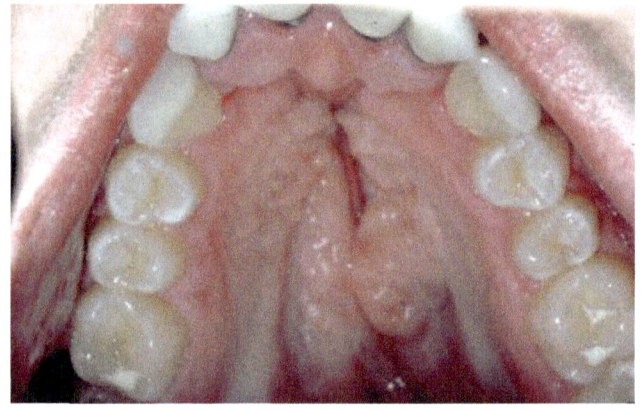

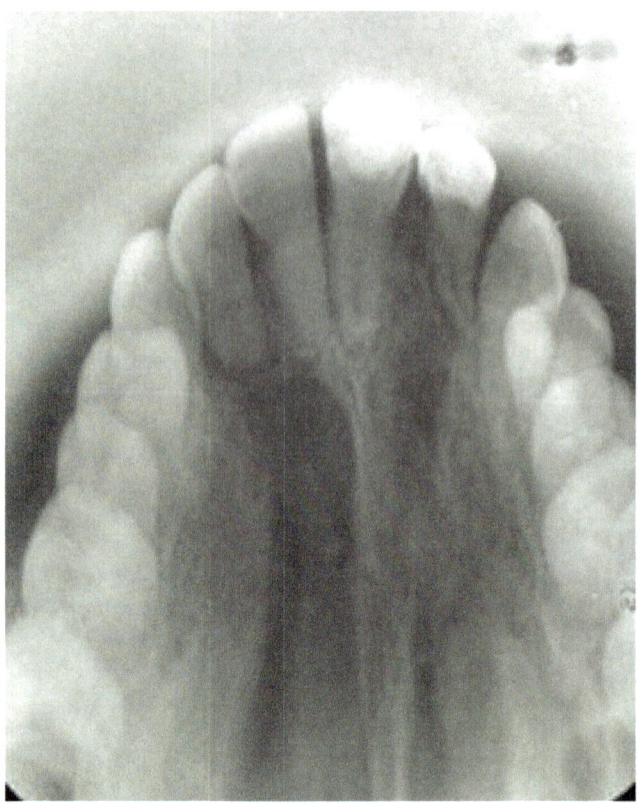

**18 years**
Occlusal radiographic view
showing covered bony palatal cleft with excellent alveolar bone

**18 years**
Very small fistula poses no functional problem.

## 9.31 Serial Dental Casts

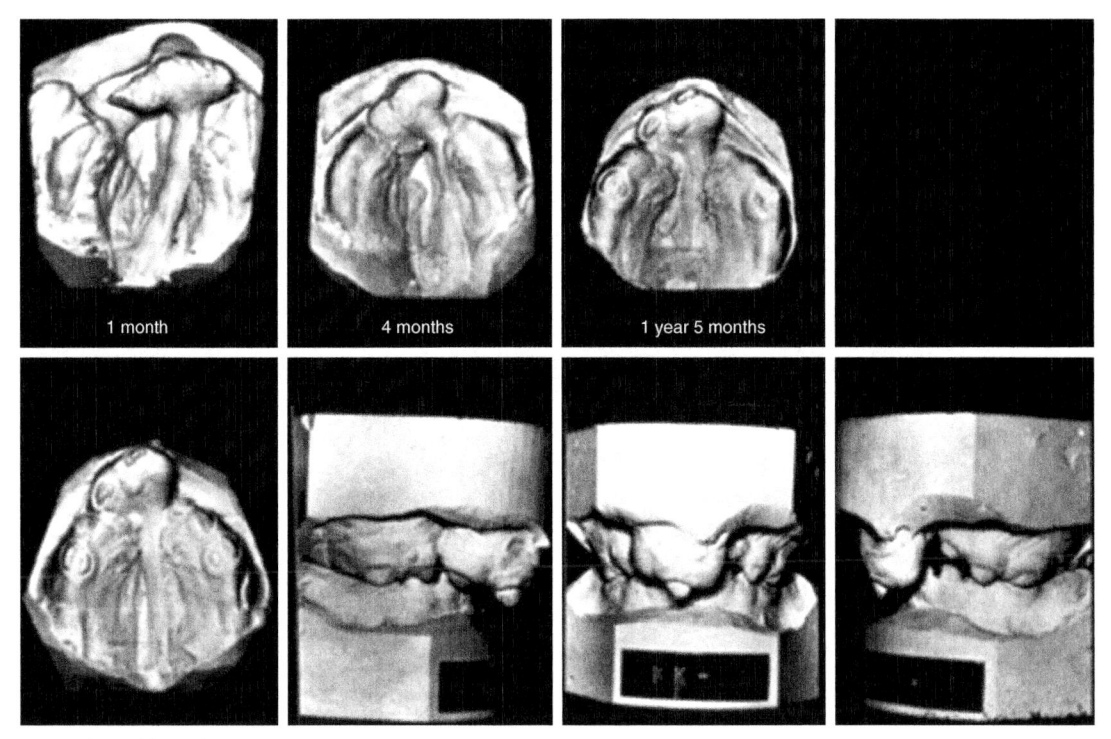

1 month

4 months

1 year 5 months

1 year 11 months

- Large premaxilla
- Right palatal segments overexpanded
- Head bonnet-caused molding
- Premaxilla forward of both palatal segments—cleft space reduced

*1 year 5 months*: Premaxilla forward of both palatal segments.

*1 year 11 months*: Protruding premaxilla, severe anterior overbite and overjet.

**Note the spontaneous movement of the premaxilla into the arch.**

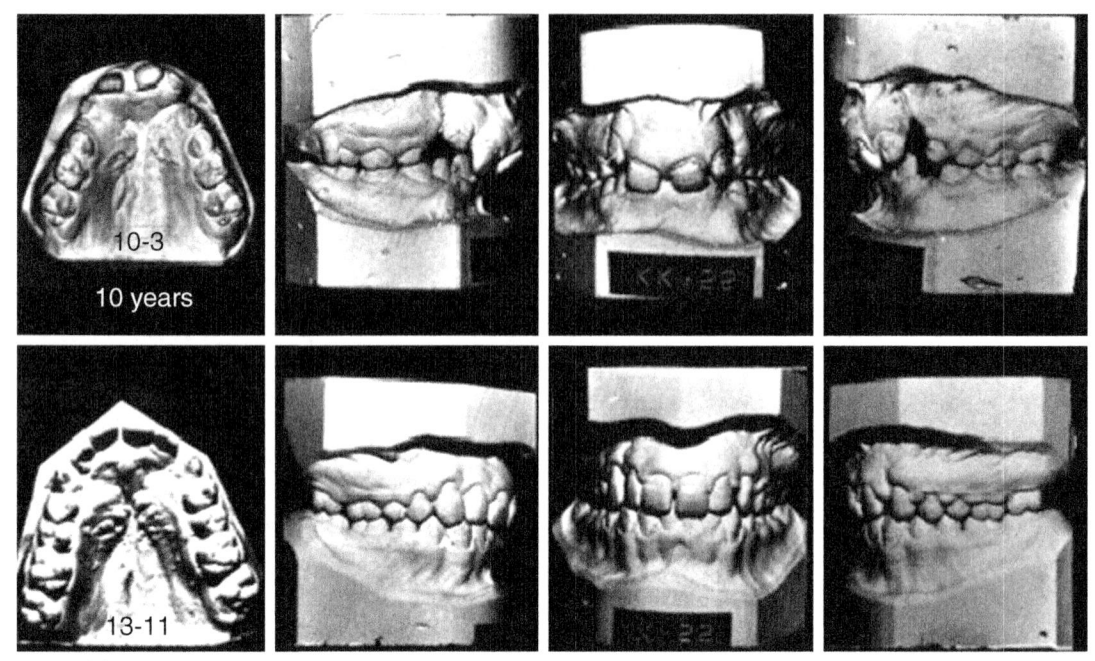

Good right and left buccal occlusion without orthodontics. After secondary alveolar bone grafts at 8 years of age. Final occlusion and after secondary alveolar bone grafts enables the anterior teeth to be perfectly aligned.

## 9.32 Superimposed Outlines of Selected Serial Palatal Casts

Note that the premaxilla remains in the same spatial area over time, even as the palatal segments increase in size.

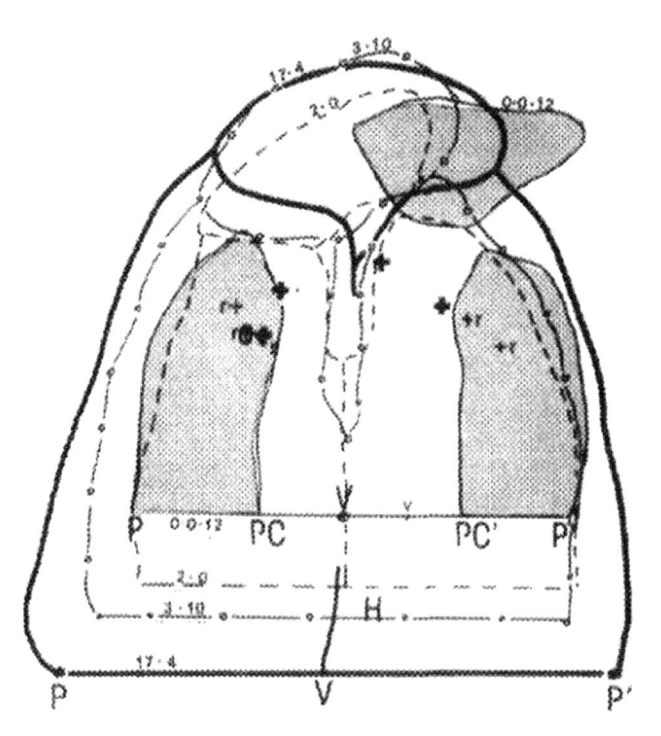

Superimposed on the rugae and registered on the vomer point.

Shows very little change in the position of the premaxilla.

Most growth changes occur posteriorly and in palatal width.

## Serial Dental Images
Von-Langenbeck + Modified Vomer Flap

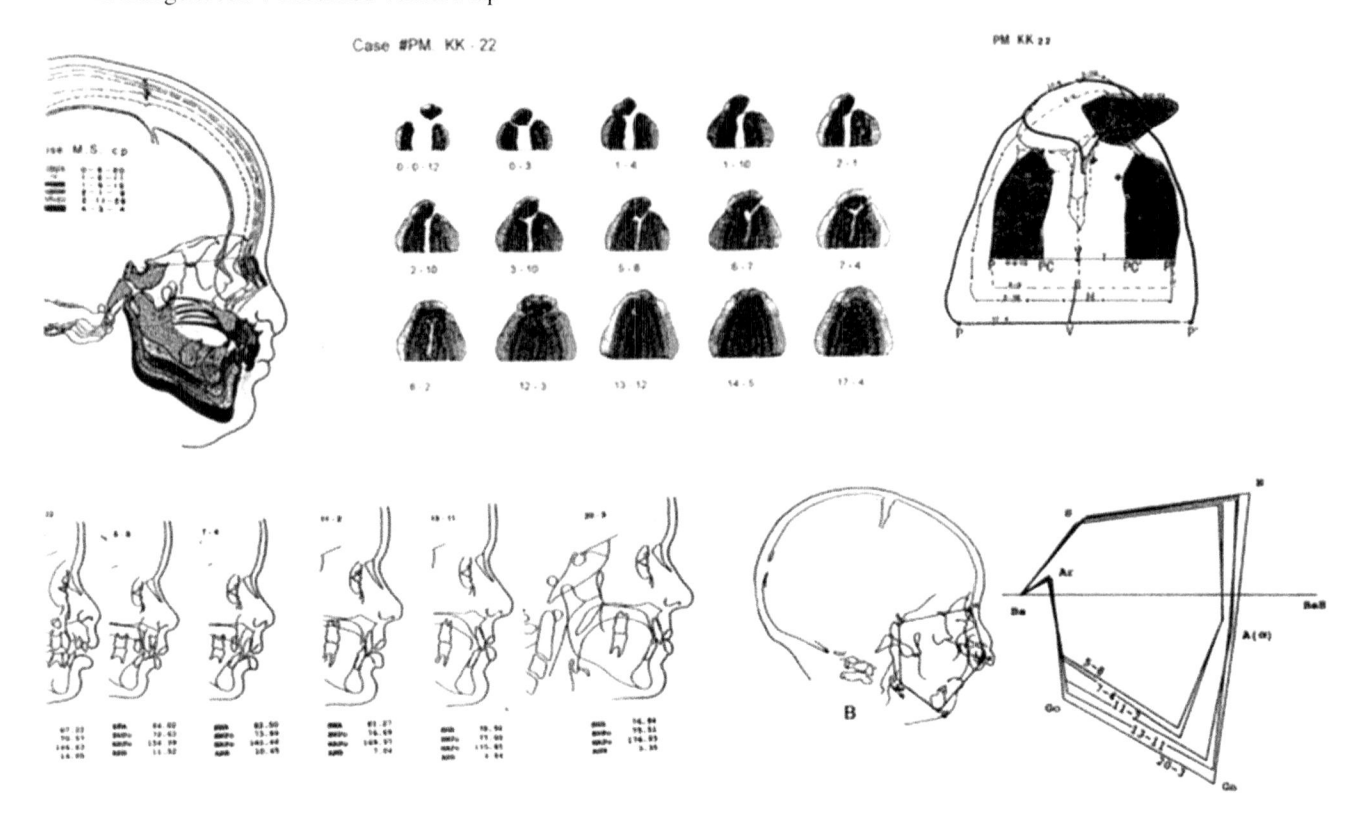

Palatal closure at 8 Years.

## 9.33 Palatal Growth

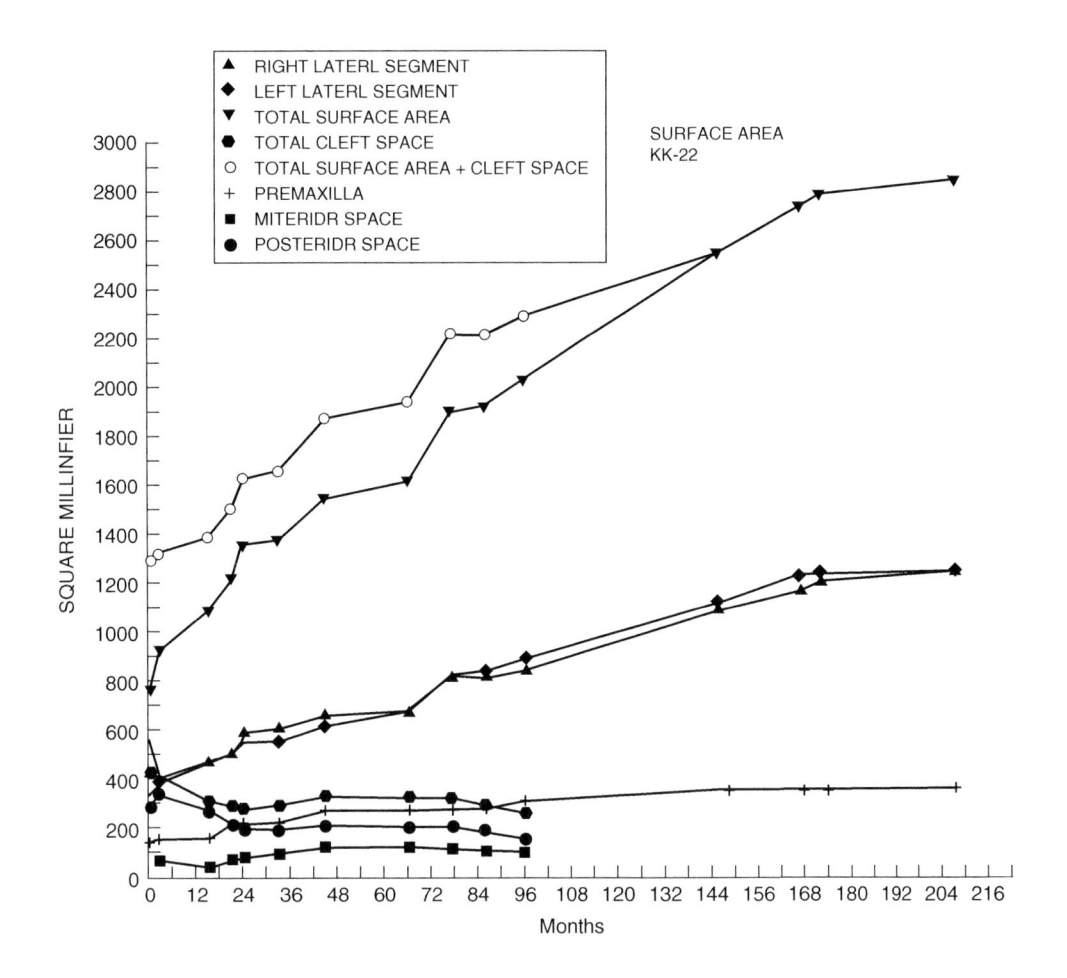

Both palatal segments develop at the same rate to the same extent.

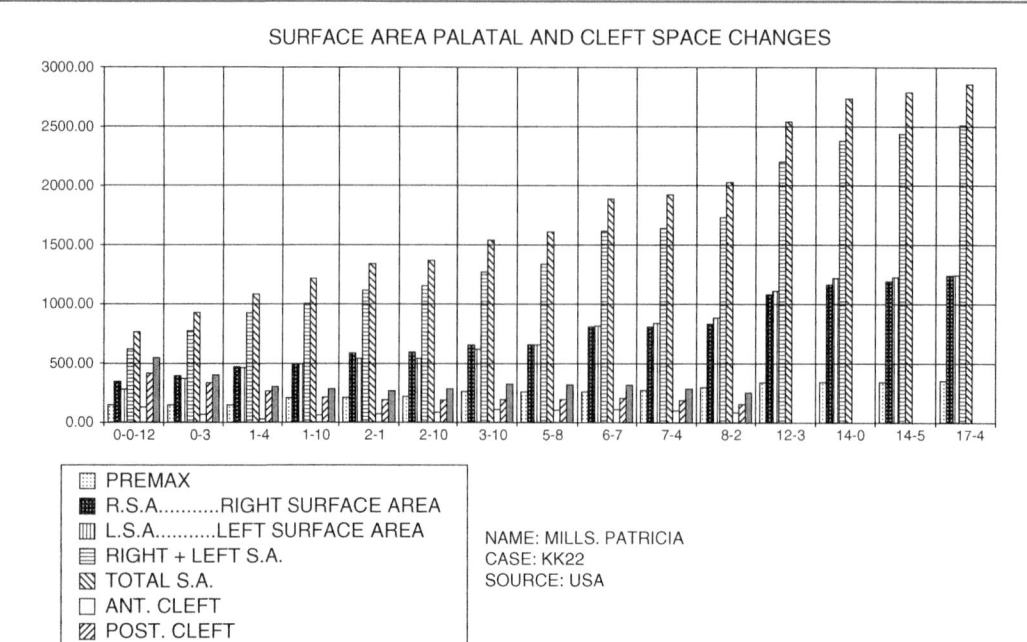

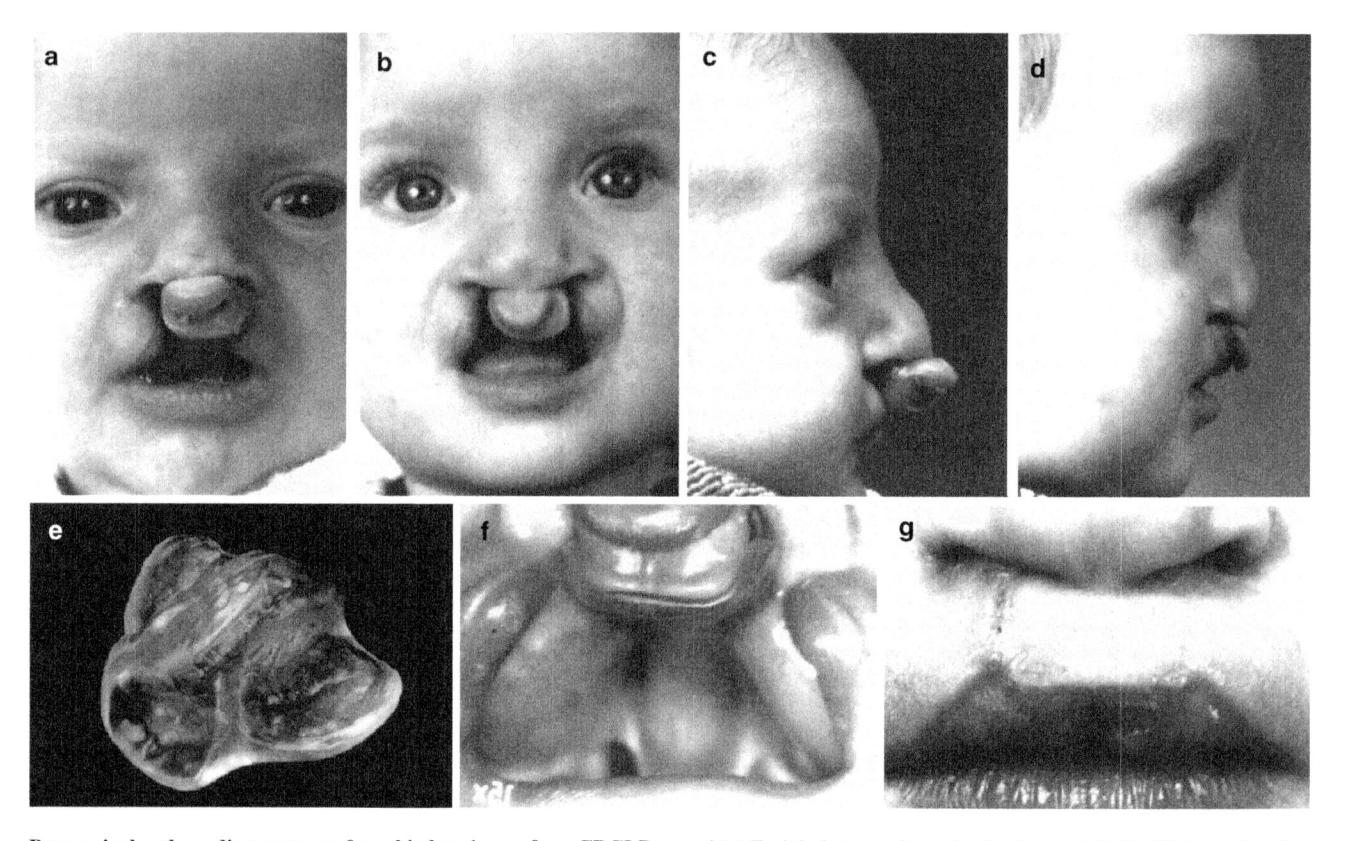

**Presurgical orthopedic treatment from birth to 1 year for a CBCLP at the University of Nijmegen** (Courtesy of AM Kuijpers-Jagtman). Lip closure at 1 year of age. Hard palatal cleft is closed between 6 and 9 years of age together with bone grafting of the alveolar cleft. (**a**), (**b**), and (**c**) Facial photographs and palatal cast at birth; (**d**) 6 months after wearing PSOT appliance; (**e**) Presurgical orthopedic appliance; when placed on the palate; (**f**) wearing appliance (**g**) 8 weeks after lip closure.

## 9.34 Zurich Switzerland: Rudolph and Margaret Hotz Procedure

### 9.34.1 Cases by Wanda Gnoinski DDS, Orthodontist

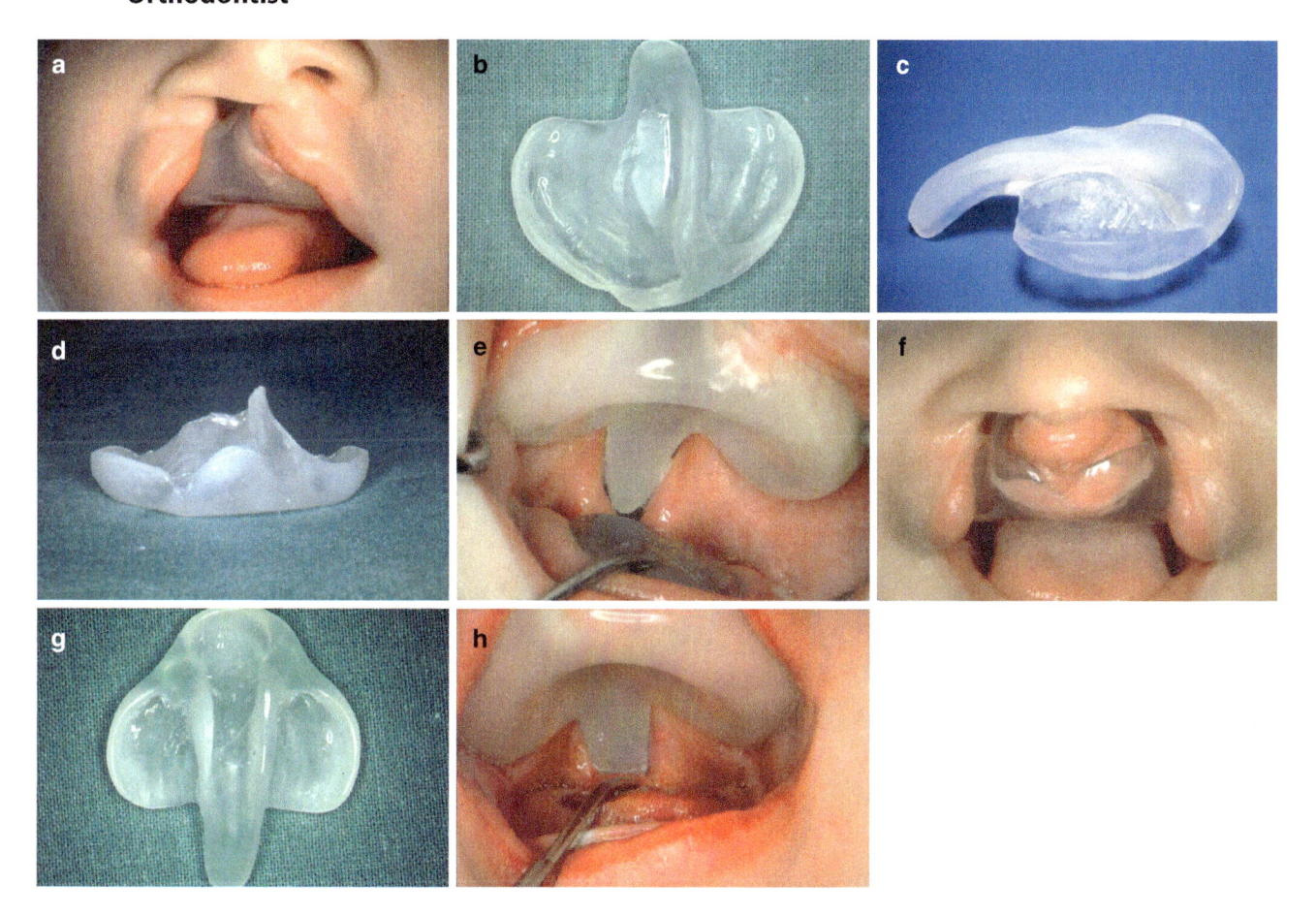

Presurgical orthopedic appliances used in complete unilateral (**a–e**) and bilateral (**f–h**) cleft lip and palate. The palatal acrylic extends posteriorly to the uvulae. (Courtesy Wanda Gnoinski, Zurich University Dental Clinic, Cleft Palate Institute)

# Presurgical Orthopedics

## 10.1 A Historical Perspective of Cleft Palate Orofacial Growth and Dentistry

"In the later 1960's and early 1970's, the period when primary bone grafting and maxillary orthopedics were in vogue, an objective of much neonatal clinical treatment for cleft lip/palate was to "make things anatomically correct" soon after birth. The goal was to align maxillary segments as early as possible and then to stabilize this segment relationship with autogenous bone. With little supporting data, the proponents of this treatment philosophy claimed many benefits from maxillary orthopedics, such as stimulating palatal growth, preventing maxillary malformations associated with a dental cross-bite. They further stated that aiding surgical repair of the lip and palate improved infant feeding and weight gain, satisfying the psychological needs of the parents, and improving speech development. This treatment philosophy was readily accepted because of its strong emotional appeal to the parents. It was hoped that well-documented clinical research which would determine the validity of the claims would soon be forthcoming.

Unfortunately no supporting literature has ever been published to support the benefits. More recently a prospective study from Holland has shown that the costs/benefits do not support the use of PSOT.

More recently, a new PSOT called nasoalveolar molding with gingivoperiosteoplasty (NAM+GPP) has been introduced. As the surgeon believes a different knife will make a better "cut", this procedure has been hailed as being better than POPLA. Unfortunately, no long term benefits have been reported."

*Samuel Berkowitz, D.D.S., M.S. Cleft Palate Journal: Vol. 74, Number 5, Page 564 (1978)*

## 10.2 Brophy Procedure 1920

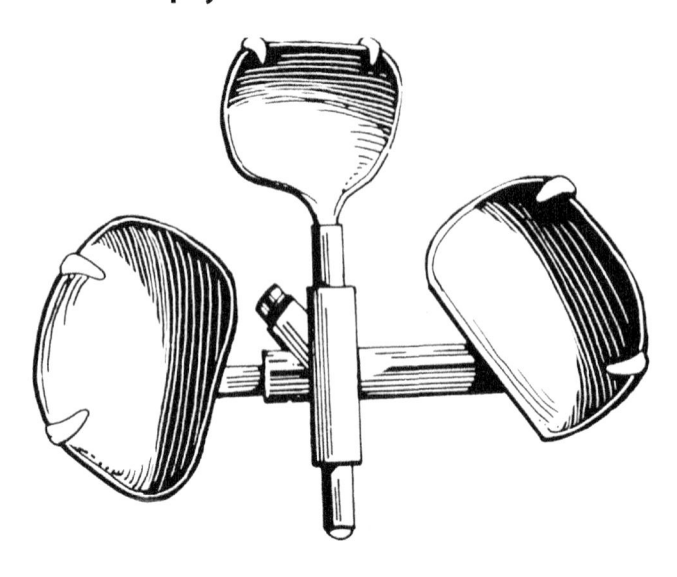

Brophy premaxillary retraction appliance attached to palate (1920–1930)

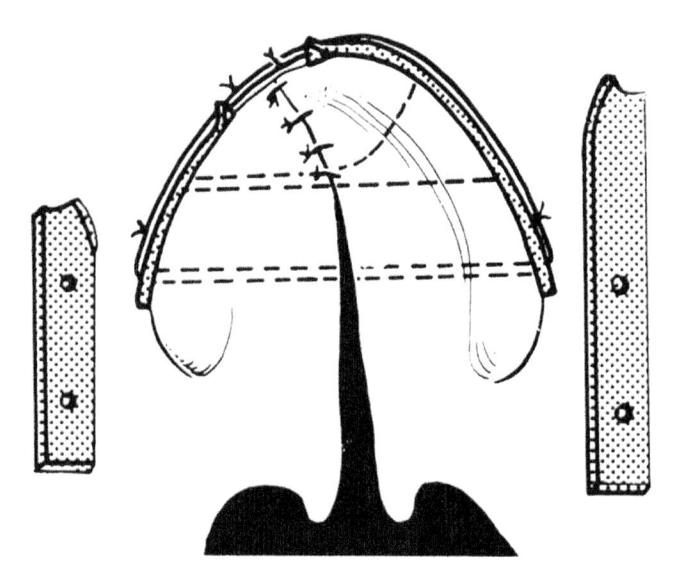

Brophy UCLP presurgical orthopedic appliance. Metal plates were placed lateral to the palatal segments. Transverse wires connecting the plates are tightened, drawing the segments together.

## 10.3 Prior Use of Presurgical Appliances

Placing tension on the steel wires brings the segments together closing the cleft space. Many of the unerupted teeth were devitalized by the wires penetrating the dental sacs within the alveolar segments. Surgical palatal cleft closure was performed during the first year. This appliance therapy has been abandoned because of the deleterious effects on midfacial growth. It cannot be determined whether the surgery, the appliance, or both led to palatal and midfacial deformity.

Along with Burstone and McNeil, they expanded the use of presurgical orthopedic appliances believing it stimulates palatal growth while aligning the segments. Many other unproven claims were made to support the use of these appliances.

Courtesy of D.R. Millard Jr. *Cleft Craft, Vol. III.* Boston, MA: Little, Brown & Co; 1980:266)

## 10.4 Controlling the Protruding Premaxilla

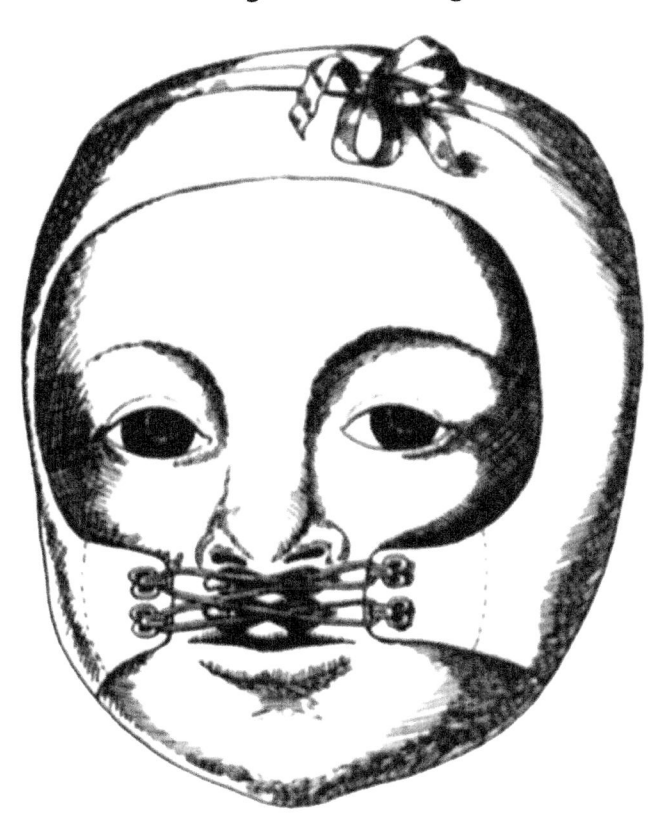

In 1968, German Johan Philip Hofman presented a headcap with cheek extensions armed with corset hooks at the sides of the lip.

When laced with tension, this apparatus could serve both to press on the premaxilla and to relieve the tension of the bilateral cleft closure.

Similar appliances are in use today.

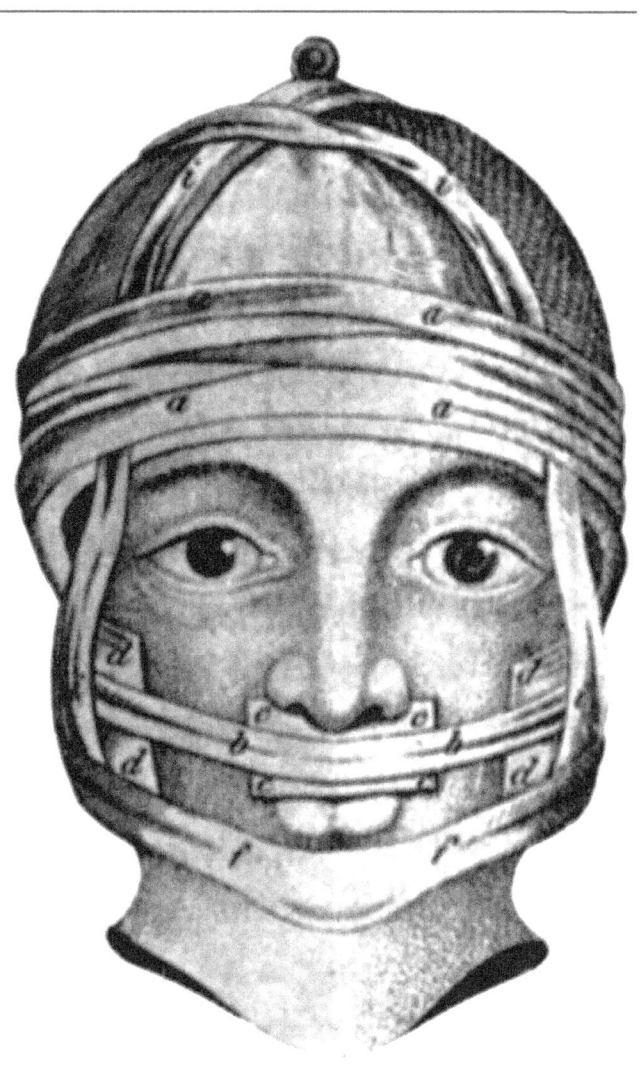

External force to retract (ventroflex) the protruding premaxilla

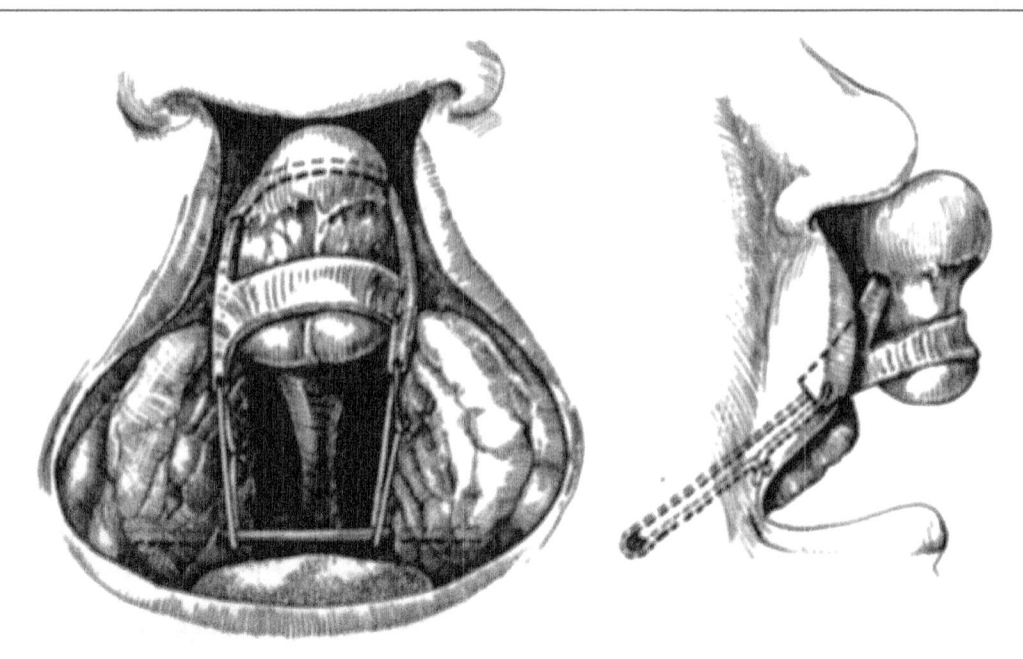

An intraoral appliance to retract the premaxilla by ventroflexion.

The rubber bands were looped around Georgiade's posterior traverse Kirschner wire exerting the required tension to cause retropositioning of the premaxilla.

**In 1970, P.J. Desault devised a rather elaborate cloth compression bandage which he applied against the projecting premaxilla for 11 days preoperatively to exert steady backward pressure. This is a description of Desault's bandage on a 5-year-old bilateral cleft lip. Similar appliances are being used on a newborn child:**

*In order to bring the protuberance to a level with the lip, and to depress the projecting portion of the premaxilla. The good effects of this bandage in compressing the parts in question were so obvious that its use was continued until the operation was performed.*

# Presurgical Orthopedics with Lip Adhesion and Periosteoplasty (POPLA)

# 11

The Latham–Millard presurgical orthopedics with periosteoplasty and lip adhesion (POPLA) was introduced in 1980. Latham had been working with Georgiade, a plastic surgeon, at Duke University Medical School. Galen Quinn, orthodontist, had been using a similar appliance in the 1970s prior to Latham's arrival.

Although a number of introductory papers were published, no follow-up longitudinal study was forthcoming. Latham wrote to Millard suggesting "a better way of handling the bilateral cleft lip and palate case." Latham came from England having studied with James Scott, an anatomist, who believed that the cleft palatal segments were diminished in size due to their detachment from the nasal septum, thus losing their growth impetus. This hypothesis has not been proven.

## 11.1 Latham–Millard Presurgical Orthopedics with Periosteoplasty

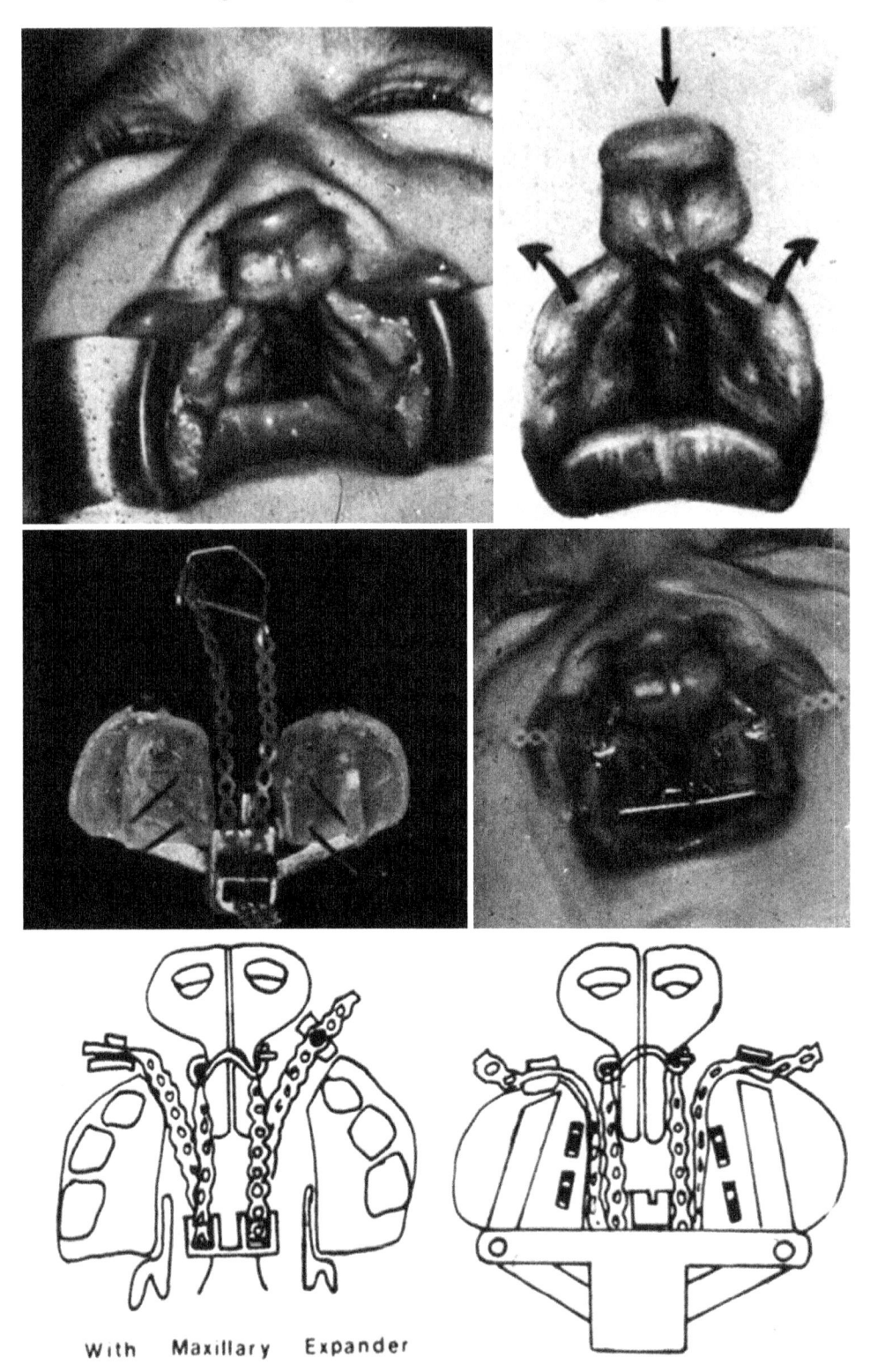

With Maxillary Expander

Millard:

A more sophisticated and effective harnessing of tension than can ever be achieved with a lip adhesion is possible through the use of an intra-oral appliance developed by Ralph A. Latham of London, Ontario, in 1984.
This appliance repositions the protruding premaxilla while expanding the lateral maxillary segments in bilateral complete clefts. A premaxillary stainless steel pin, 0.7 mm in diameter and in the form of a self-retraining clip, is inserted through a previously drilled hole in the posterior stem.
Forces generated from the continuous elastic chain bring the premaxilla back bodily without tipping. The lateral palatal segments are widened at the same time in order to reposition the retruded premaxilla.

## 11.2 Latham–Millard Procedure

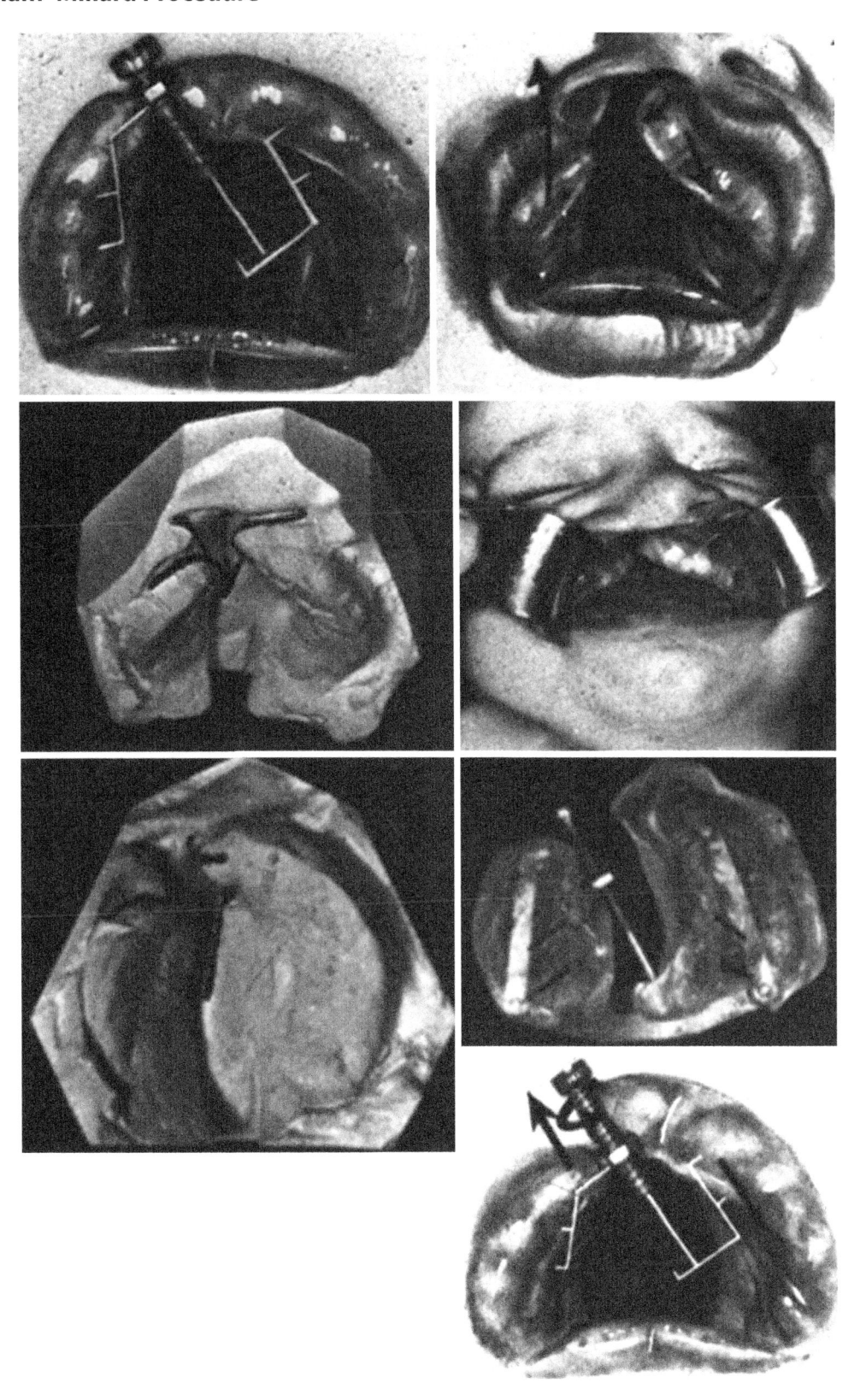

### 11.2.1 CUCLP

Latham's presurgical orthopedic appliance is pinned to the hard palate for stabilization.

Metal control mechanism to activate movement of palatal segments. The premaxillary portion of larger segments is moved palatally while the cleft segment is advanced palatally.

## 11.3 Pre-Surgical Orthopedic Periosteoplasty with Lip Adhesion (POPLA)

### 11.3.1 Periosteoplasty

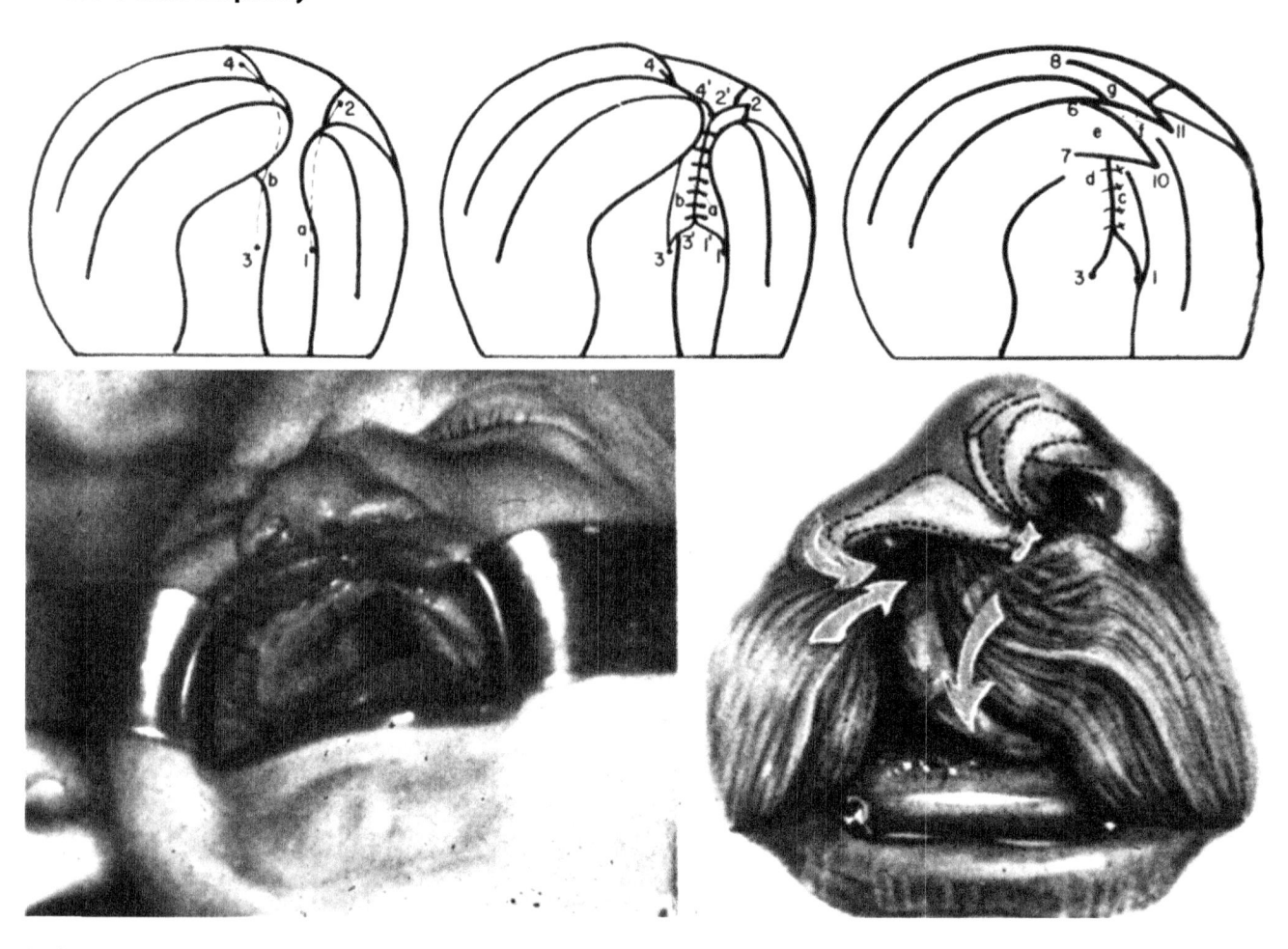

Periosteoplasty: Surgery closes the cleft alveolus creating a "tunnel" lined with periosteum. A bony bridge of various thickness in most instances will span the cleft.

## 11.4 The Latham Pinned Appliance

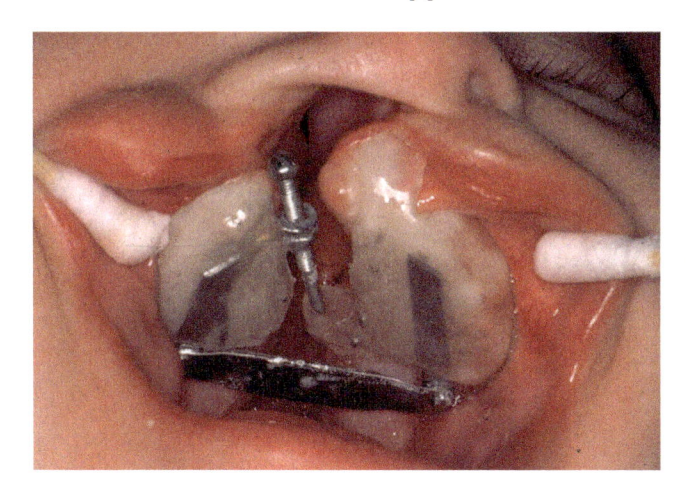

Presurgical orthopedic appliances pinned to the palate. Turning the screw on the bar moves the palatal segments.

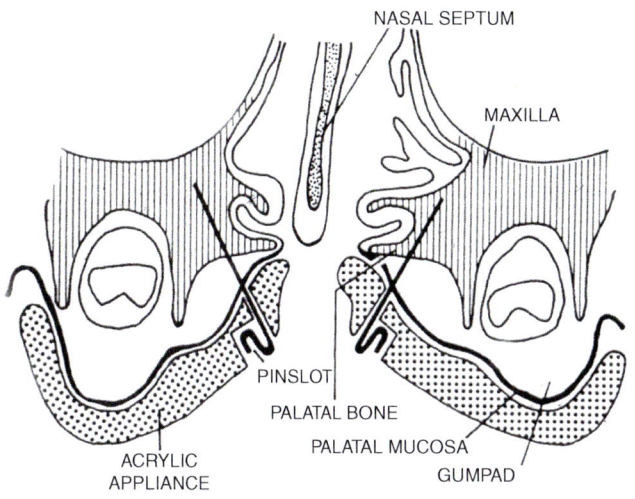

Drawing showing pinned appliance in place (Latham).

## 11.5 Complete Unilateral Cleft Lip and Palate Treated with POPLA

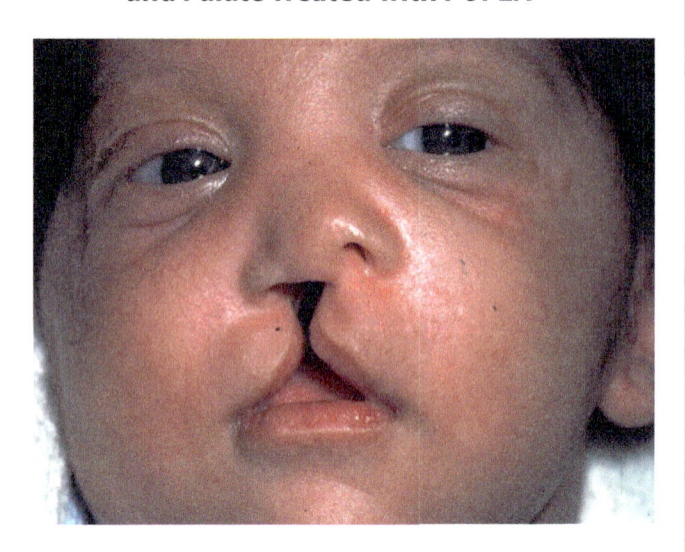

After appliance activations: Lip and nasal distortions reduce when the palatal segments are moved together.

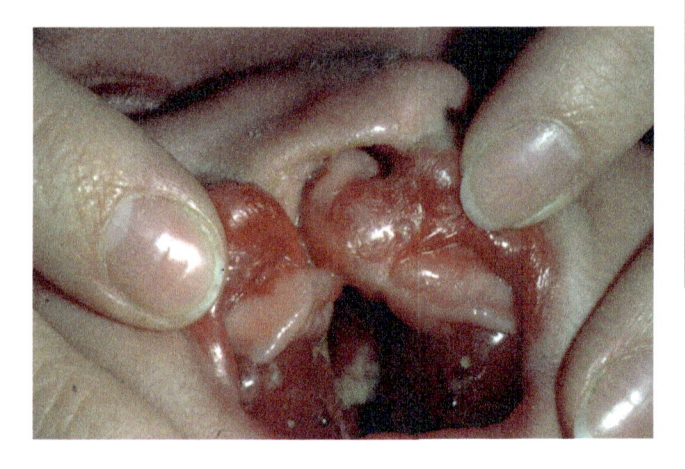

Alveolar segments in contact. Periosteoplasty is then performed.

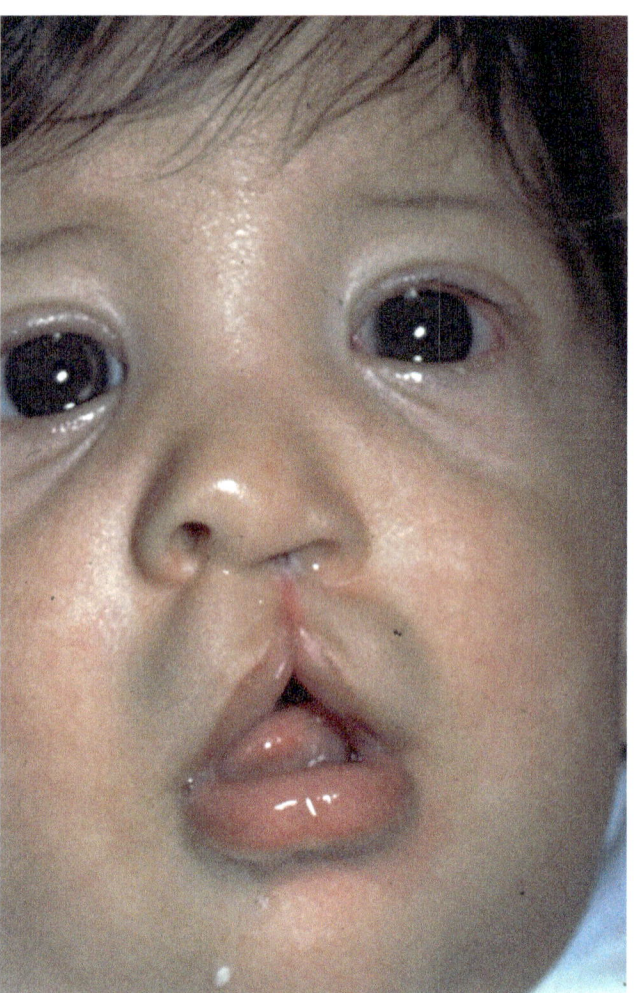

## 11.5.1 After Molding with PSOT

Lip adhesion to establish muscle continuity and mold the overexpanded palatal segments in preparation for a definitive lip surgery at 6 months of age.

There are instances when definitive lip and nose surgery can be performed without first performing a lip adhesion.

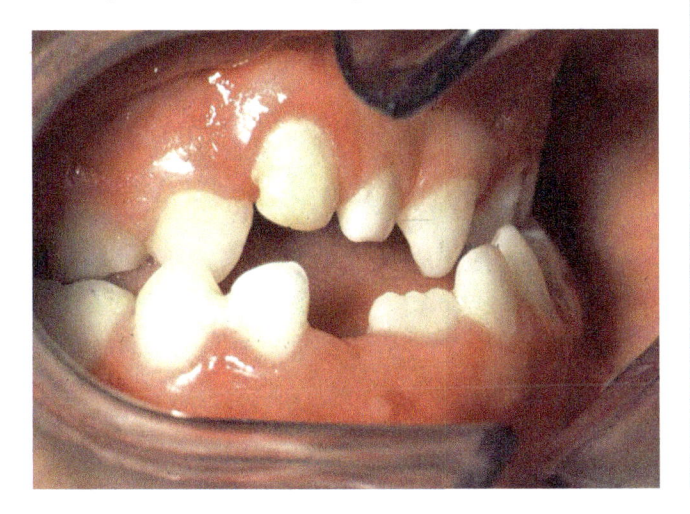

4 years of age

Intraoral view: Alveolar segments are distorted and in contact creating both an anterior open bite and anterior crossbite.

Note the obliteration of the deciduous right lateral and central incisors space. The right and left deciduous cuspids and left buccal segments. The upper to lower anterior segments are no longer congruent due to the loss of anterior teeth spaces.

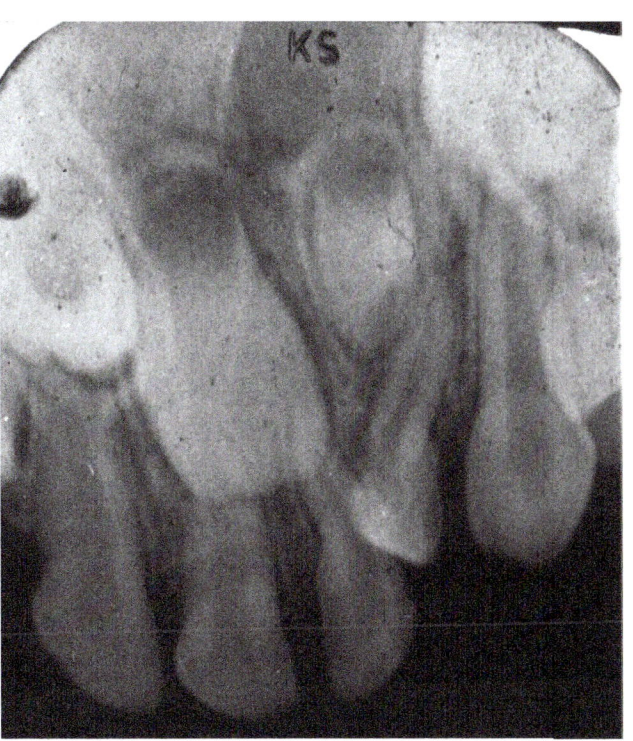

Periapical film:

Showing closure of the lateral incisor area cleft space by the palatal segments being brought into contact. There is no room for unerupted and impacted lateral incisor or a replacement tooth if it is absent.

## 11.6 Facial Photographs

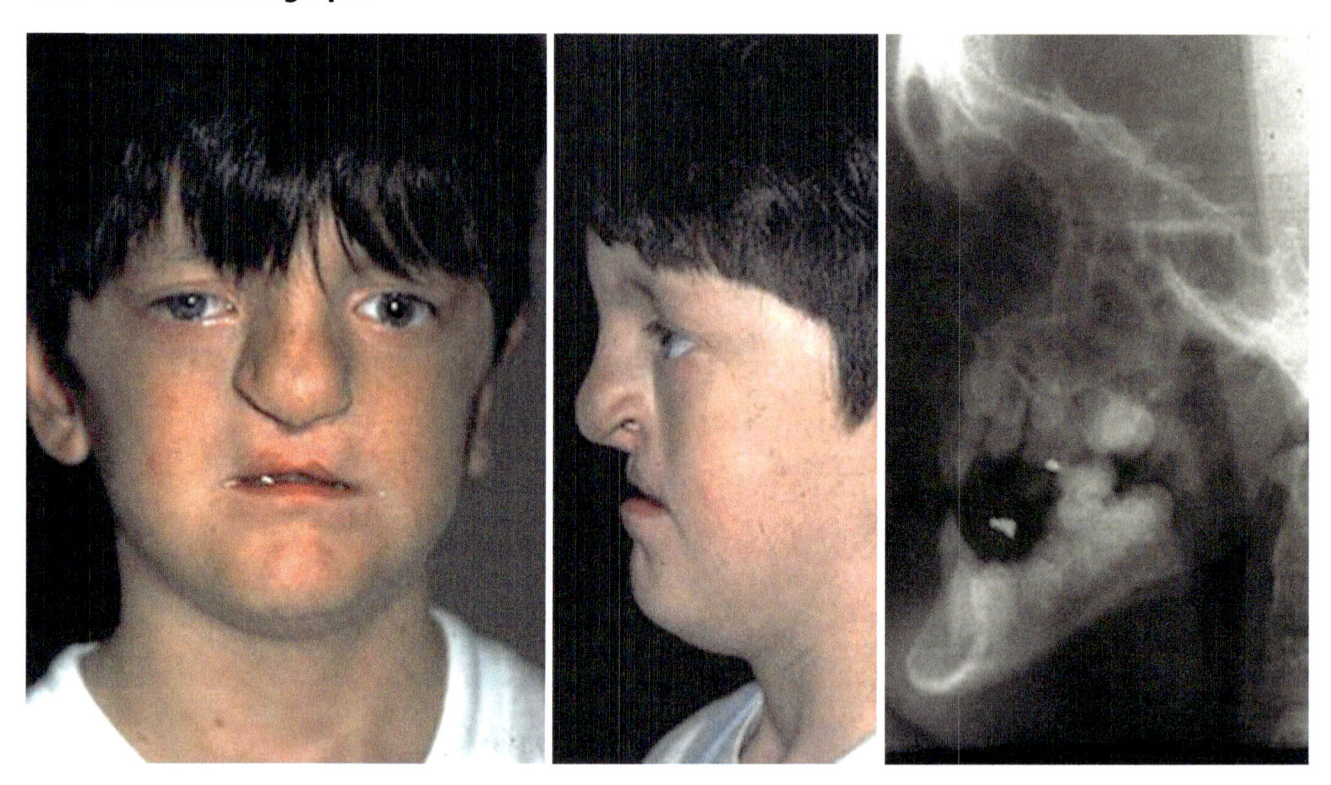

8 years—Slight Anterior Crossbite—Strong Symphysis.

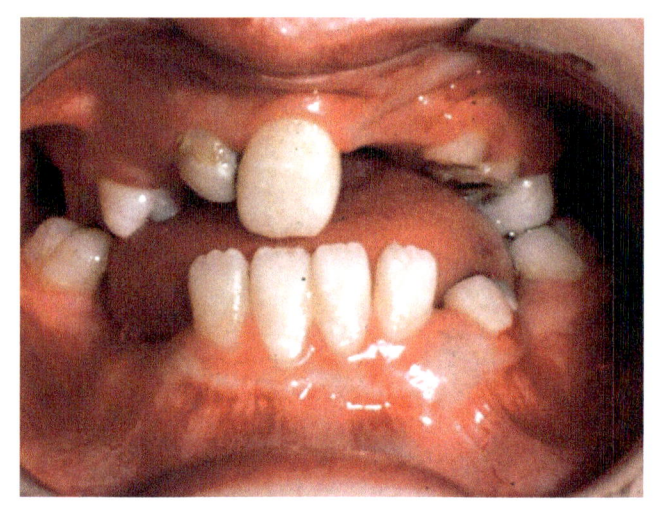

10 years—Recessive midface due to the failure of midface growth of the retruded premaxilla. Retruded premaxilla showing same missing incisor teeth.

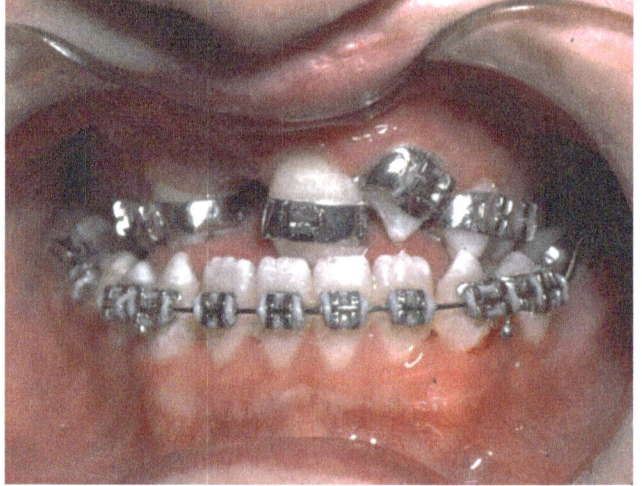

12 years—Orthodontic appliances placed to correct anterior crossbite.

Protraction facial mask with Class III mechanics was unsatisfactory in correcting this problem.

## 11.7 Facial Photographs

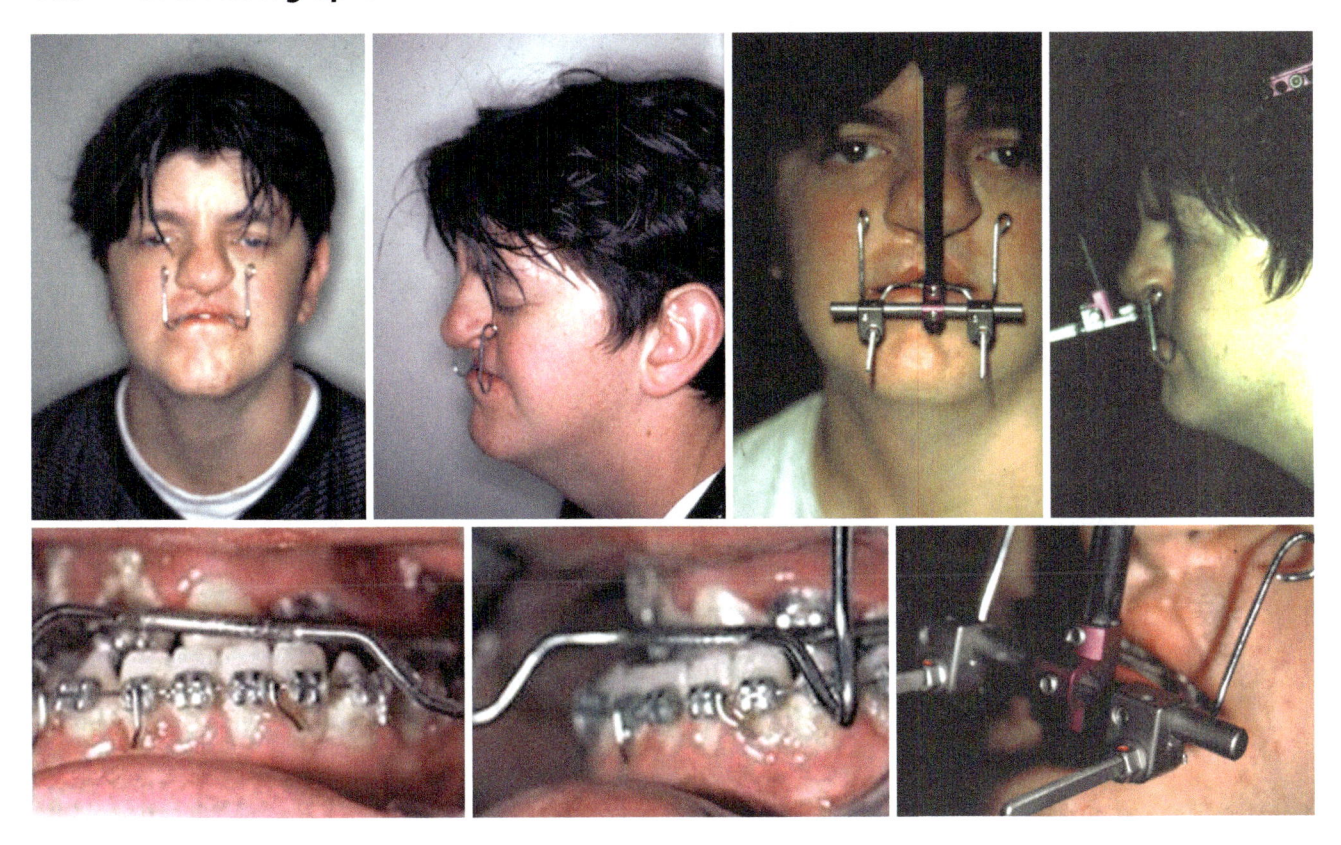

After distraction osteogenesis oral appliance in place. The head frame was removed after 3 months. Two weeks of facial advancement followed by 2-1/2 months of retention and maxillary protrusion intraoral (class 3) elastics.

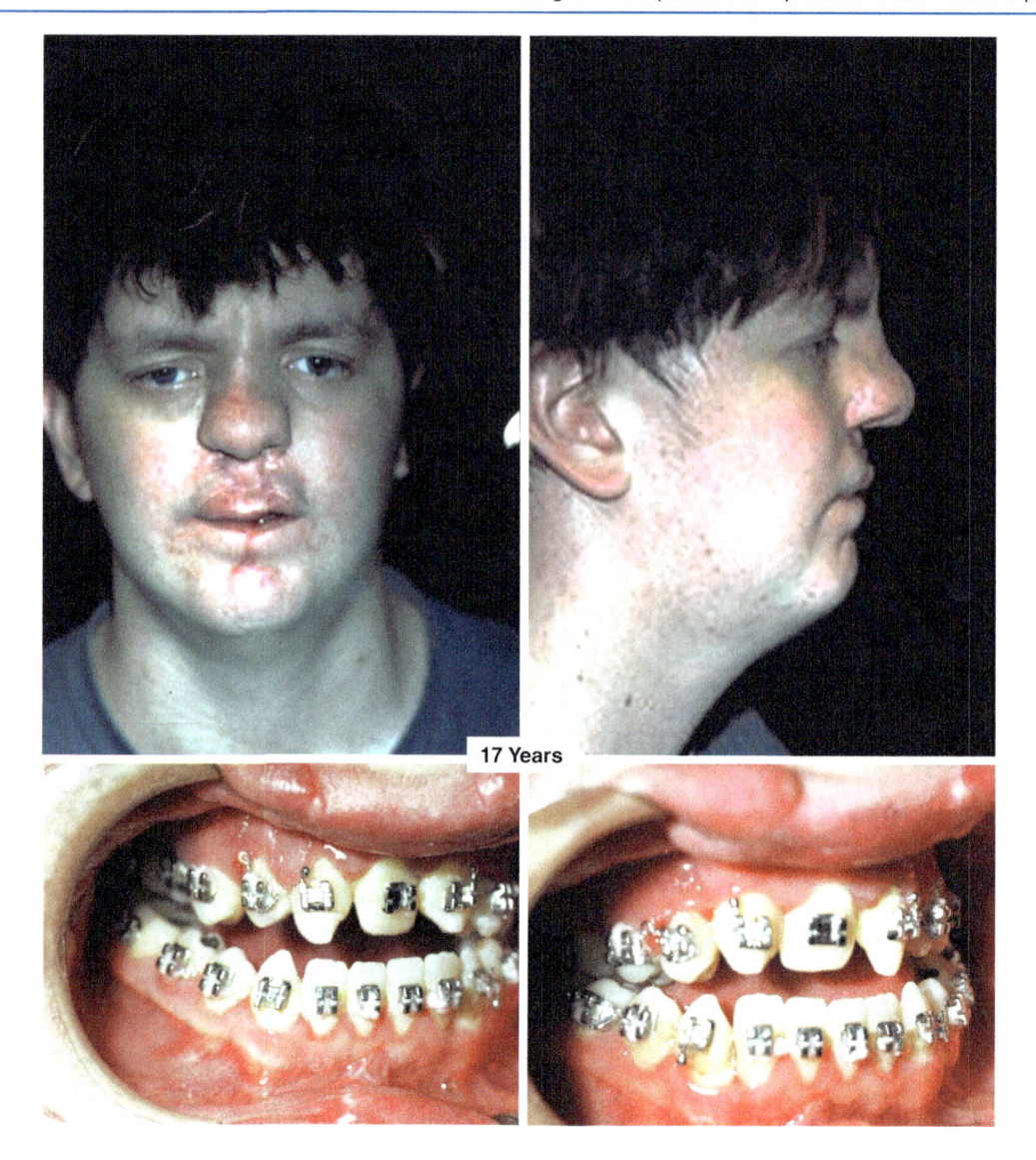

**Upper anteriors only one central incisor**
**No anterior arch congruency Anterior crossbite**
**After midfacial protraction**

Note: No maxillary lateral incisors and 1 missing central incisor. Since all of these missing teeth spaces are closed, the anterior maxillary oral mandibular arches are not congruent creating an anterior crossbite. Retarded midfacial growth coupled with normal forward growth of the lower face created a severe recessive midface.

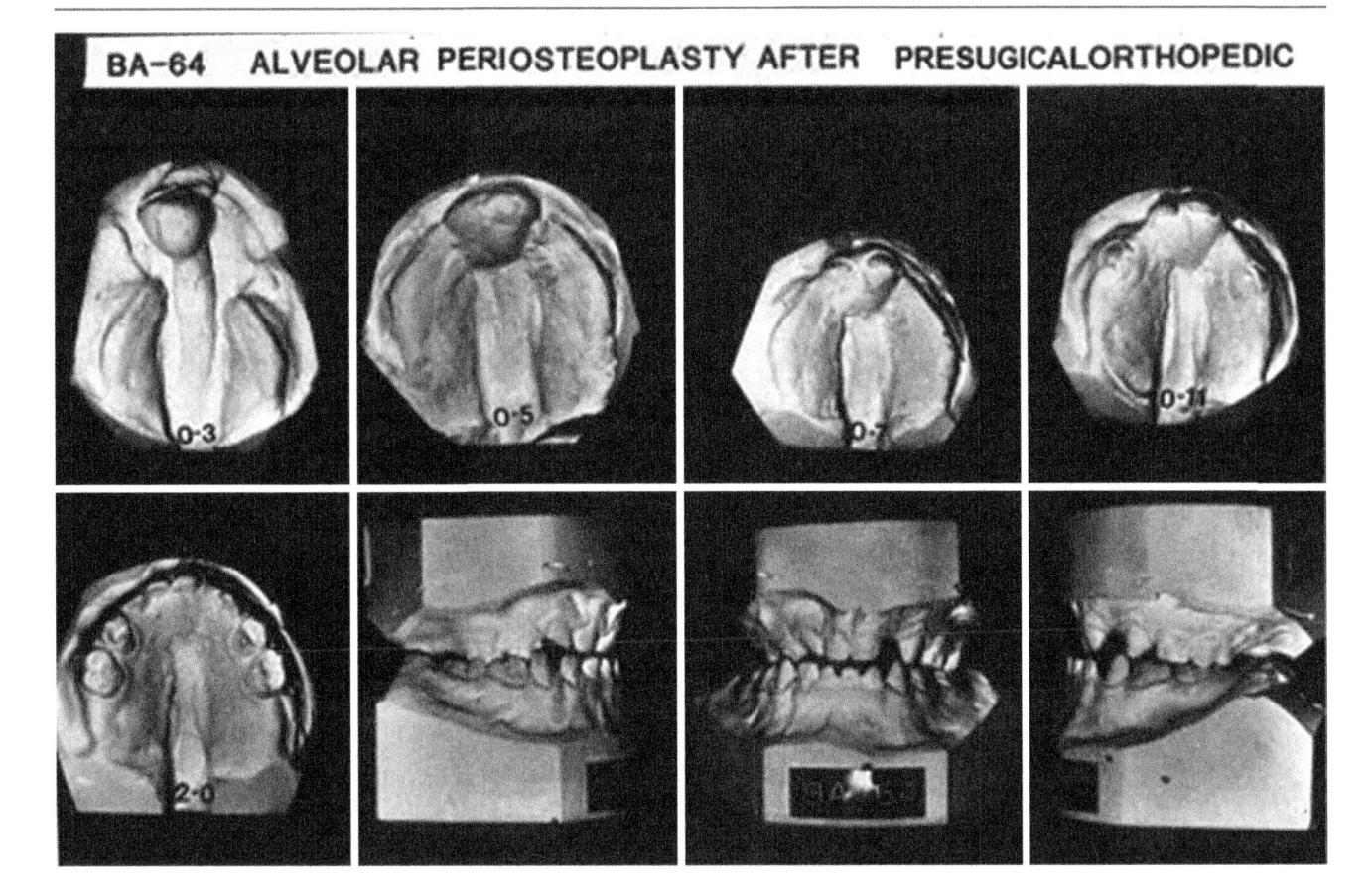

## BA-64 ALVEOLAR PERIOSTEOPLASTY AFTER PRESUGICALORTHOPEDIC

**Presurgical orthopedics + periosteoplasty + lip adhesion (POPLA)**

The premaxilla was retruded and positioned within the arch. Followed by periosteoplasty the palatal cleft was closed at 2½ years using a Von Langenbeck procedure with a modified Vomer Flap.

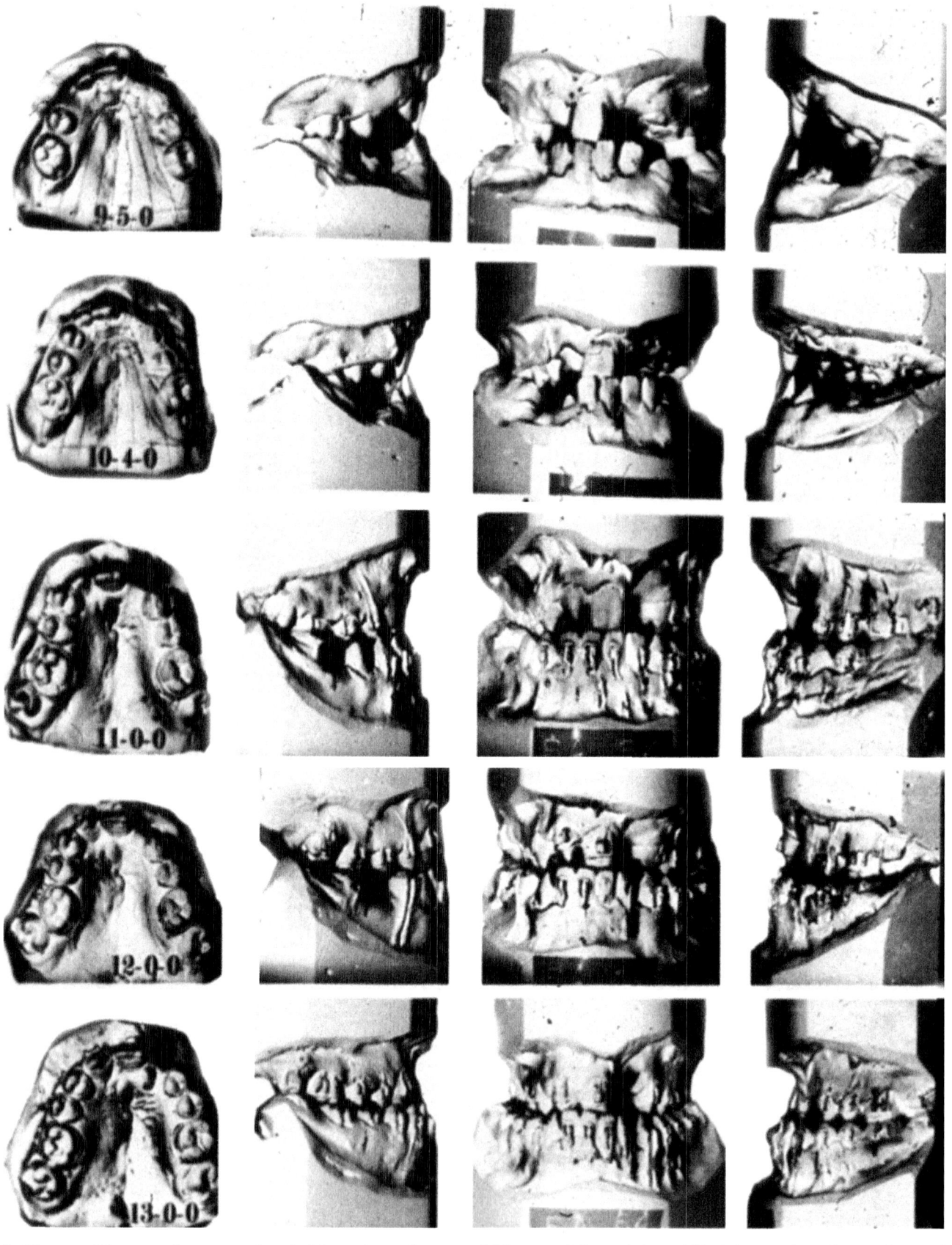

9–13 years: The use of a protraction facial mask to advance the premaxilla was unsuccessful. This was followed by midfacial retrusion due to forward growth of the upper and lower faces.

## 11.7 Facial Photographs

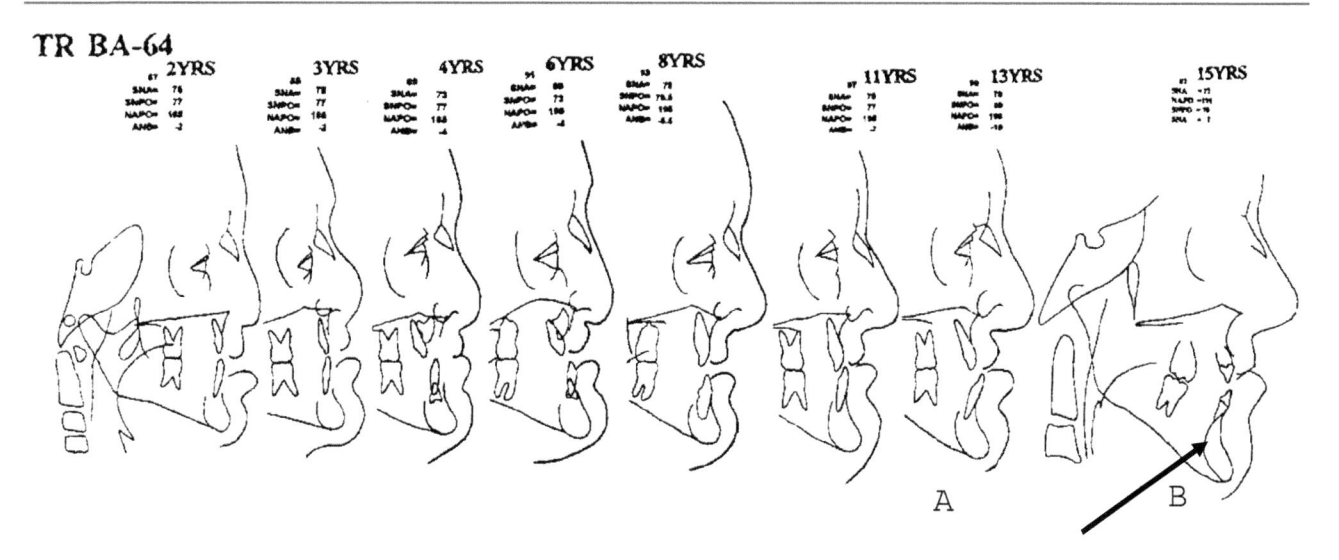

**TR BA-64**

A—After protraction facial mask—no changing profile. B—Distraction osteogenesis to tip occlusion—now hyponasality is present.

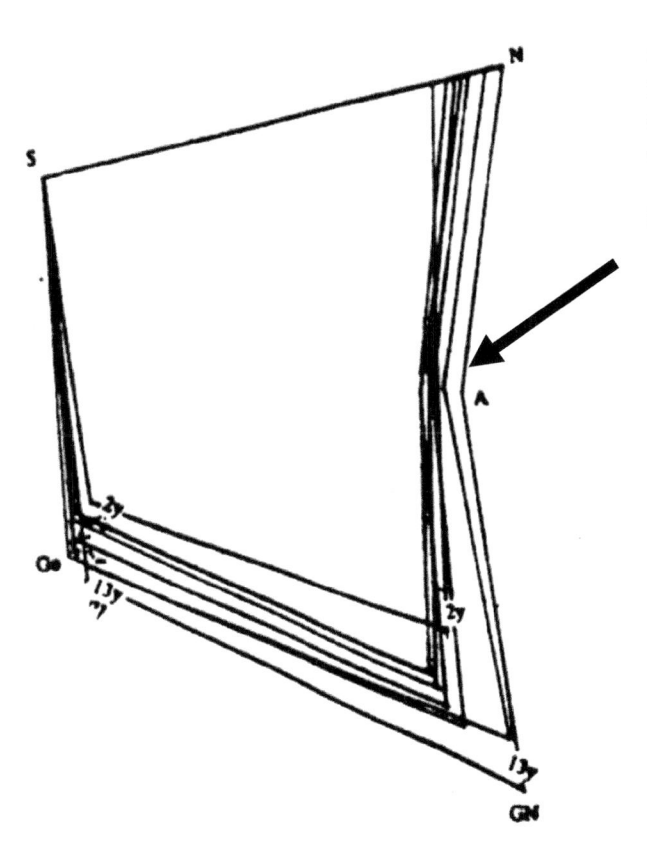

Serial cephalometric tracings showing the stability of the midfacial recessiveness even after the use of a protraction facial mask. There was a slight change in the Class I buccal occlusion since the orthopedic forces were directed to advance the retruded maxilla.

Post maxillary distraction osteogenesis. Due to severe hyponasality, maxillary advancement was discontinued.

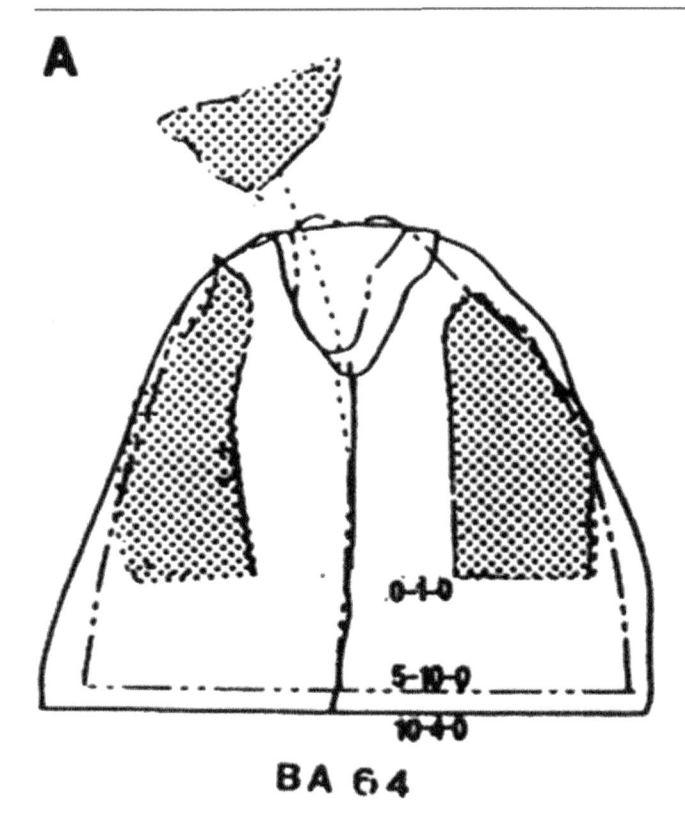

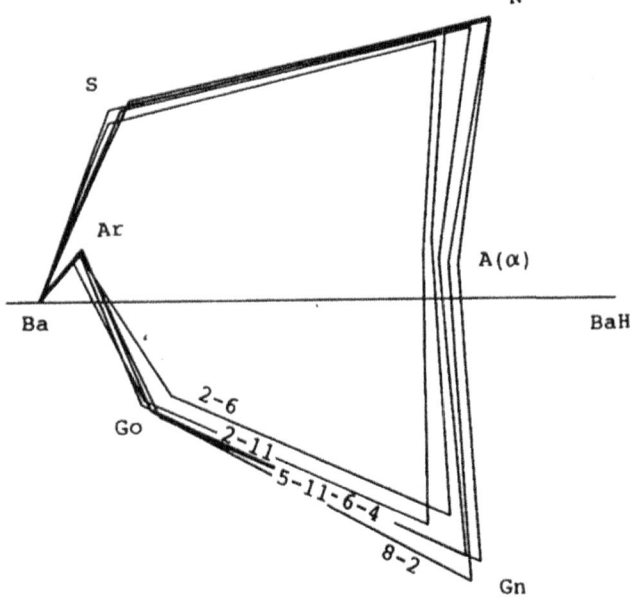

## 11.8 CBCLP: Change in premaxillary position with Latham's PSOT (POPLA)

Outline of palatal cast superimposed on palatal rugae and registered at the vomer. This shows that the protruding premaxilla at birth, once set back, does not move forward with growth or treatment. The synostotic premaxillary vomerine suture does not permit the premaxilla to grow forward along with the other facial bones. Once retruded it remains retruded.

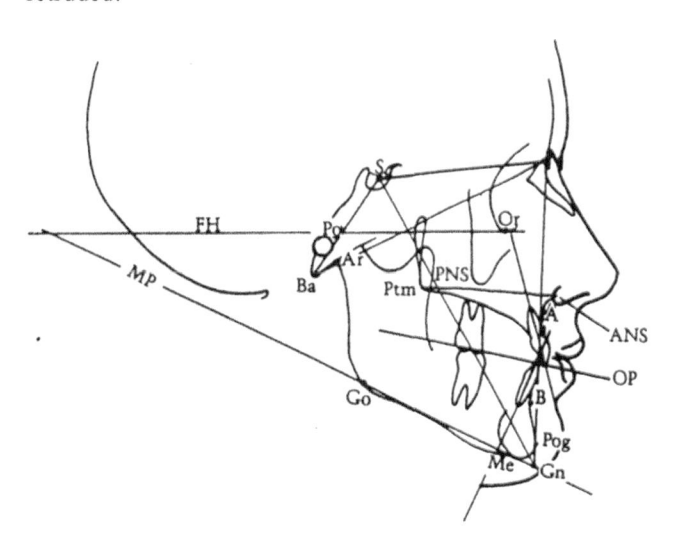

Normal Standard
**Coben Analysis: Maxillary complex growth changes.**
Case TR—BA 64

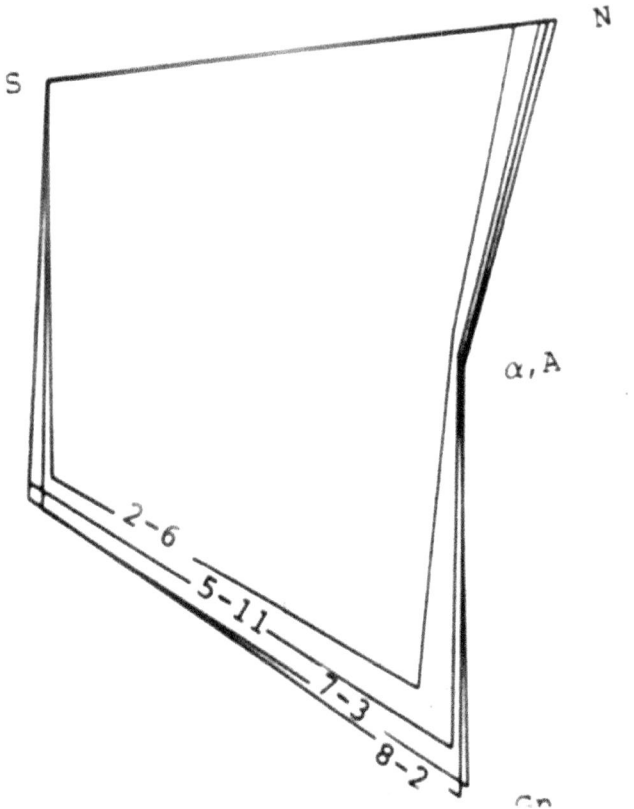

**Superimposed on the anterior cranial face—profile changes.**
Case TR—BA 64

**Profile changes showing diminished midfacial growth.**
Cat Scans of a CBCLP that had the Premaxilla Retracted with the Latham Appliance

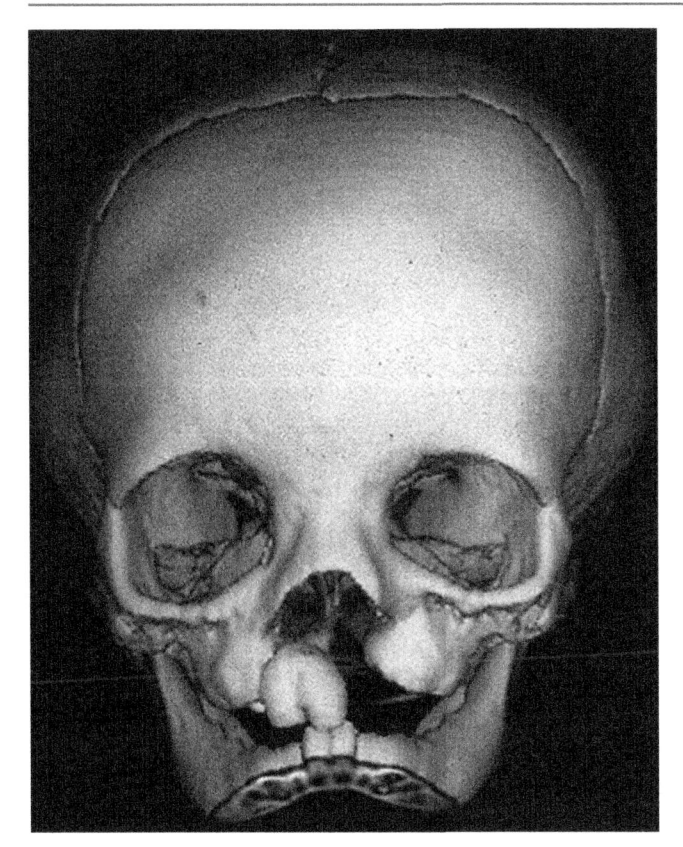

## 11.8 CBCLP: Change in premaxillary position with Latham's PSOT (POPLA)

*Frontal View*: The premaxilla is fused only with right palatal segment. The buccal segments are in good alignment since the posterior occlusion is normal.

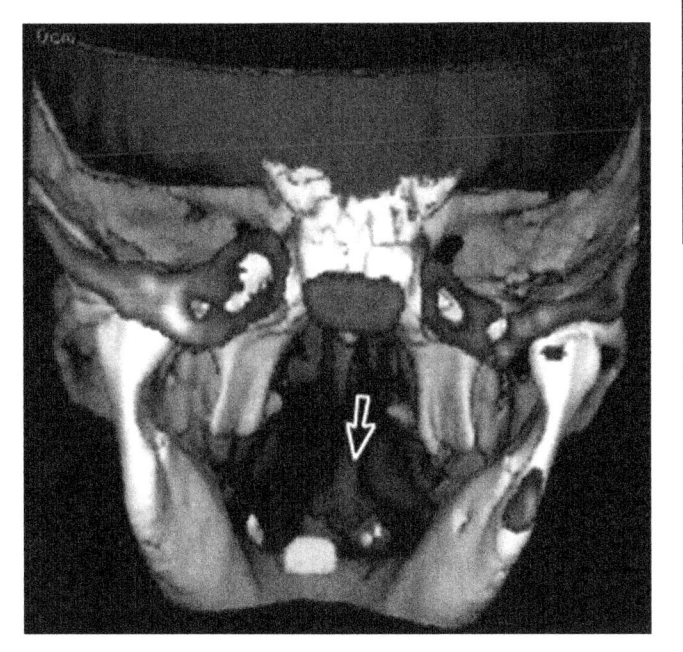

*Dorsal View*: The arrow points to the telescoped junction of the premaxilla with the vomer. There was no lateral bending of the nasal septum.

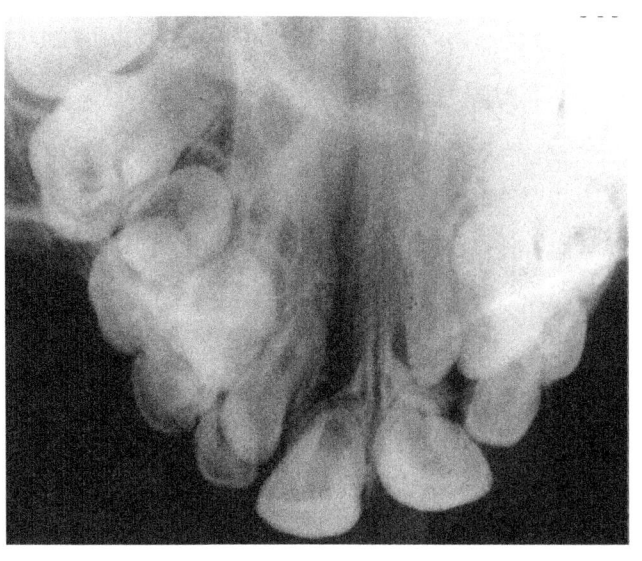

Premaxilla that was not forcibly retruded. Note the open premaxillary vomerine suture.

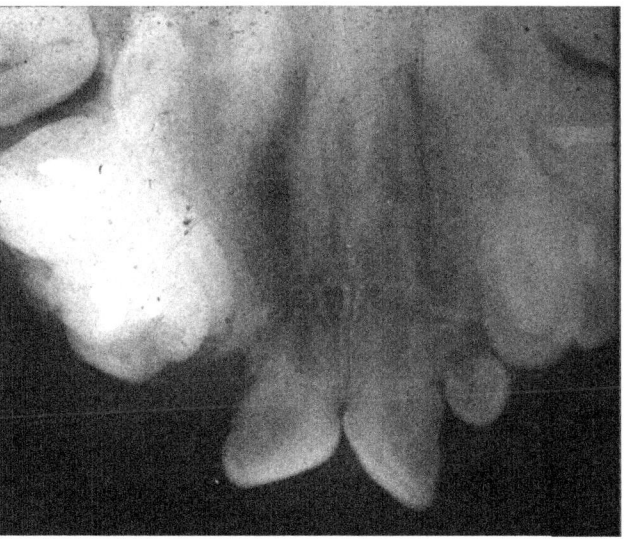

After POPLA the premaxillary vomerine suture was obliterated by synostosis caused by forceful premaxillary retrusion. This slide represents a typical case that was treated with POPLA.

## 11.9 CUCLP: Presurgical Orthopedic with Periosteoplasty and Lip Adhesion (POPLA)

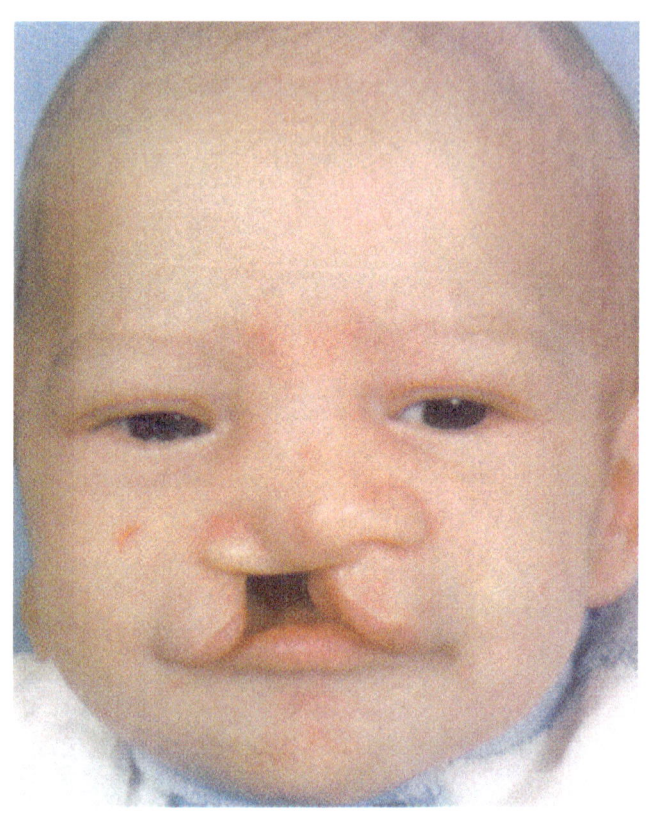

Birth

Distorted nostrils and lip due to aberrant muscle pull.

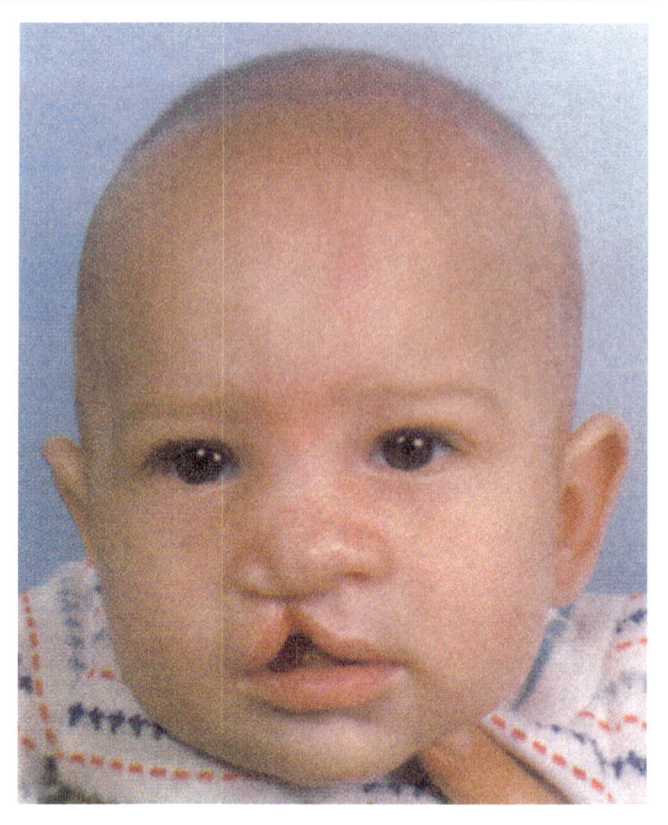

4 months

Lip adhesion reduces nasal and lip distortion.

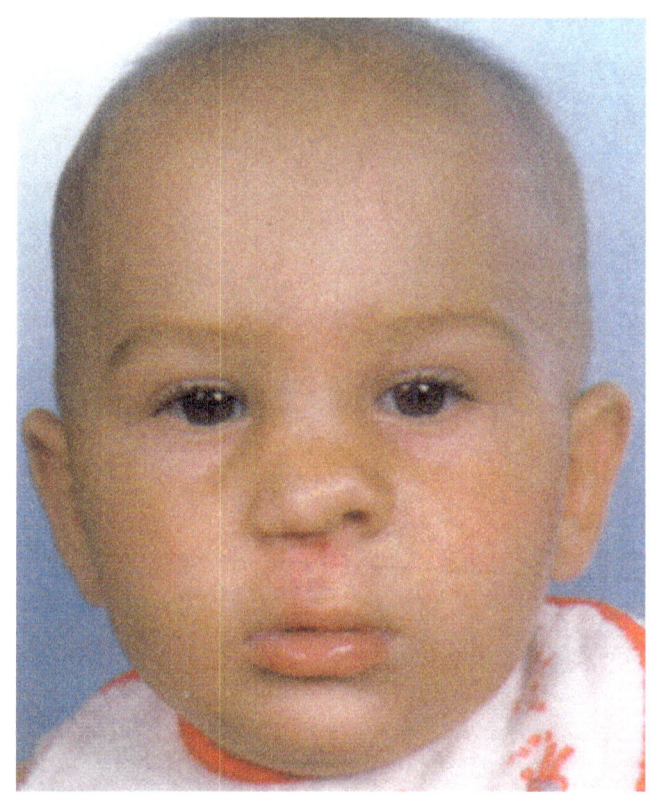

10 months

Rotation Advancement for definitive lip closure.

## 11.10 Frontal and Lateral Facial Photos

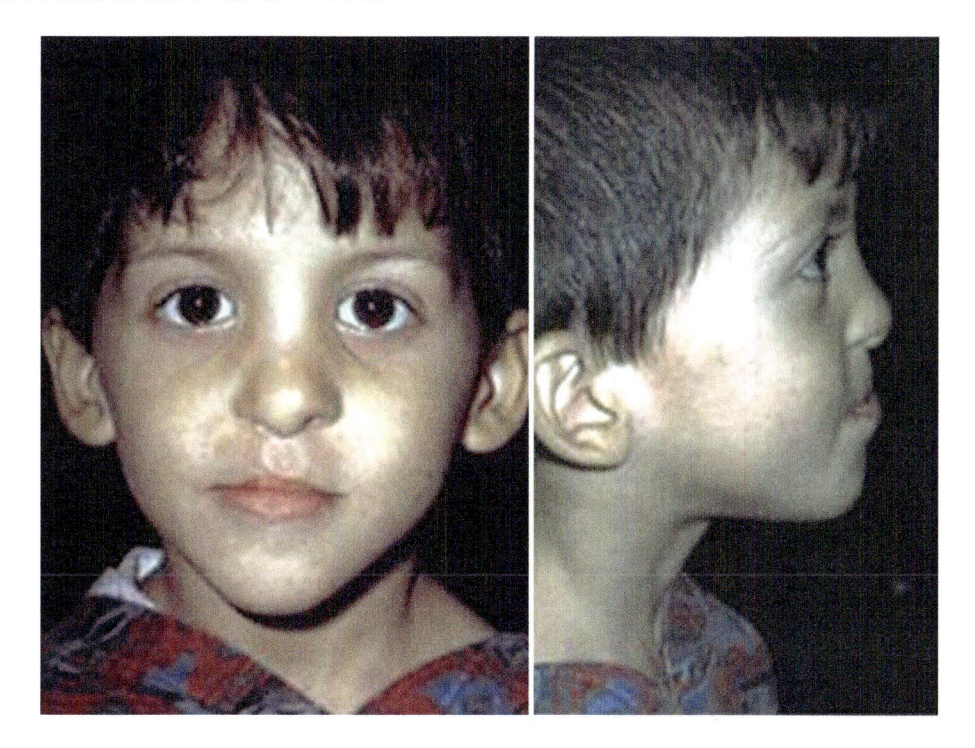

7 Years

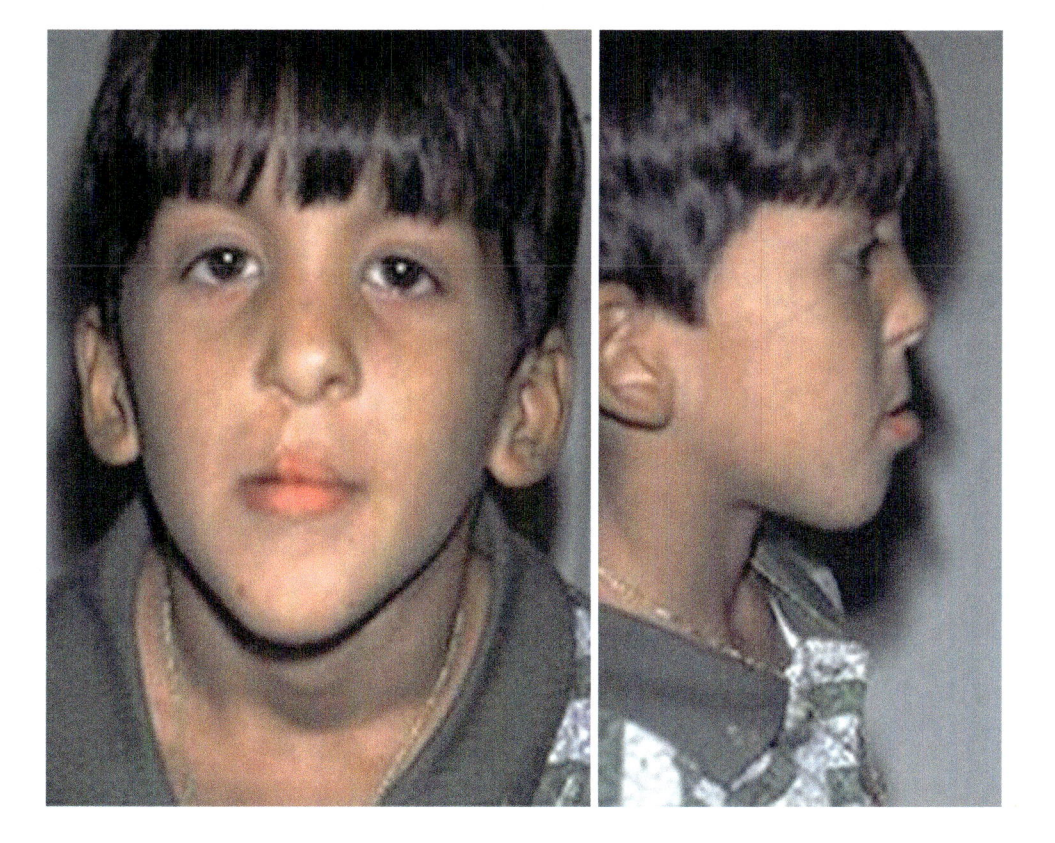

8 Years

Note that the upper lip is slightly retruded when compared to the lower lip. This is associated with the retraction of the premaxillary portion of the non-cleft palatal segment.

## 11.11 Recessiveness of the Midface Slowly Develops

Facial Changes: all faces usually look good the first 5 years

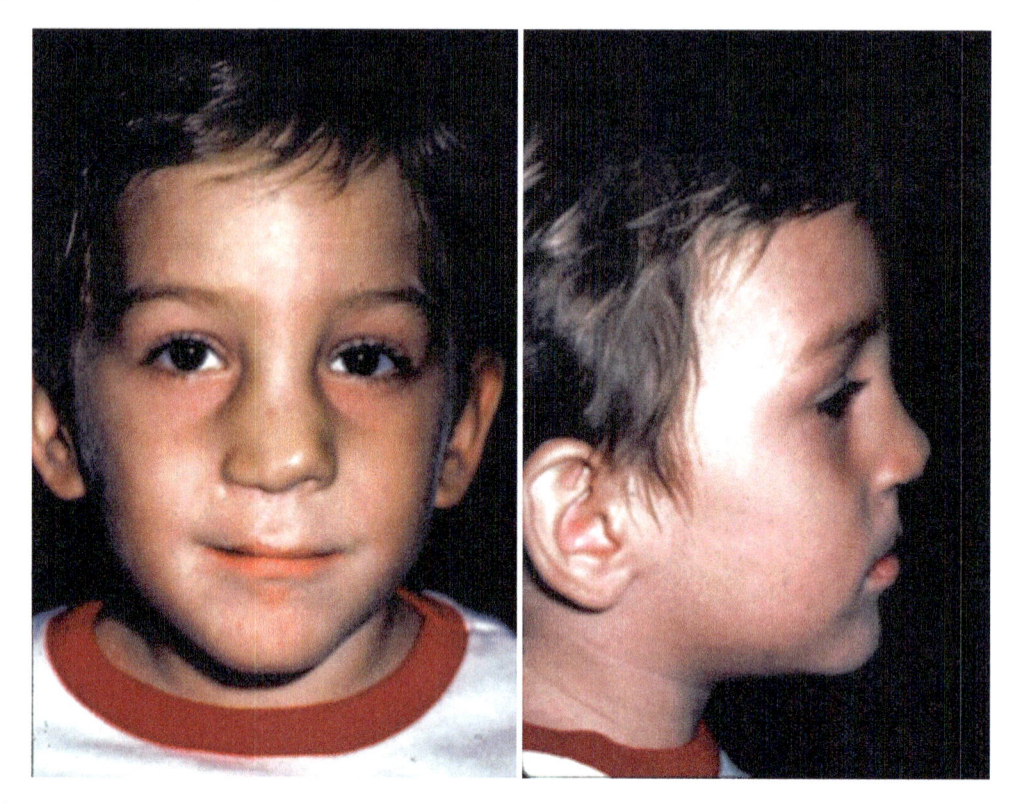

3 years 7 months

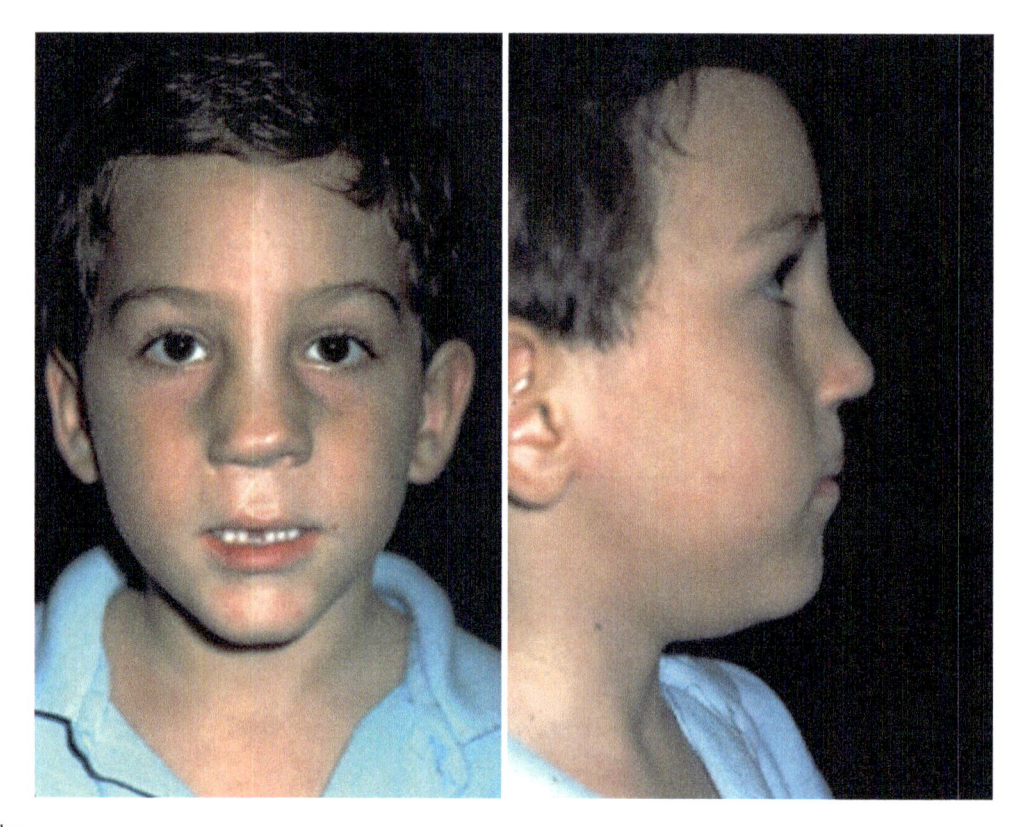

5 years 8 months

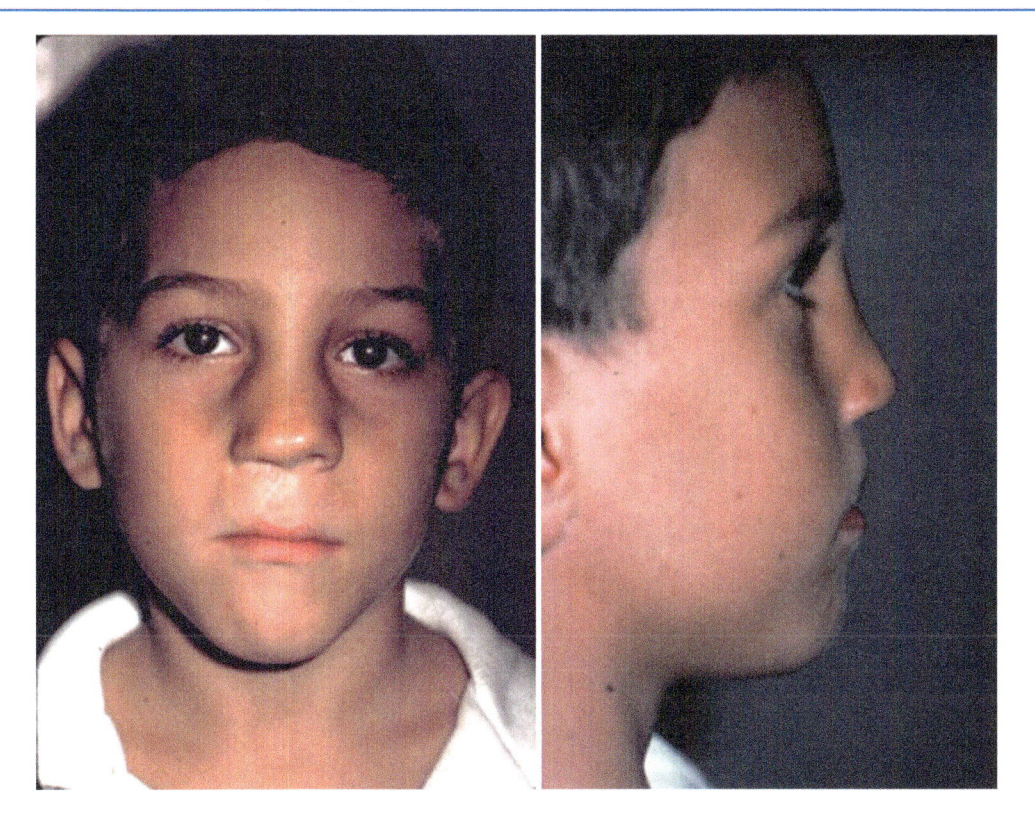

## 11.11 Recessiveness of the Midface Slowly Develops

6 years 9 months

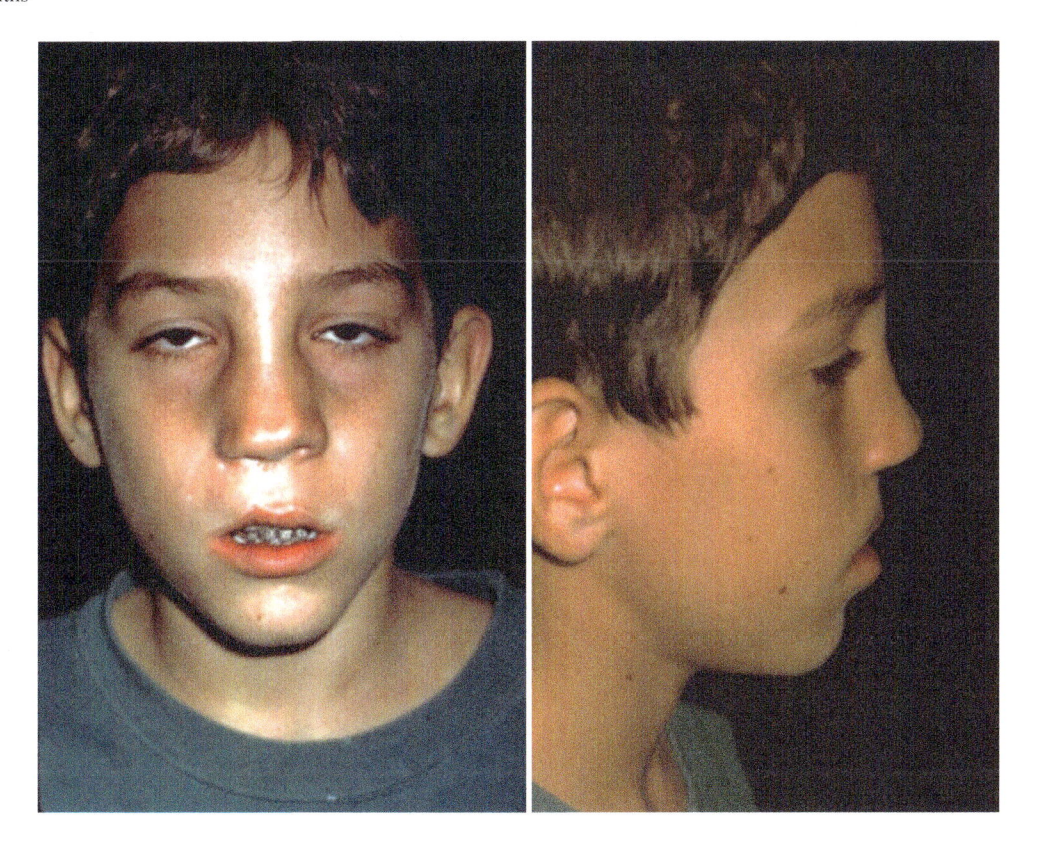

11 years

## 11.12 Loss of the Lateral Incisor Space

Poor occlusion yet the face looks good

Molding the premaxillary segment into contact with the cleft segment always closes off the lateral space

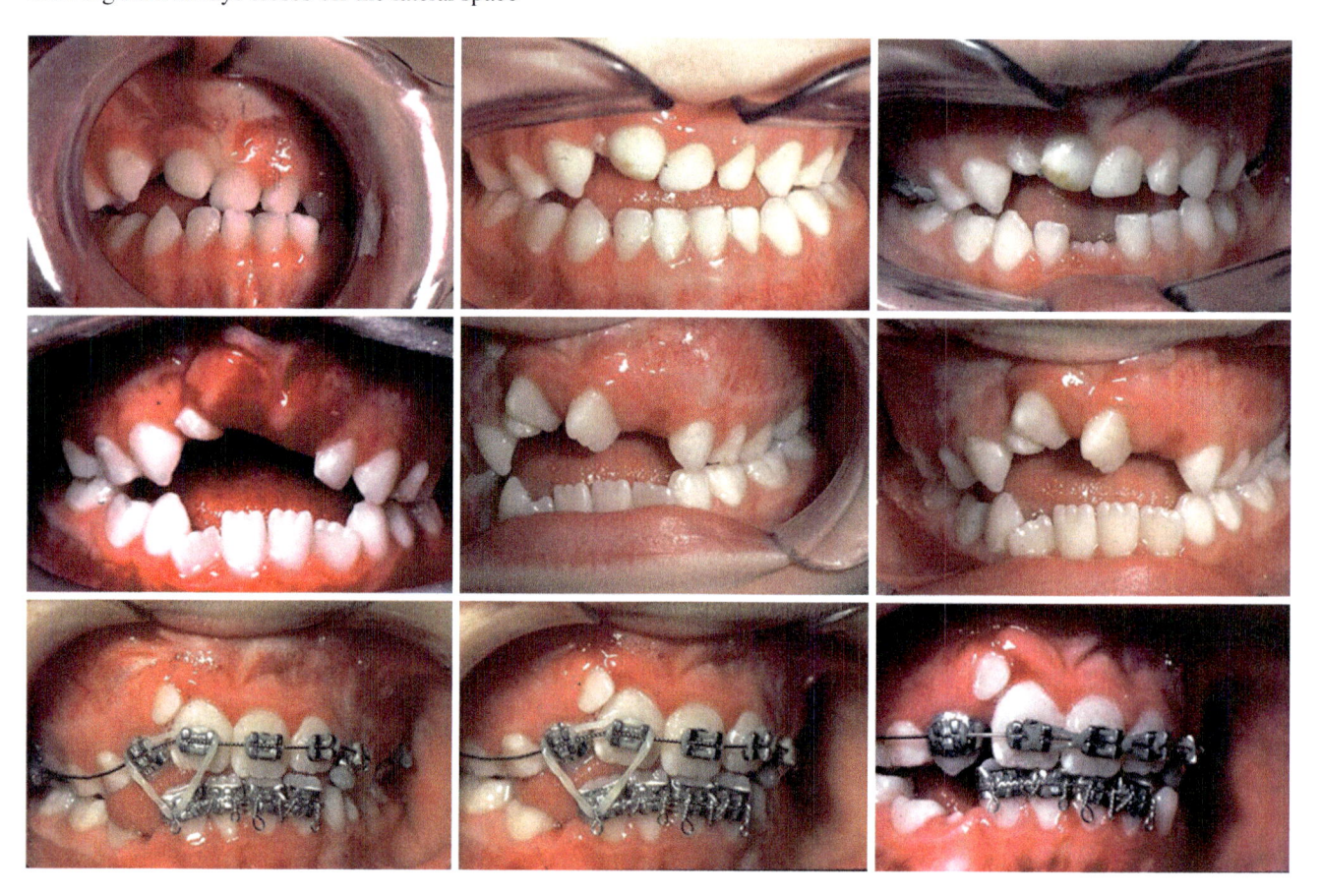

## 11.12 Loss of the Lateral Incisor Space                                                                   199

### 11.12.1 Midfacial growth retardation is now evident

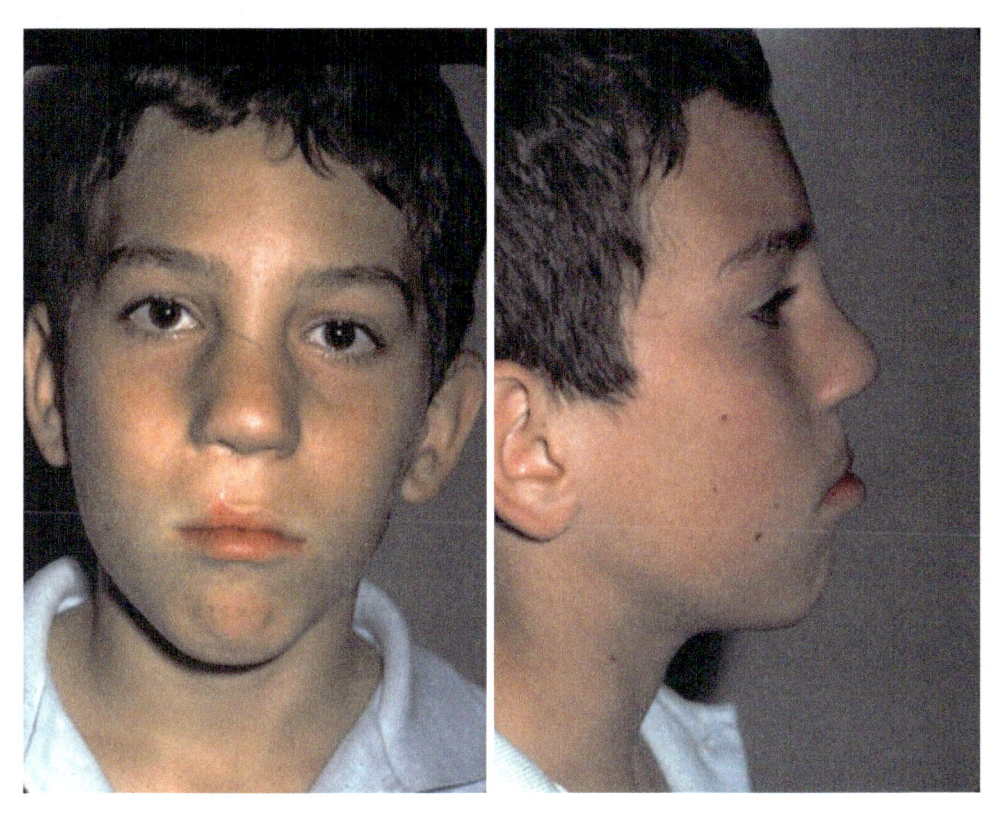

11 years 3 months—recessive midface

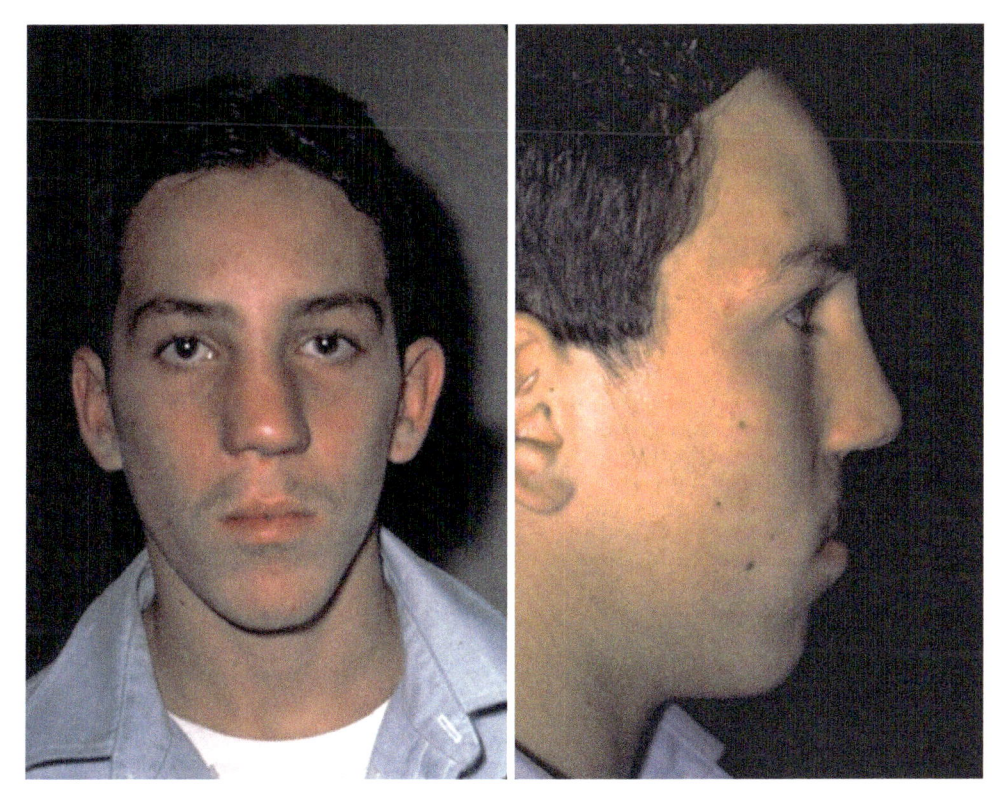

11 years 3 months

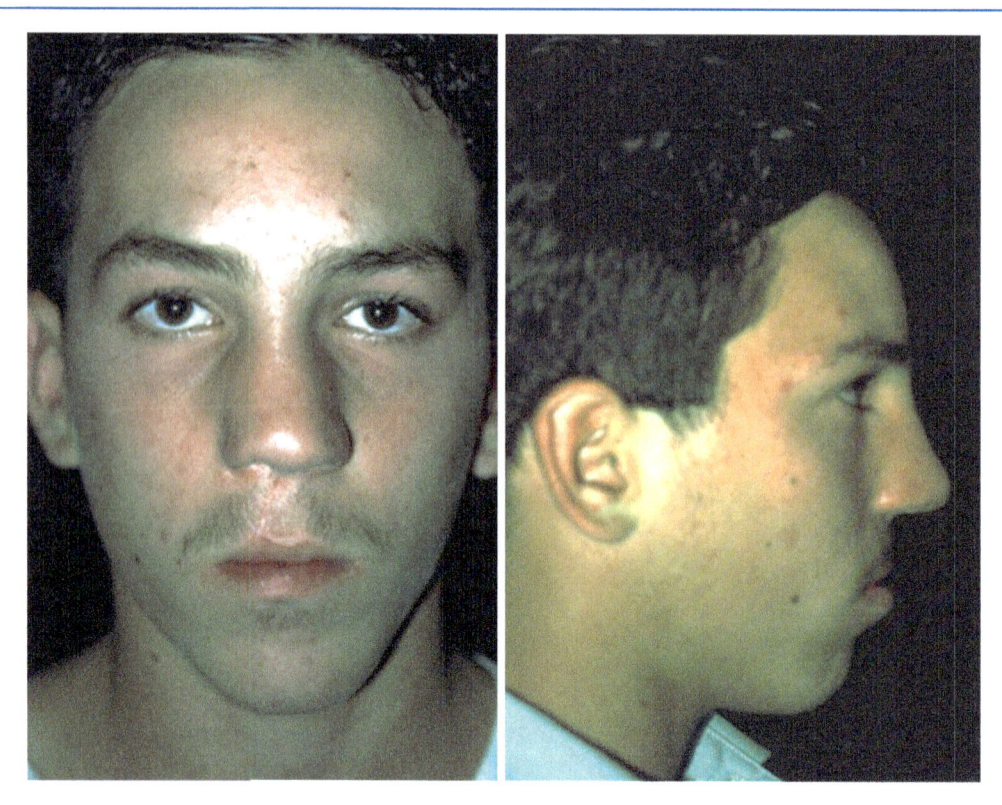

17 years: advancement of the upper teeth

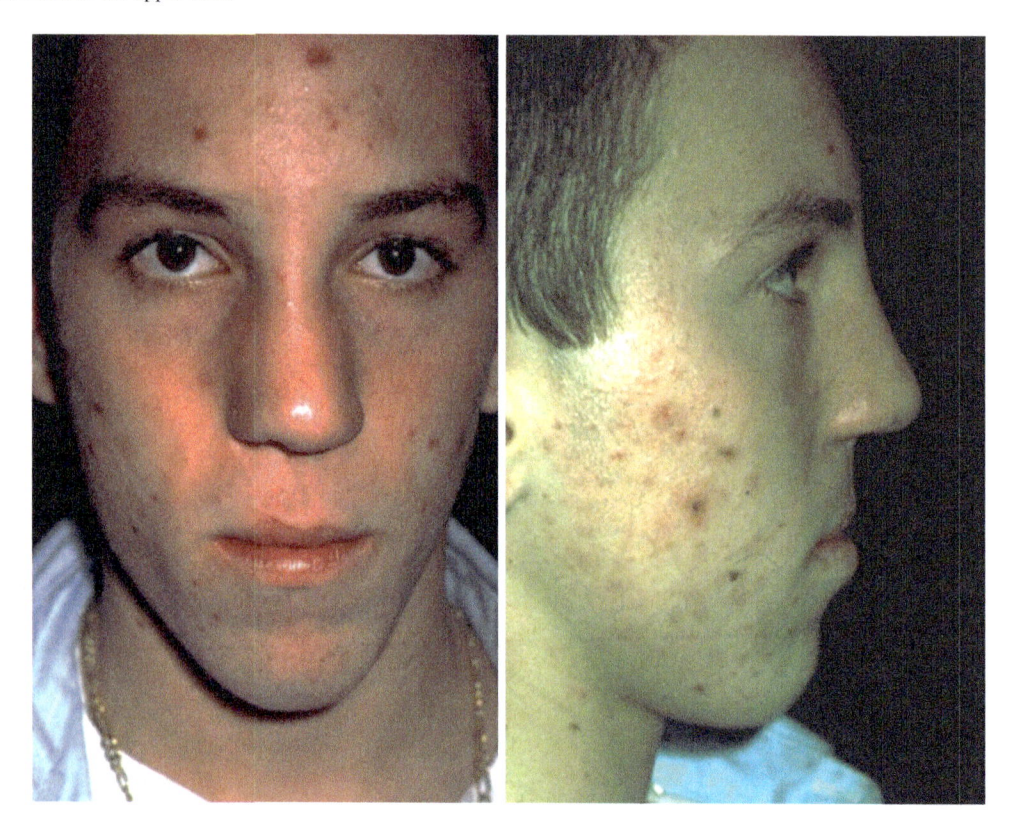

19 years

## 11.13 POPLA Treated CUCLP and Its Effect on the Facial Profile

### 11.13.1 Early Midfacial Recessiveness Due To Excessive Mandibular Growth

#### 11.13.1.1 Unpredicted Facial Growth

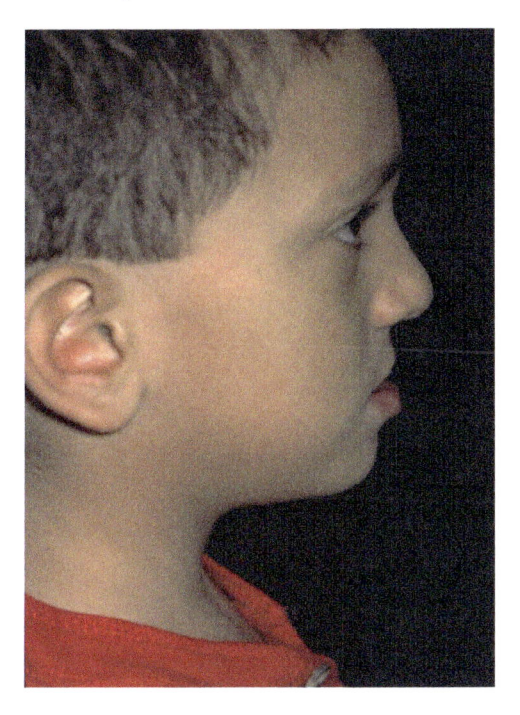

4 years

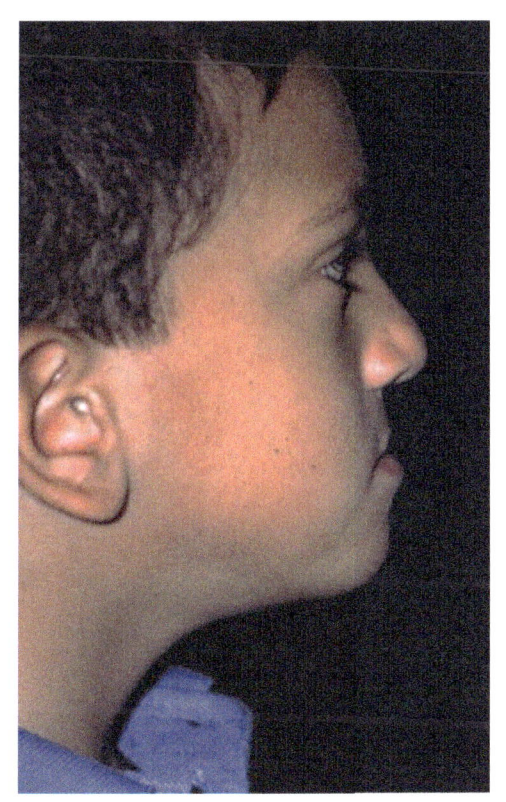

6 years

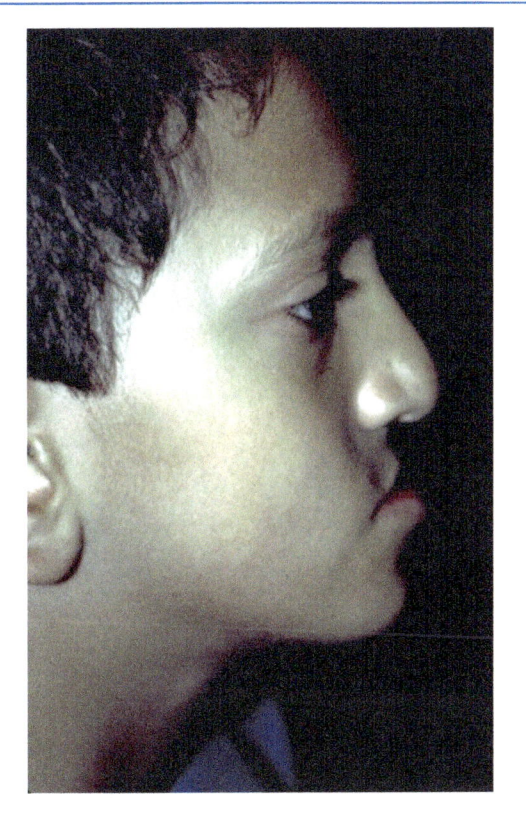

9 years

**Facial Changes** Recessive midface at 4, 6, and 9 years of age.

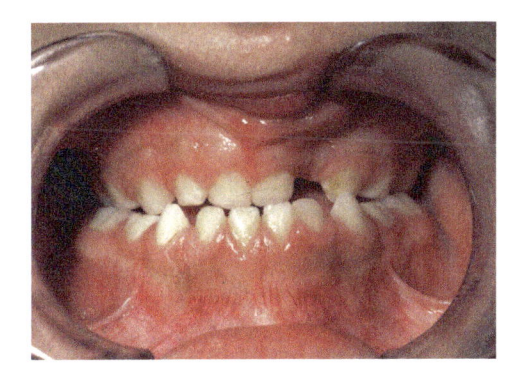

4 years

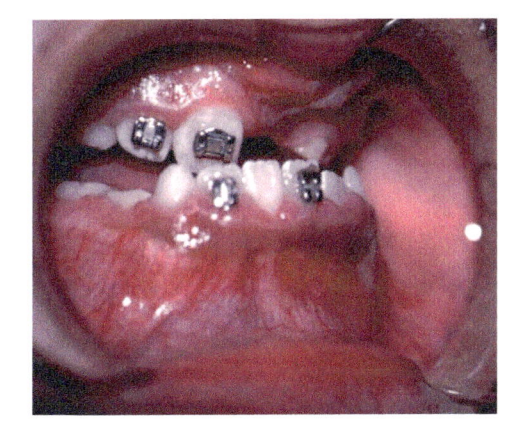

9 years

**Intraoral occlusal photographs** Showing anterior dental crossbite at 4 and 9 years of age.

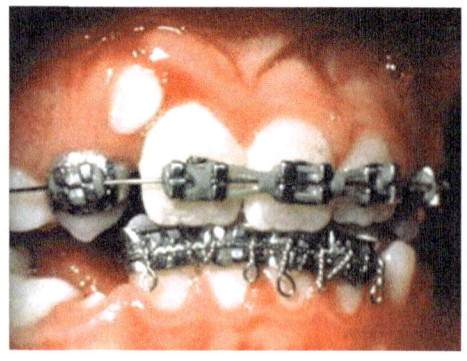

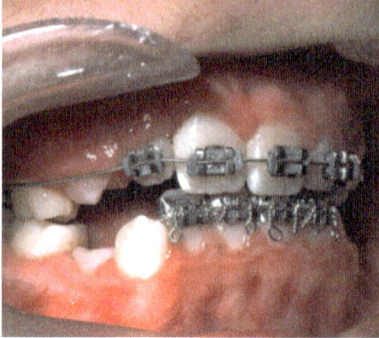

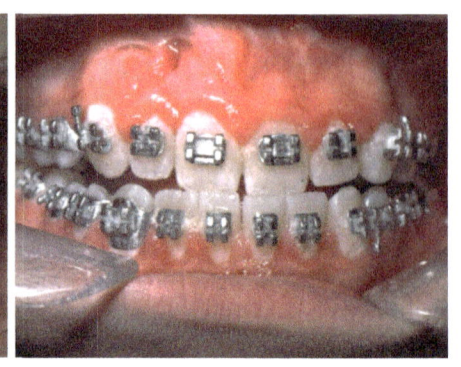

Vertical elastics used to extrude the upper anterior teeth.

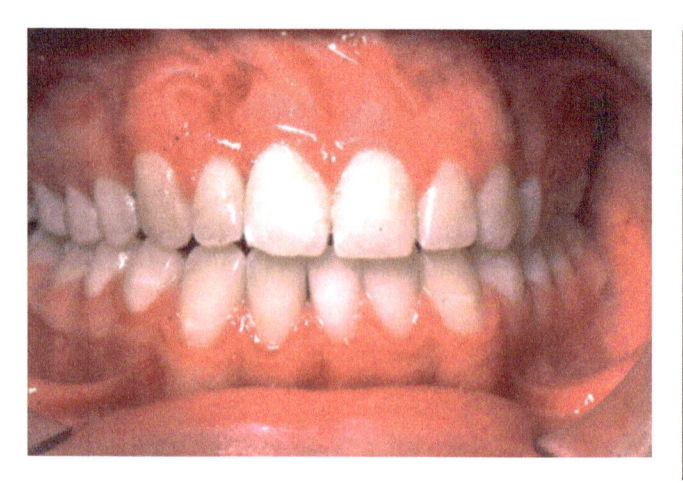

A lower incisor was extracted in order to create an overbite + overjet.

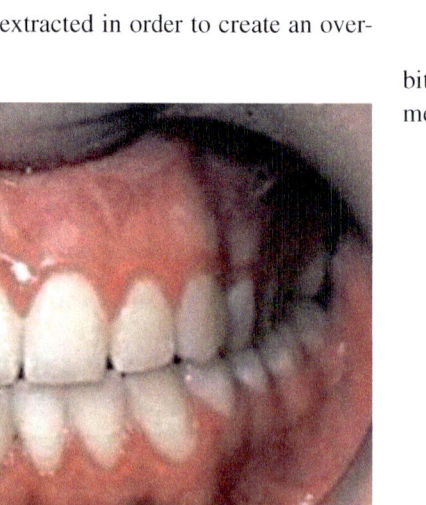

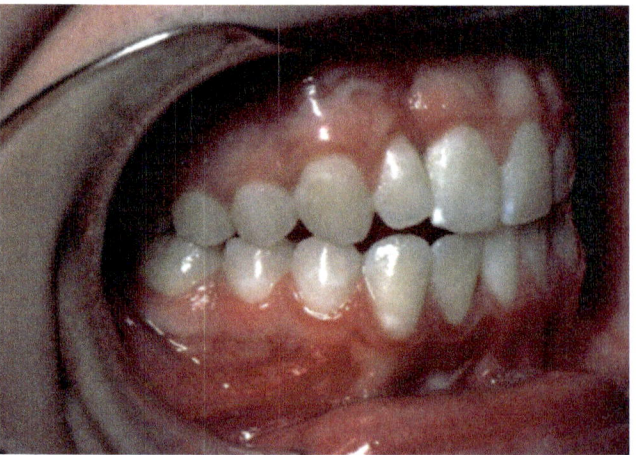

Anterior occlusion is poor due to the return of the open bite. This is caused by the displacement of the palatal segments by PSOT.

Anterior open bite returning.

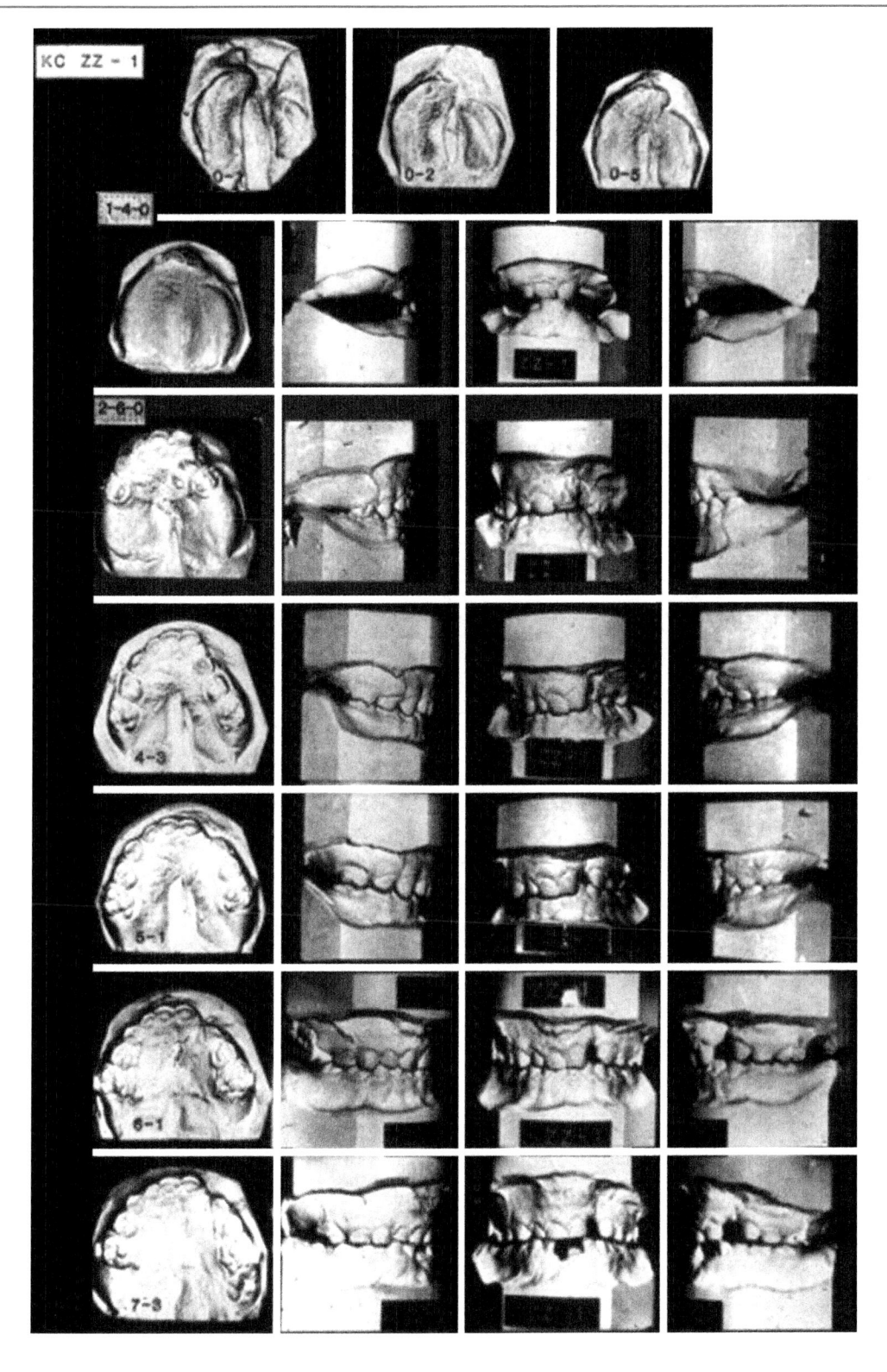

## 11.13 POPLA Treated CUCLP and Its Effect on the Facial Profile

An upper to lower congruency is dependent on four upper and lower incisor or its equivalent (a cuspid in the lateral incisor space).

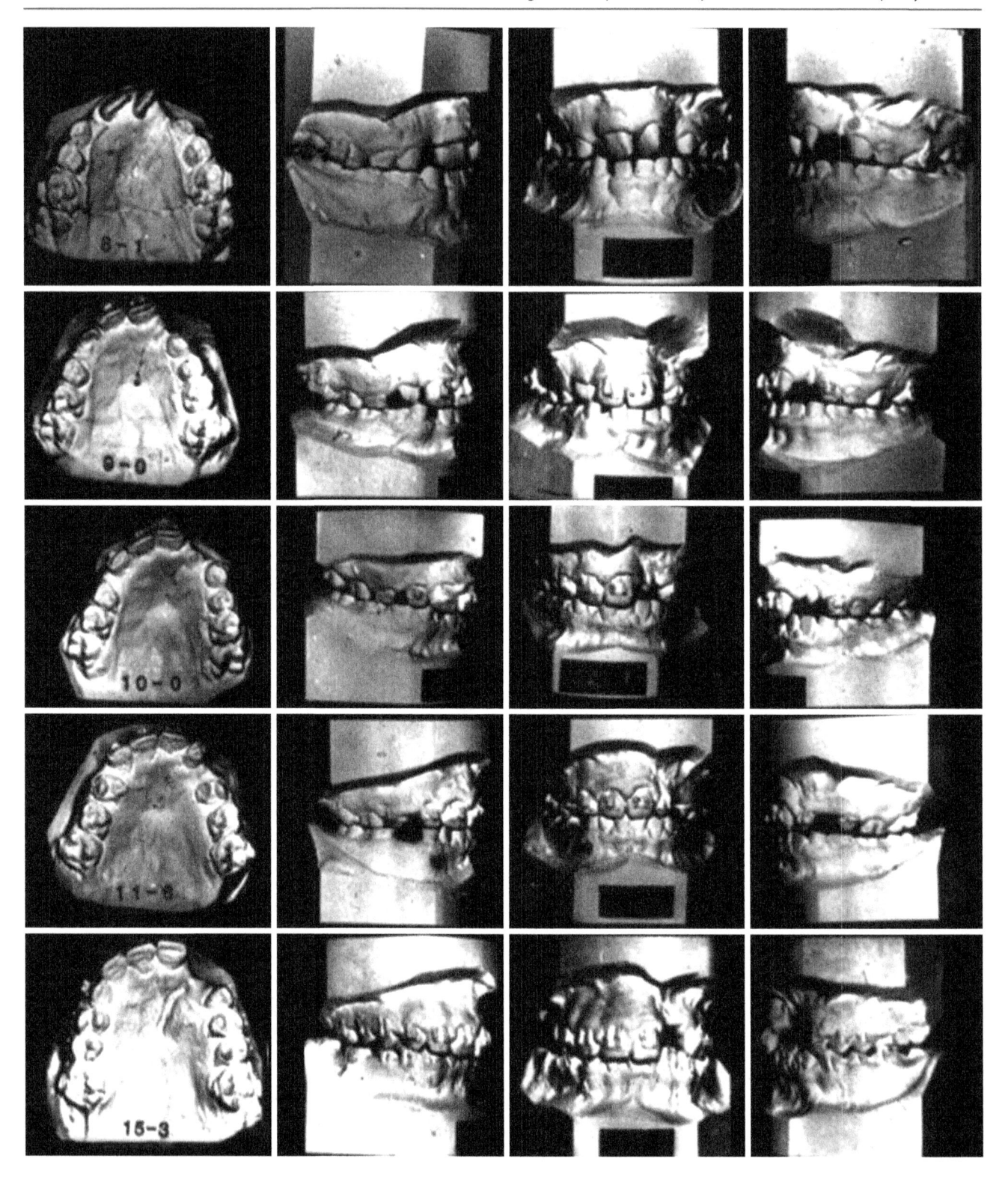

## 11 Presurgical Orthopedics with Lip Adhesion and Periosteoplasty (POPLA)

## 11.14 Miami

Rapid narrowing of the cleft space

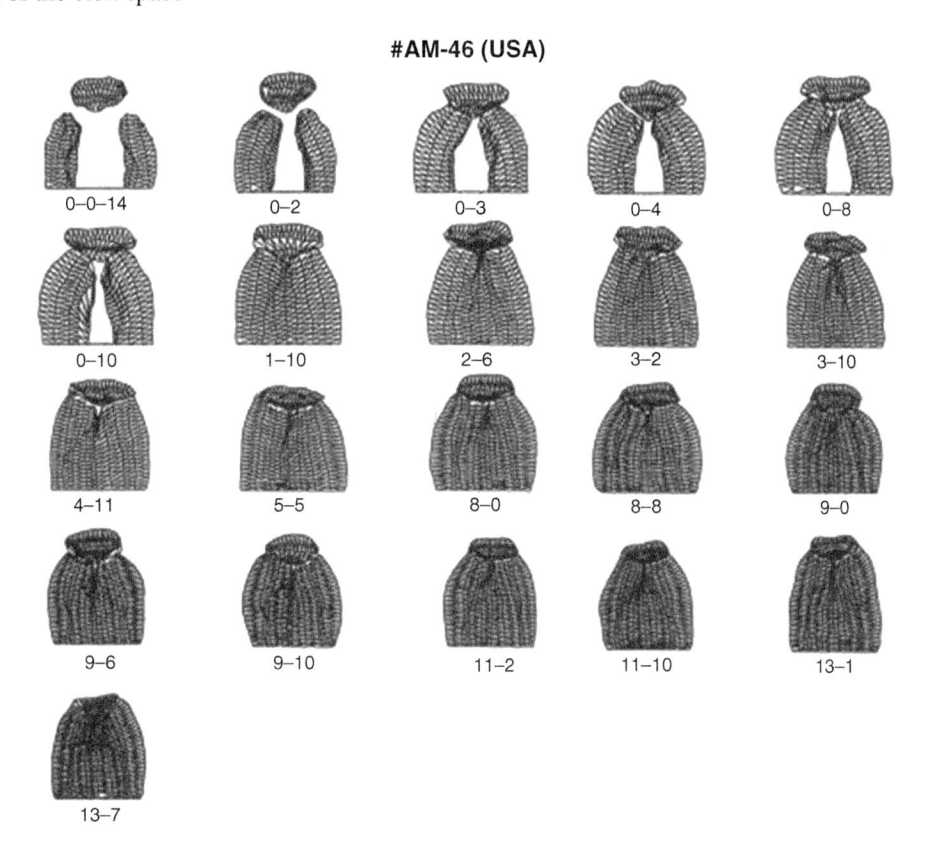

**#AM-46 (USA)**

0-0-14, 0-2, 0-3, 0-4, 0-8
0-10, 1-10, 2-6, 3-2, 3-10
4-11, 5-5, 8-0, 8-8, 9-0
9-6, 9-10, 11-2, 11-10, 13-1
13-7

Non-PSOT. Narrowing of the cleft space resulted in molding plus palatal growth.

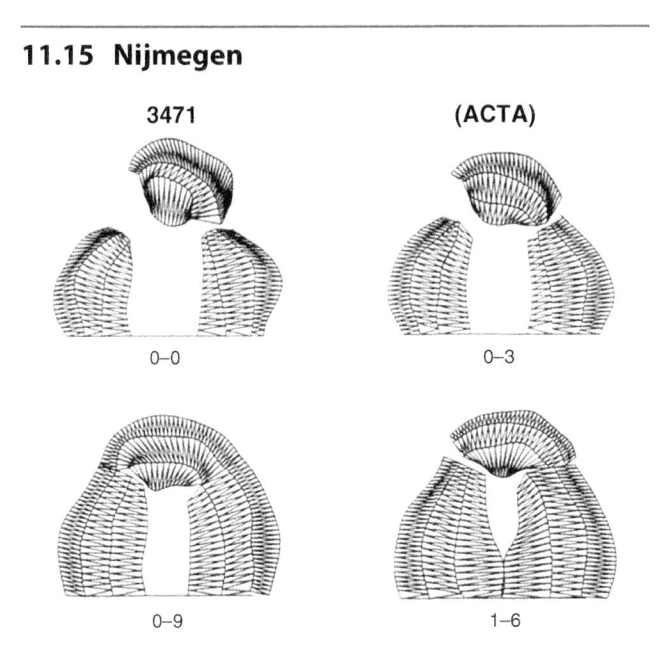

## 11.15 Nijmegen

**3471**  **(ACTA)**

0-0, 0-3
0-9, 1-6

PSOT prevents cleft space from narrowing. Appliance was removed at 1–4 years resulting in molding of palatal segments.

## 11.16 Maxillary Protraction Facial Mask

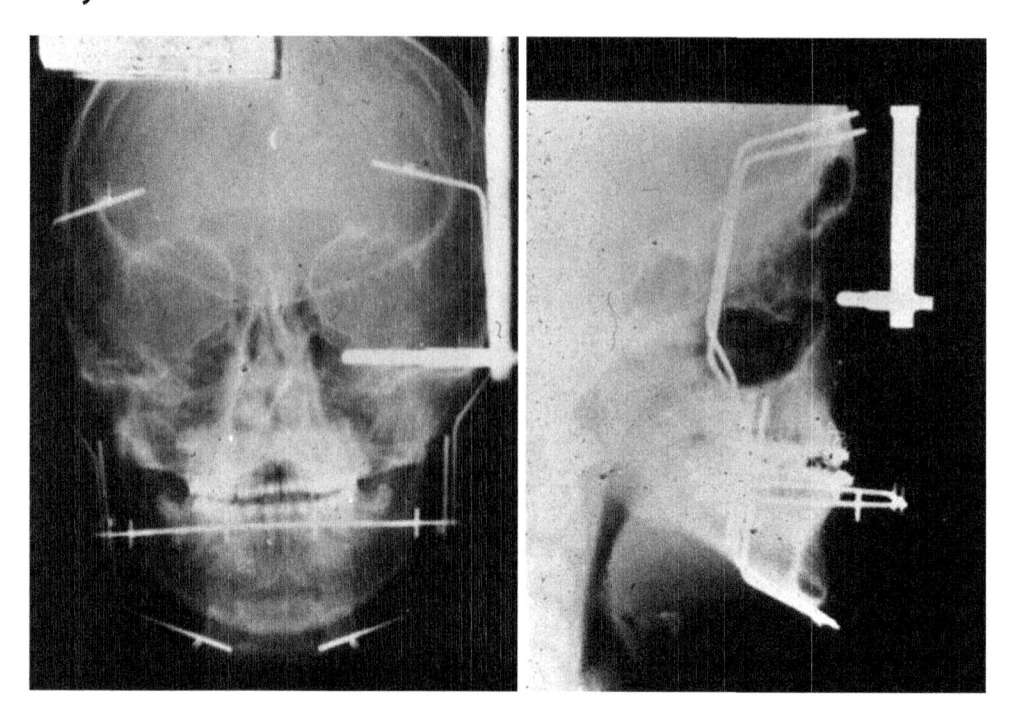

Protraction facial mask to advance maxilla orthopedically—worn 12 h per day.

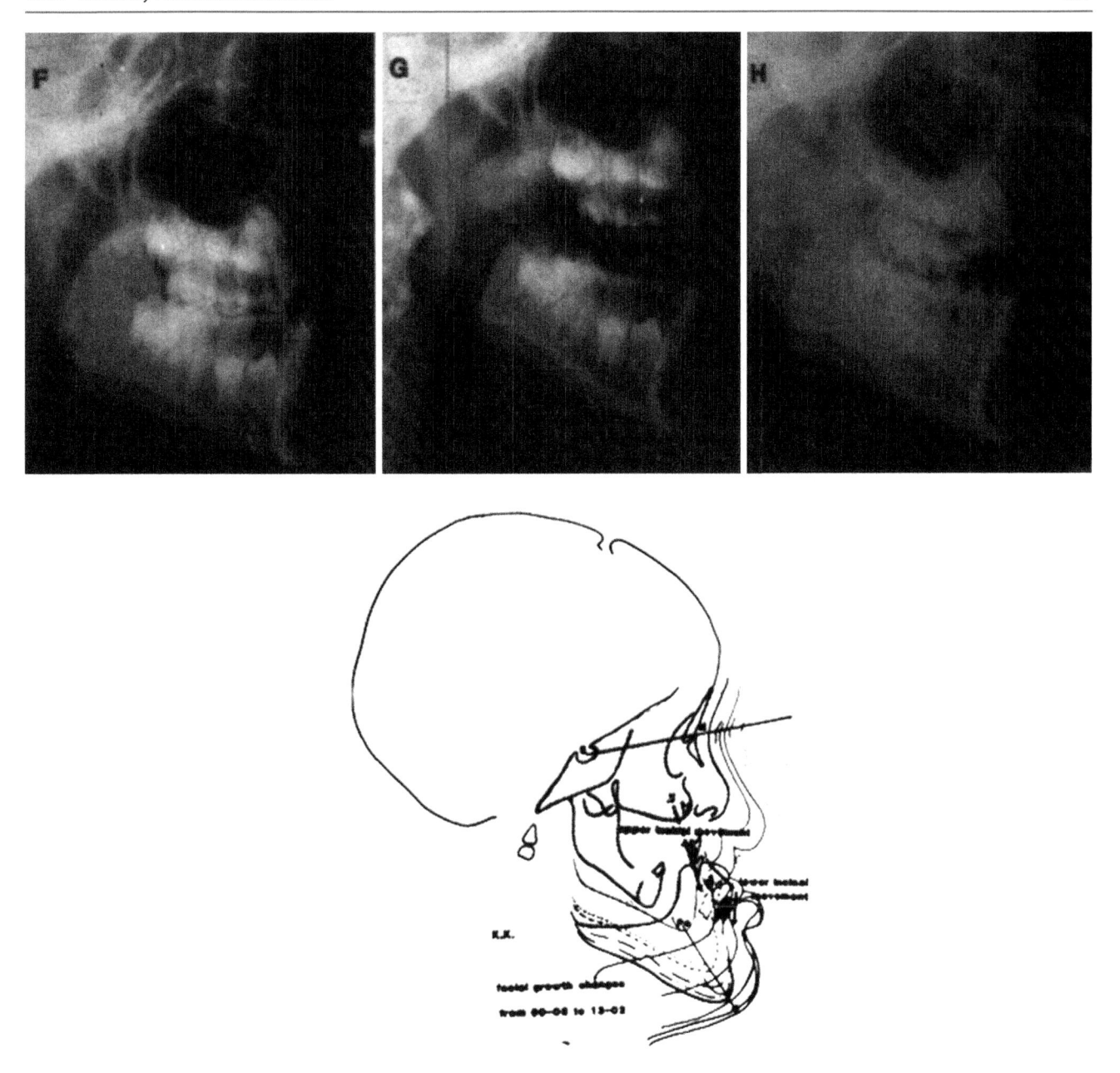

## 11.16 Maxillary Protraction Facial Mask

Good maxillary mandibular relationship

## 11.17 Lateral Head X-Rays Show Good VPC

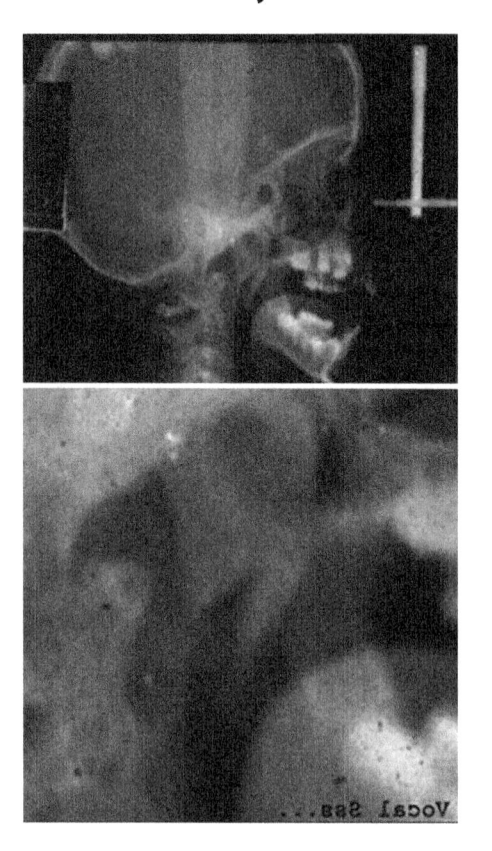

Vocal Sss…

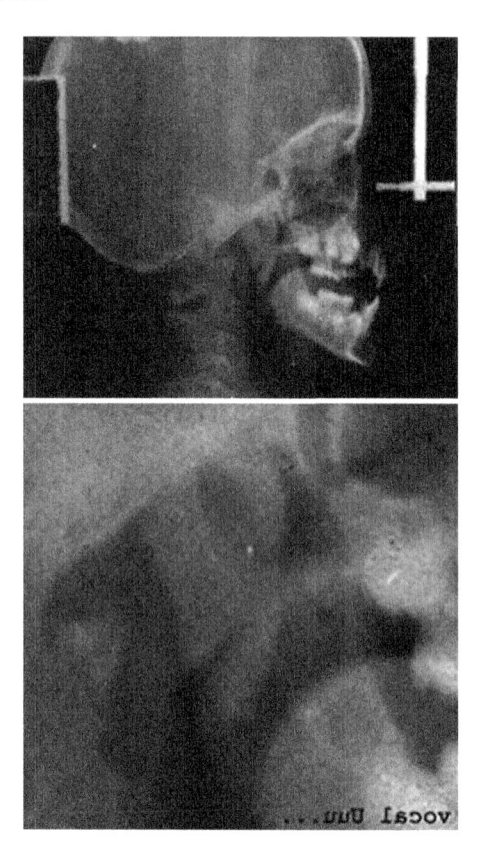

VOCAL Uuu…

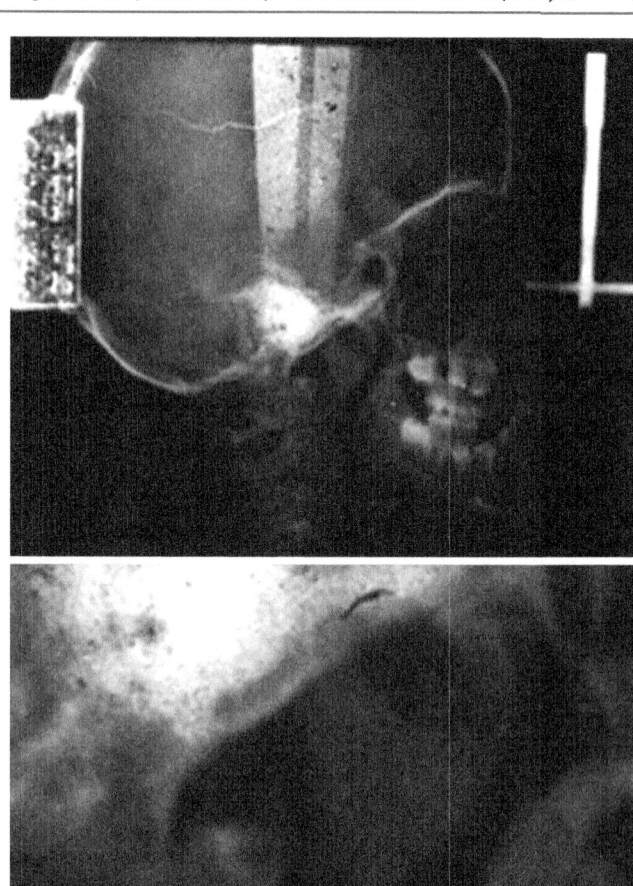

Velum at rest

## 11.18 Skeletal and Soft Tissue Profile Changes

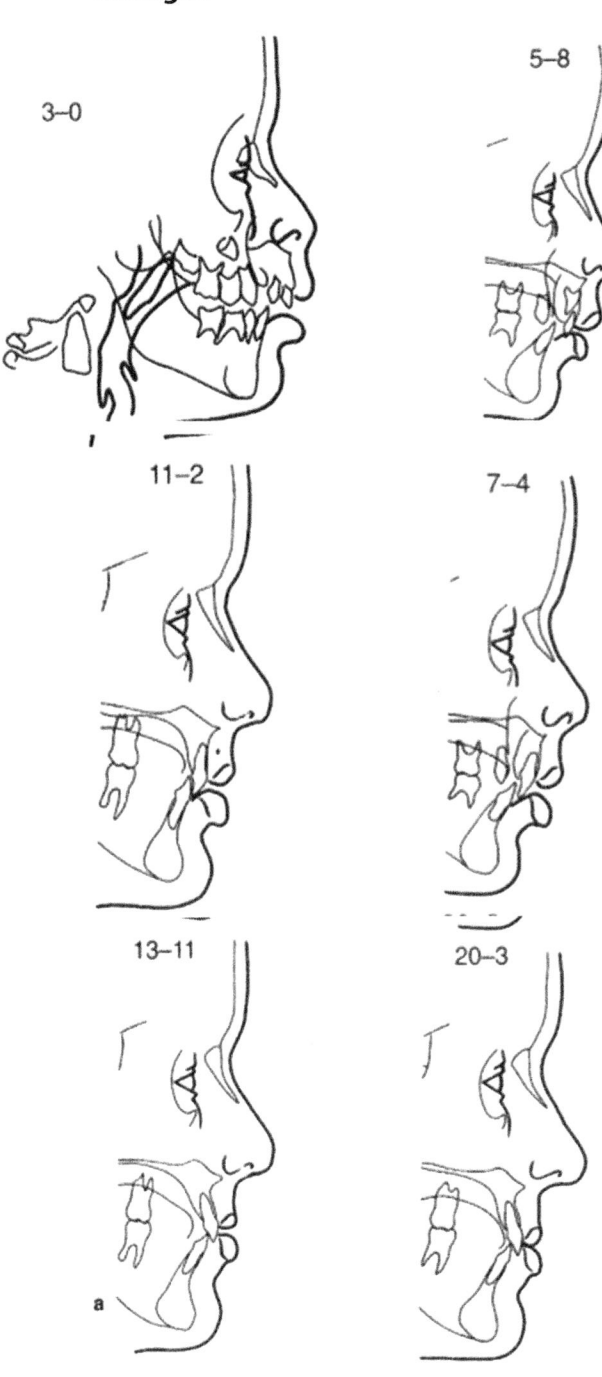

Facial profile is markedly improved by 11 years.

## 11.19 Superimposed Polygons

Facial growth changes and profile changes

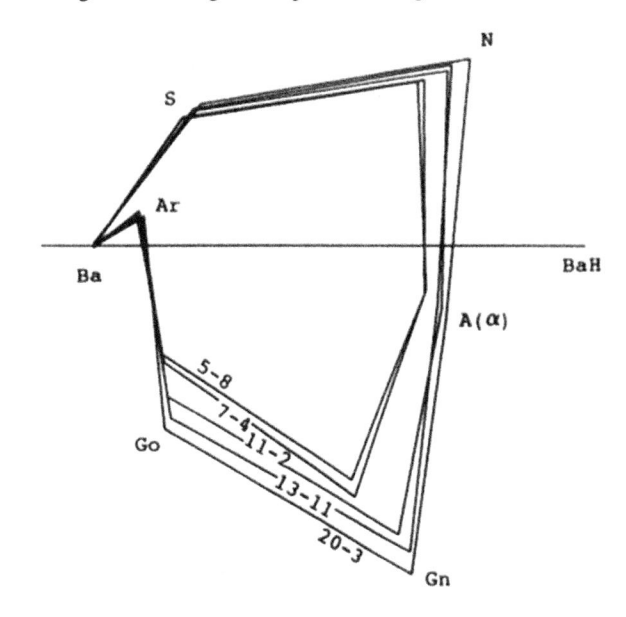

Coben analysis
Profile changes

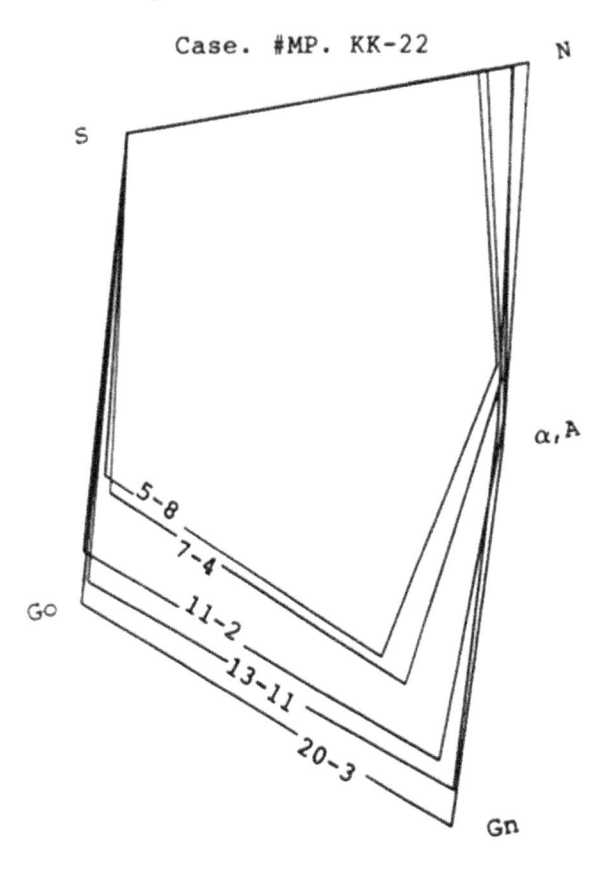

Midfacial growth is retarded. Upper and lower facial growth flattens the facial profile.

## 11.20 CBCLP Case Which Required Midfacial Advancement at Adolescence

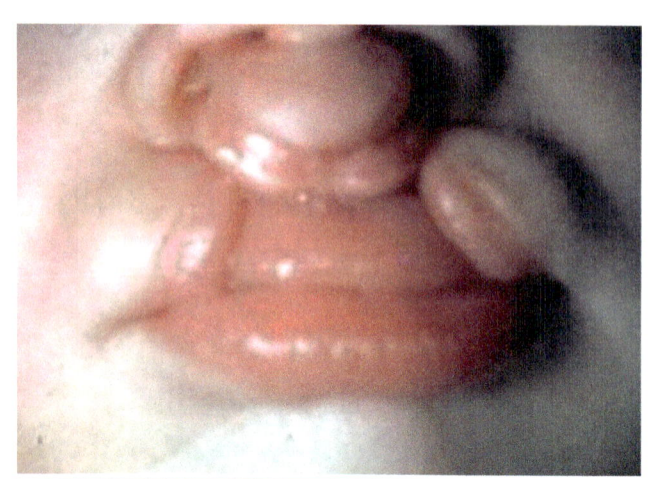

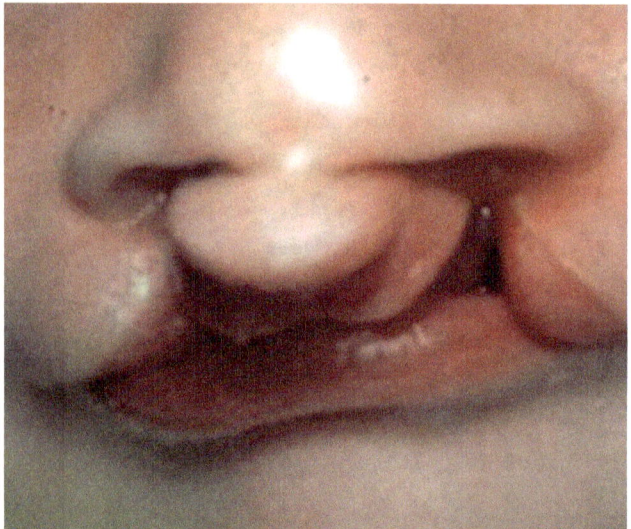

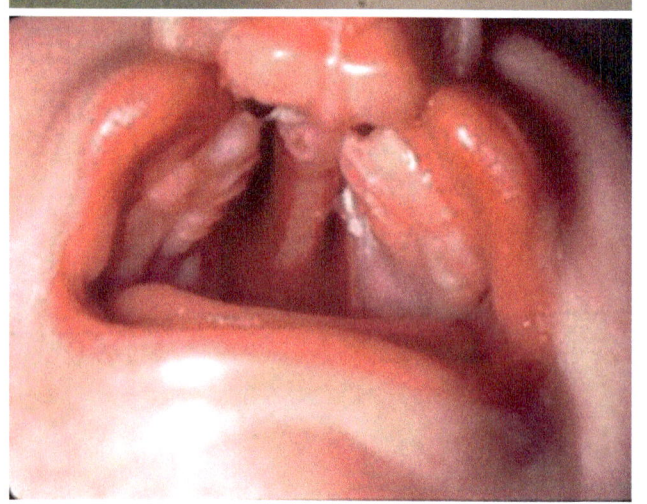

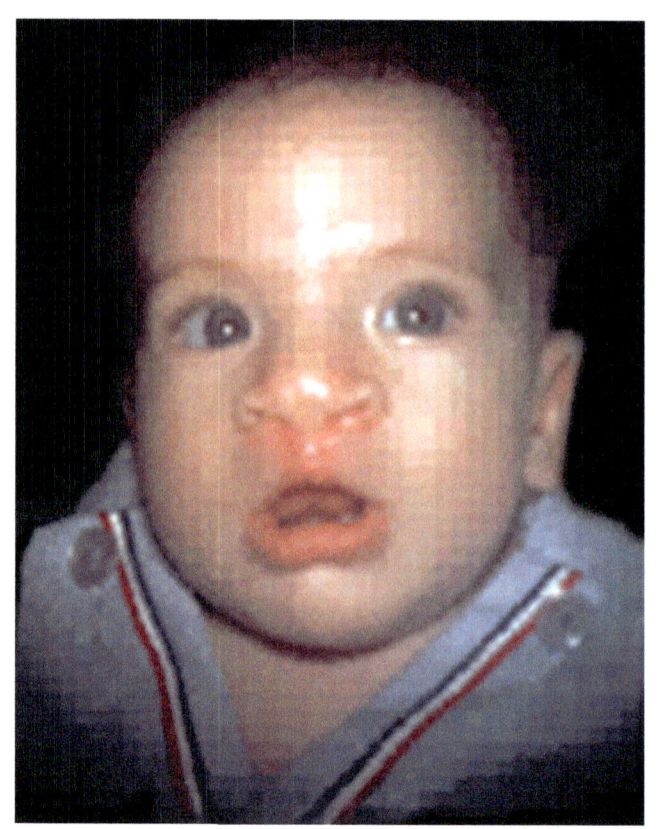

11.21 CBCLP: Ideal Treatment Results

## 11.21 CBCLP: Ideal Treatment Results

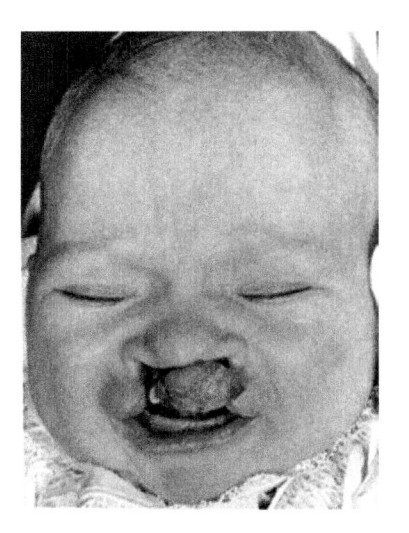

(**a**) 1 month

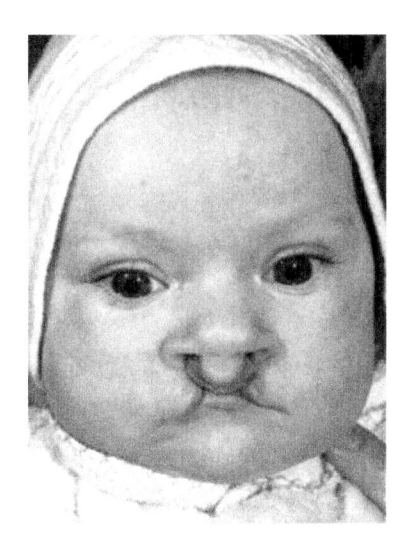

(**b**) 2 months after head bonnet and strap

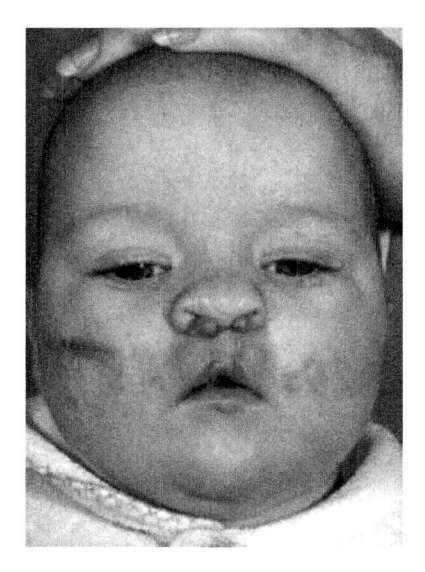

(**c**) 6 months

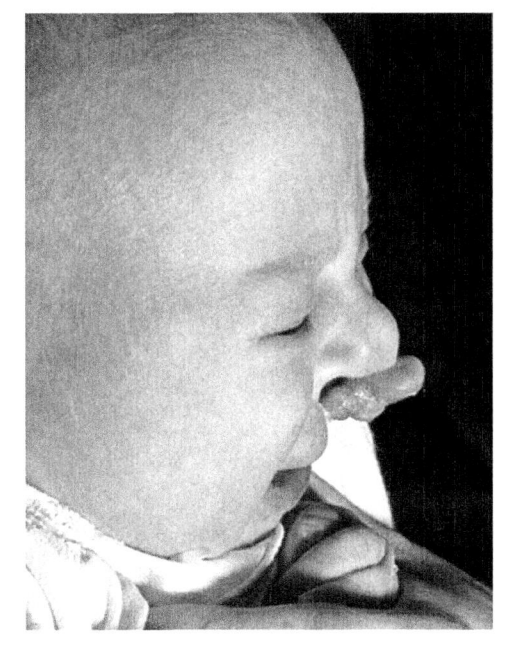

(**d**) 1 month

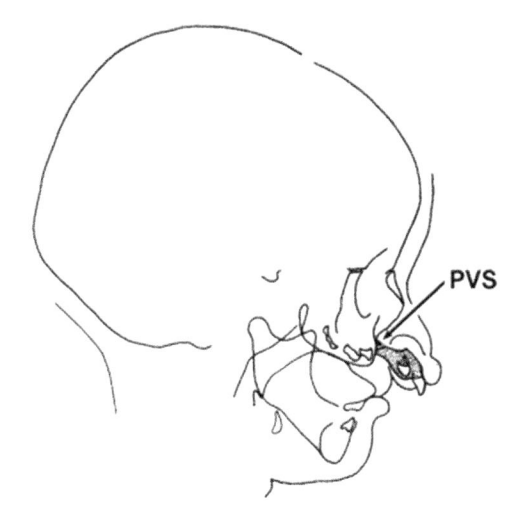

(**e**) Example

Lip united with banked forked flap.

a, b, d, e: Protruding premaxilla due to excessive growth at the premaxillary vomerine suture (PVS).

18 days

25 days

4 months

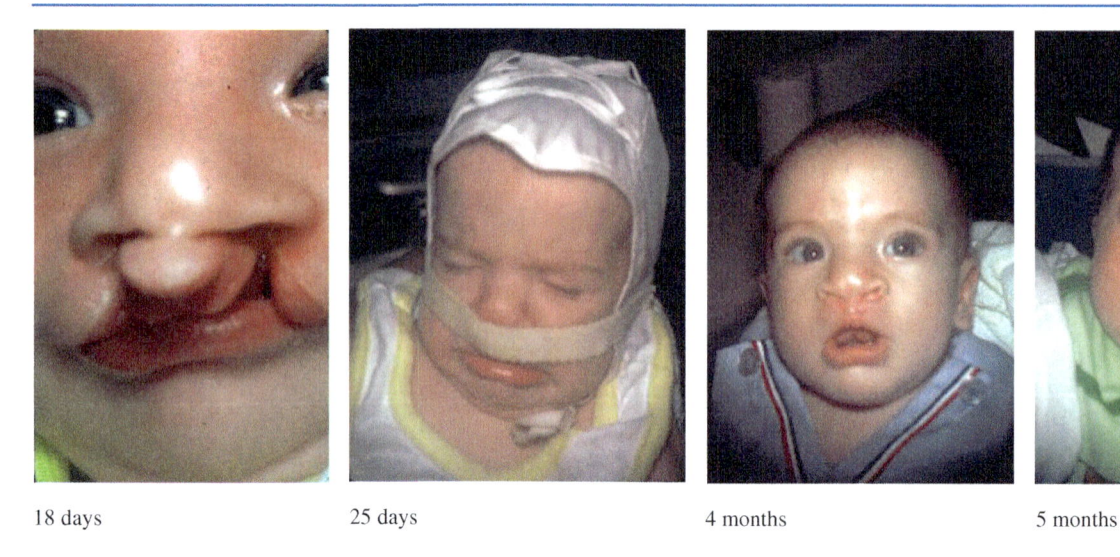

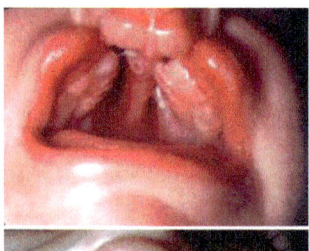

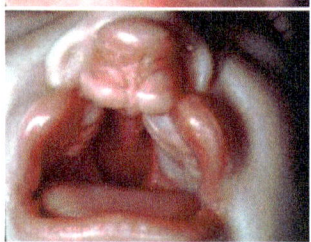

5 months

Head Bonnet—to ventroflex premaxilla and mold lateral palatal segments

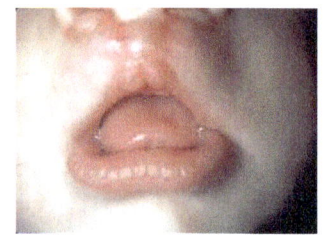

4 months—Banked fork flap

## 11.22 Progressive Changes in Facial Profile Leading To a Flattened Midface

Protruding premaxilla even when ventroflexed
 "good!"

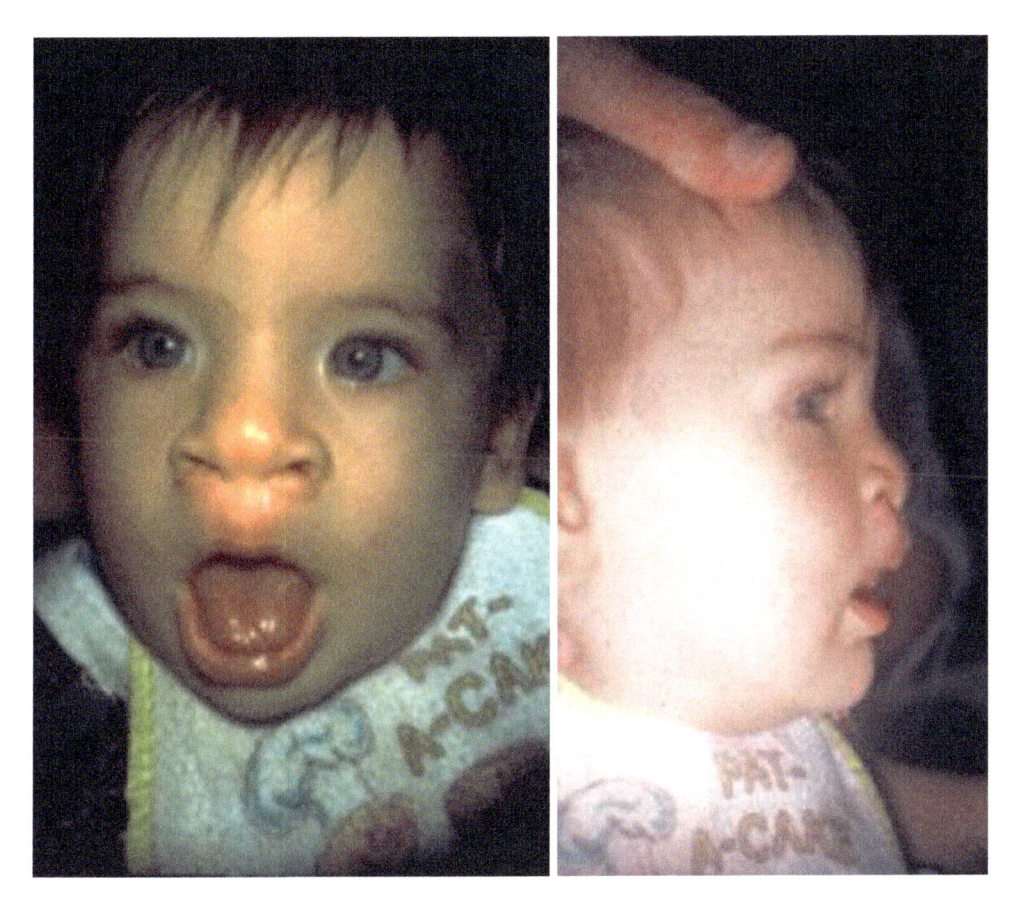

8 months

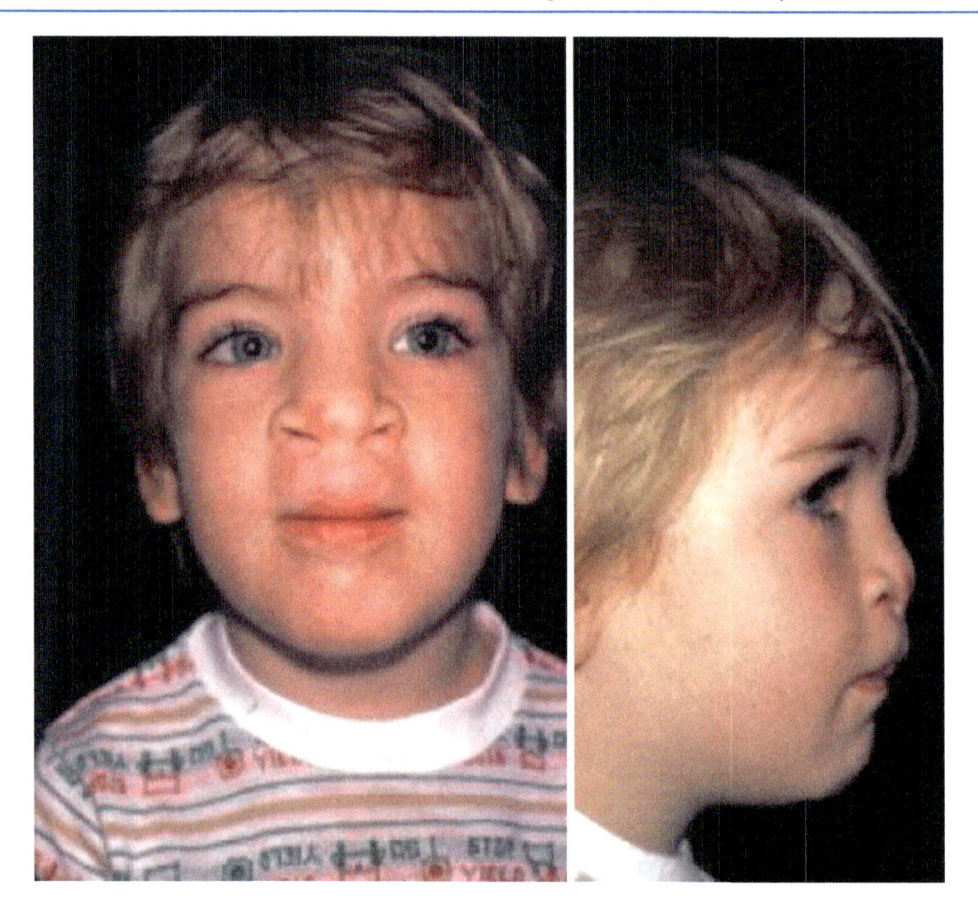

2 years

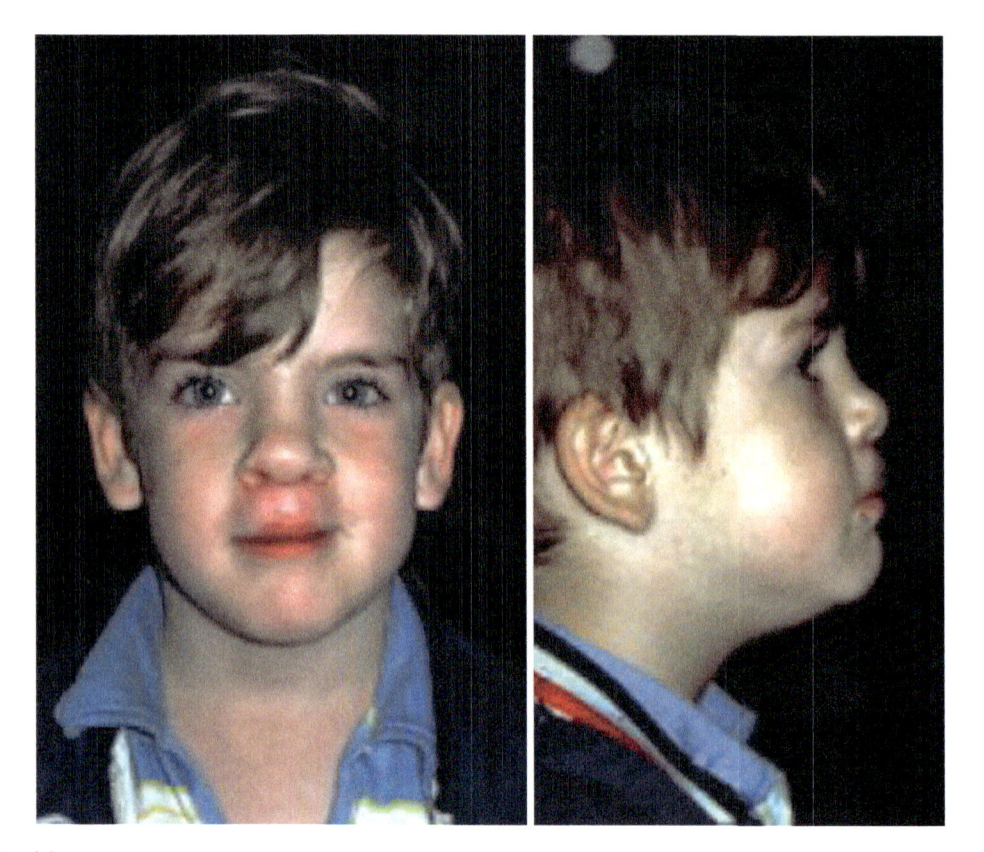

4 years Nasal revision

## 11.23 Nasal Revision

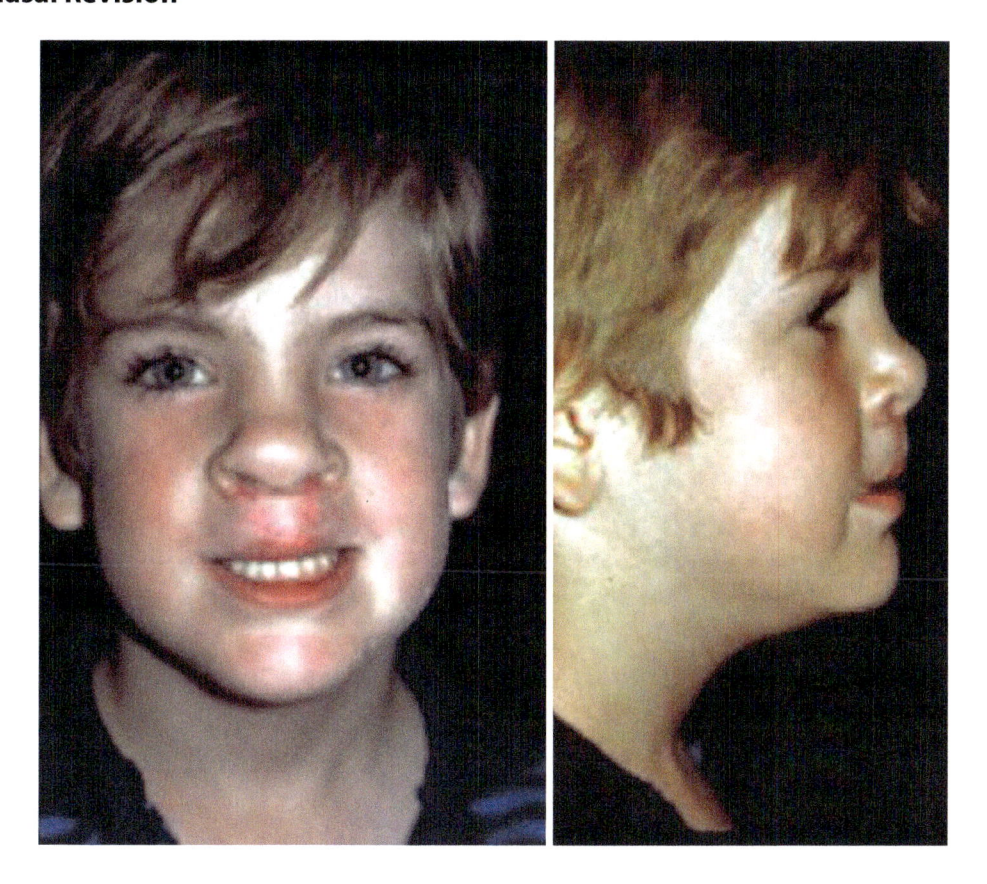

5 years

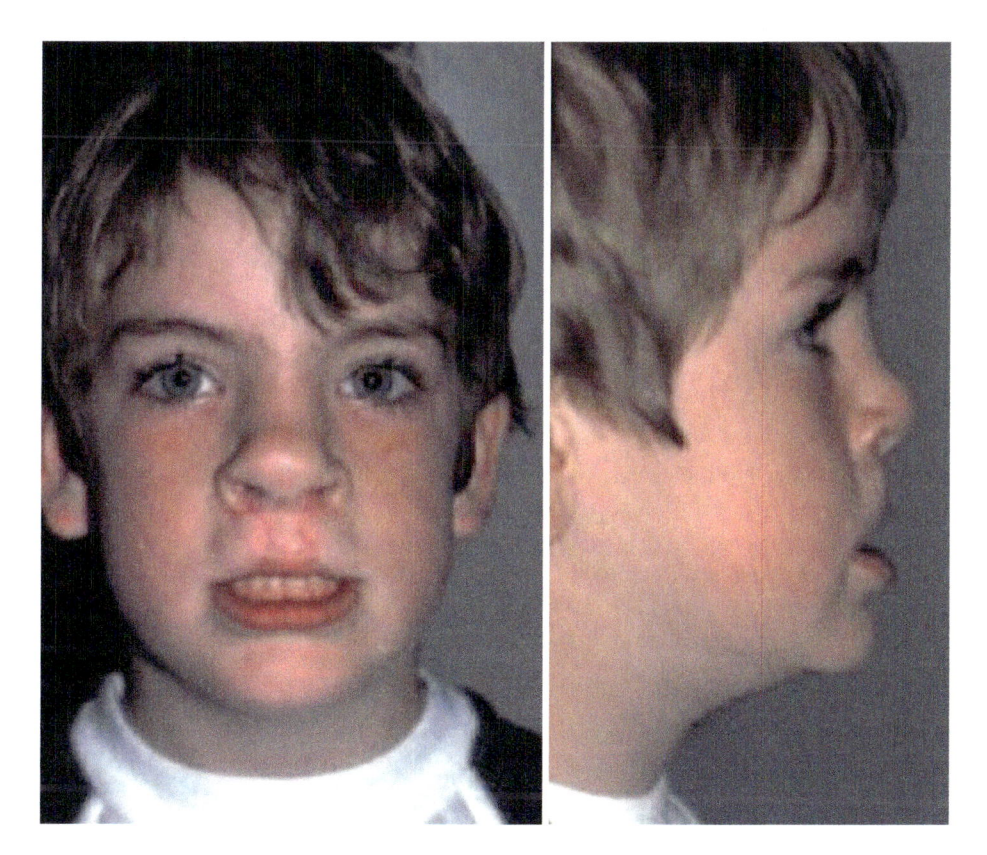

6 years

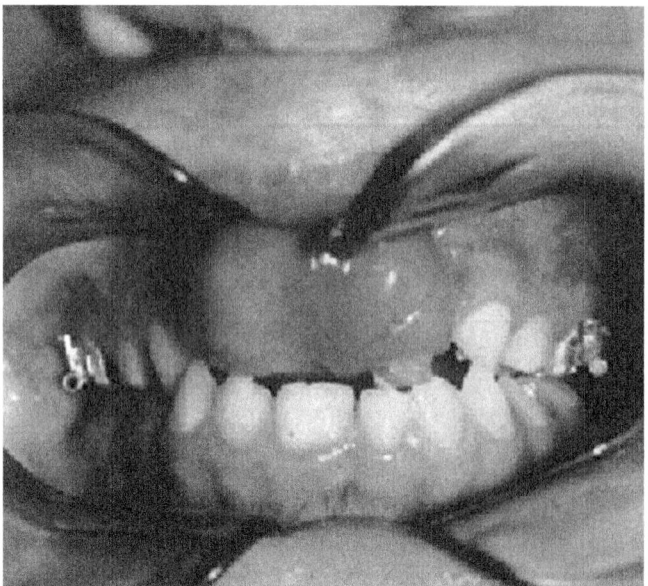

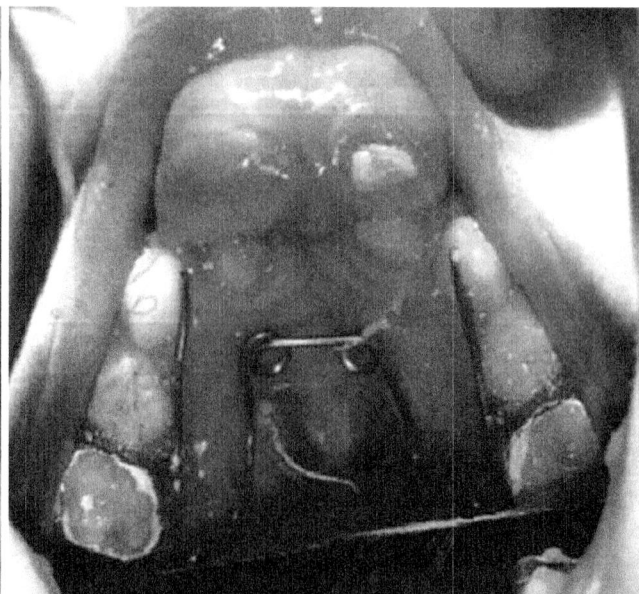

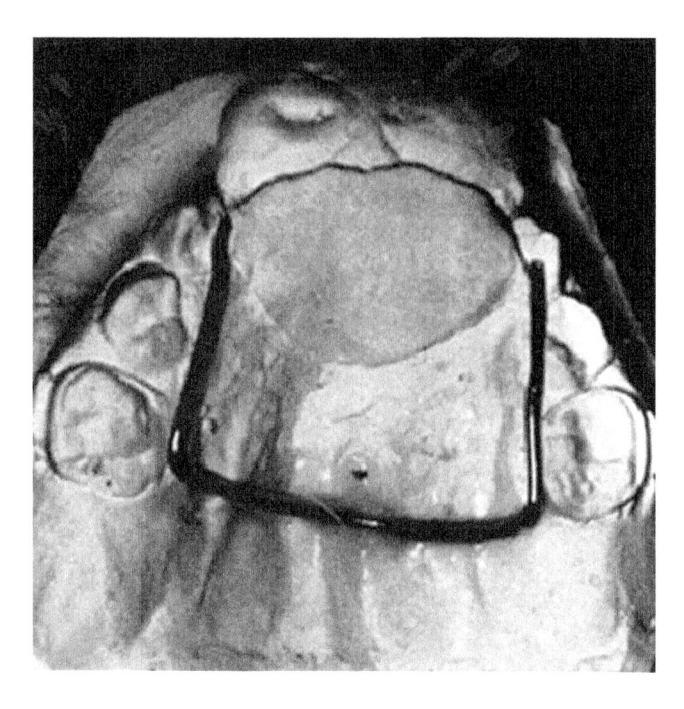

The oversized premaxilla is due to the developing permanent maxillary incisors. The buccal crossbite had been corrected which allows for the premaxilla to be spontaneously aligned within the arch. The expansion was maintained with a fixed retainer.

## 11.23 Nasal Revision

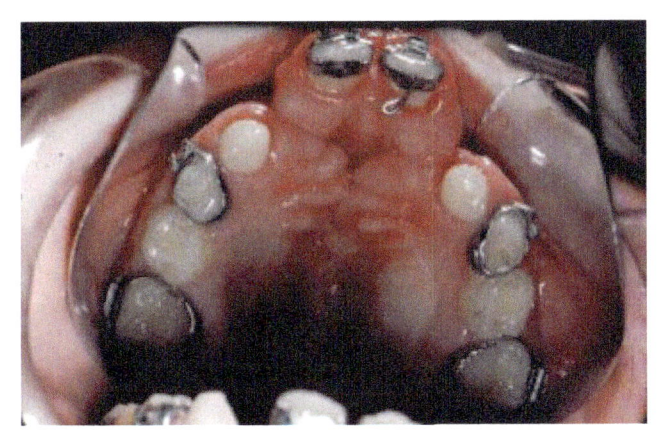

9 years

Developing anterior crossbite

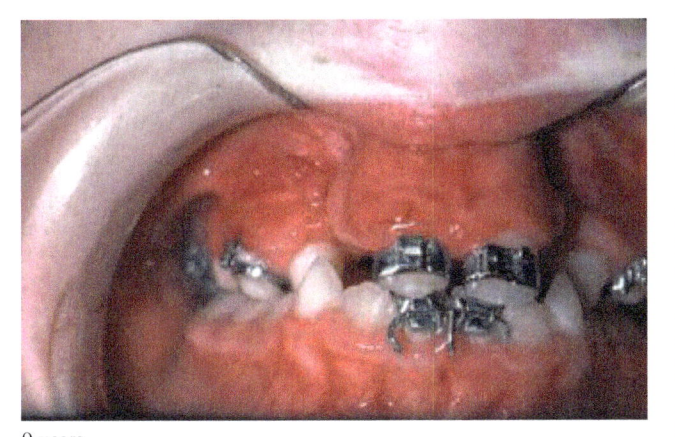

9 years

Attempting to advance the maxillary anterior teeth

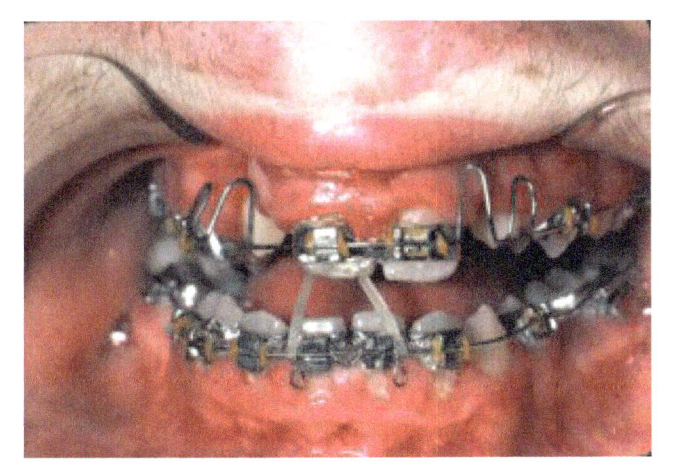

12 years

Prior to Lefort I maxillary advancement

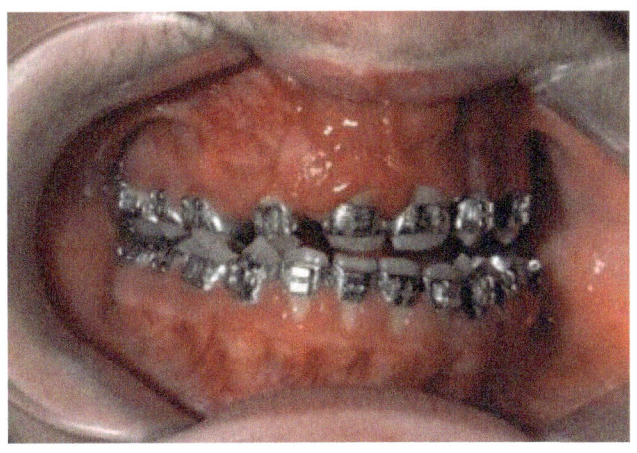

13 years

After maxillary surgical advancement Orthodontic retainers

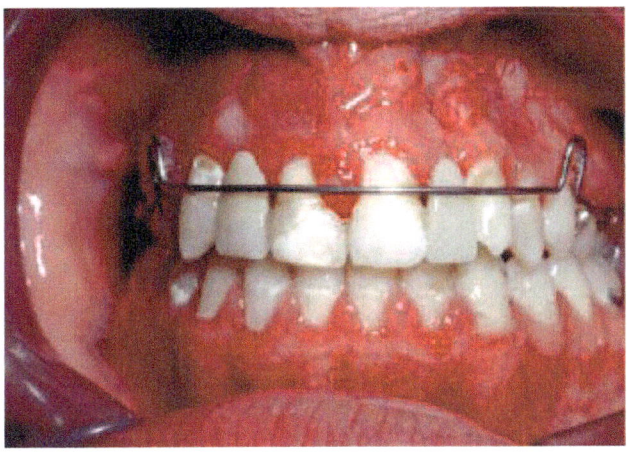

20 years

Failure of orthodontics to correct anterior crossbite

## 11.24 Recessed Mid-face With Concave Facial Profile After Surgery

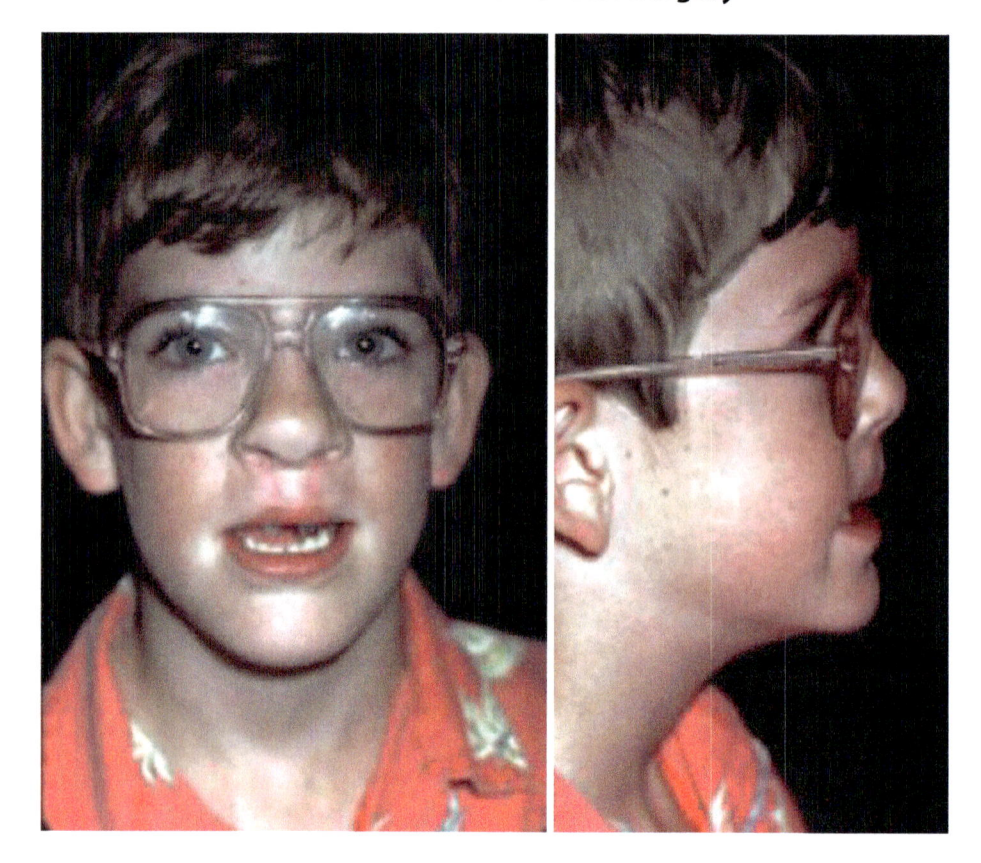

8 years

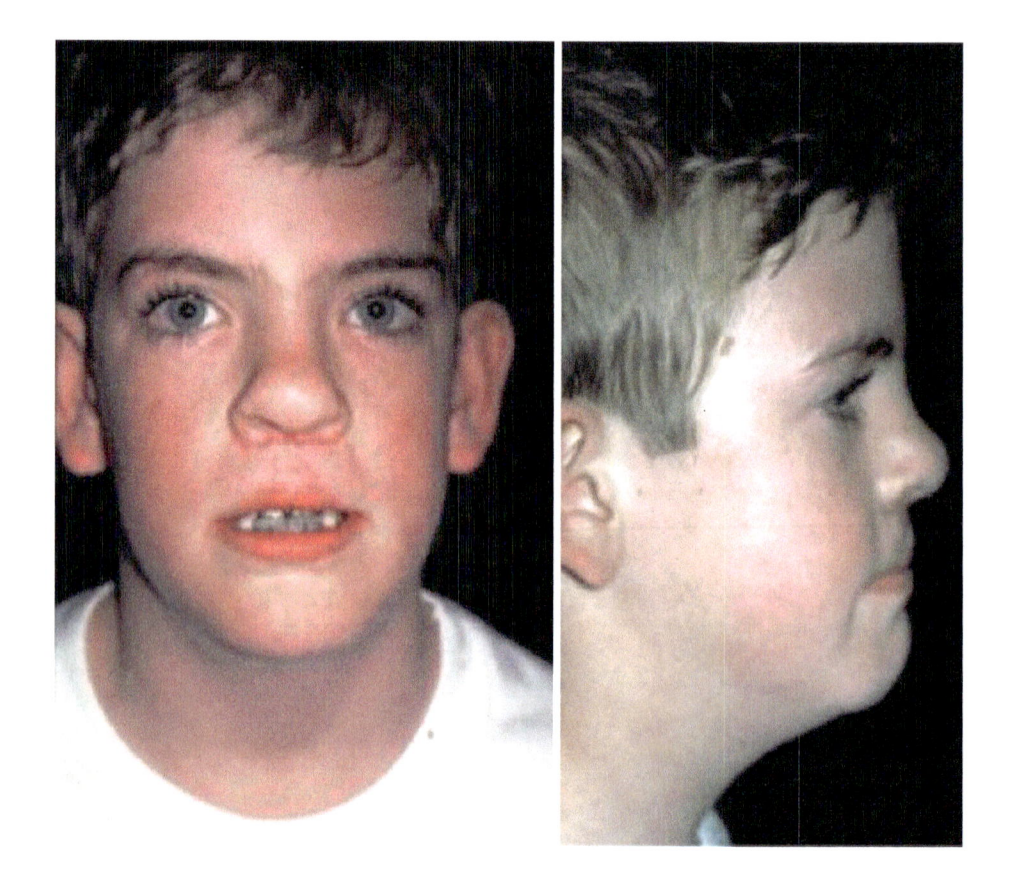

9 years

## 11.24 Recessed Mid-face With Concave Facial Profile After Surgery

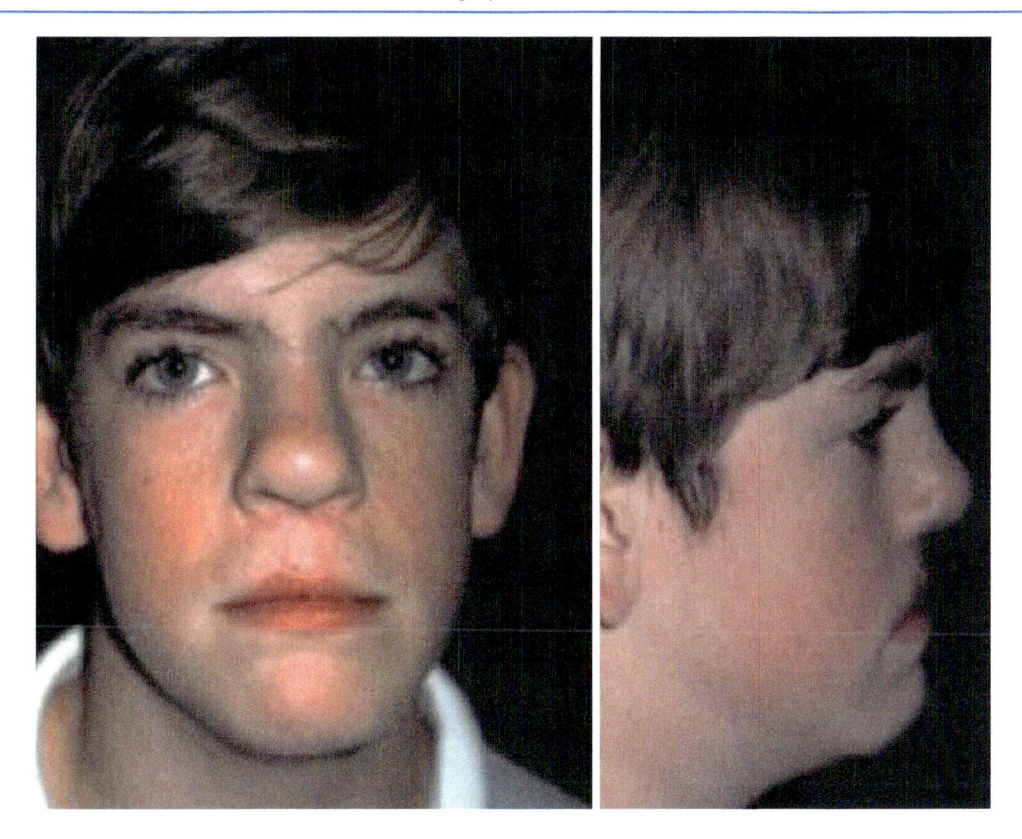

12 years

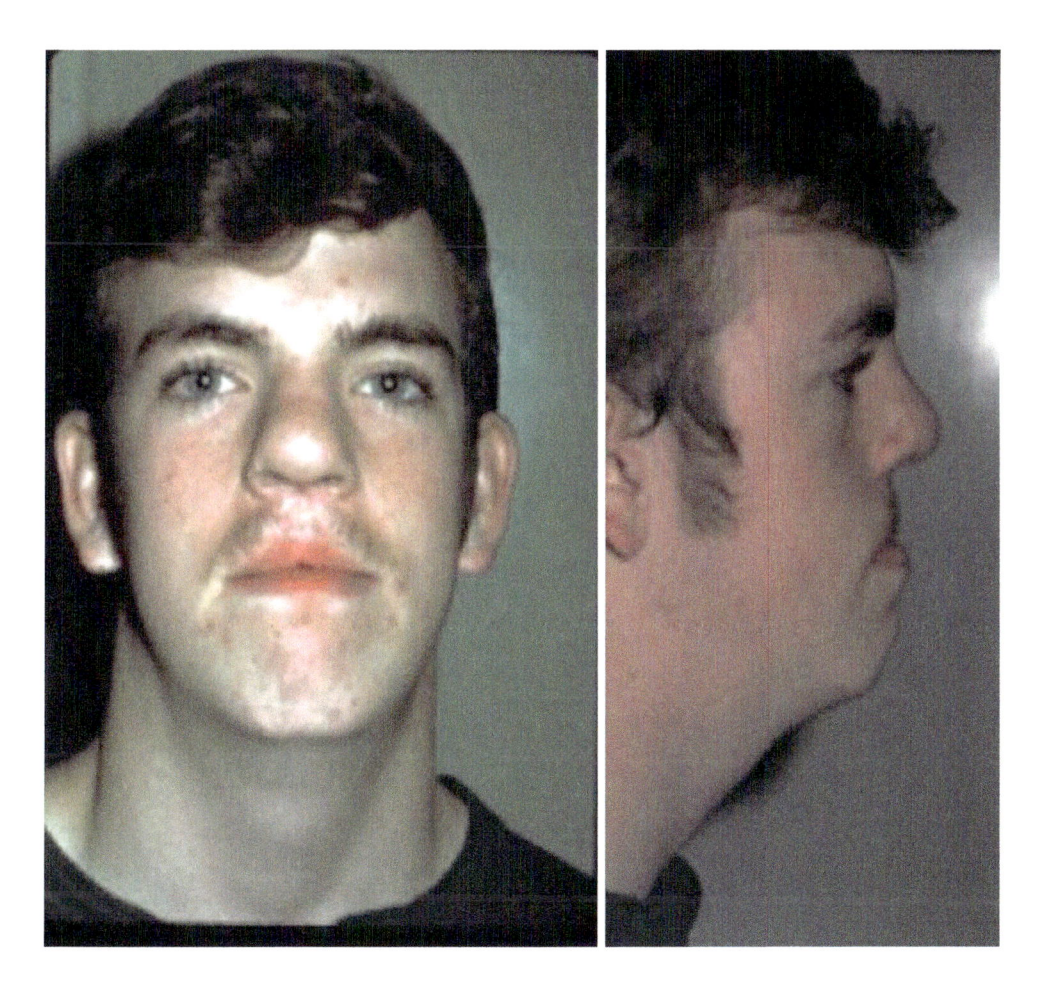

16 years

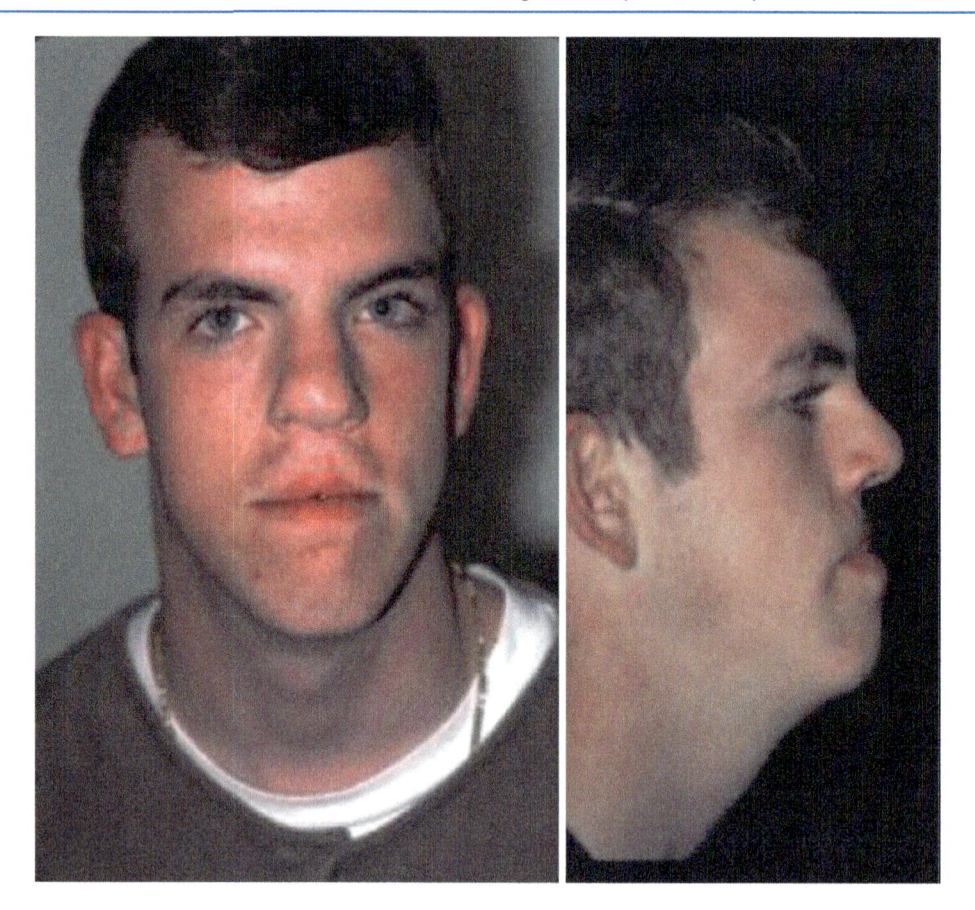

17 years

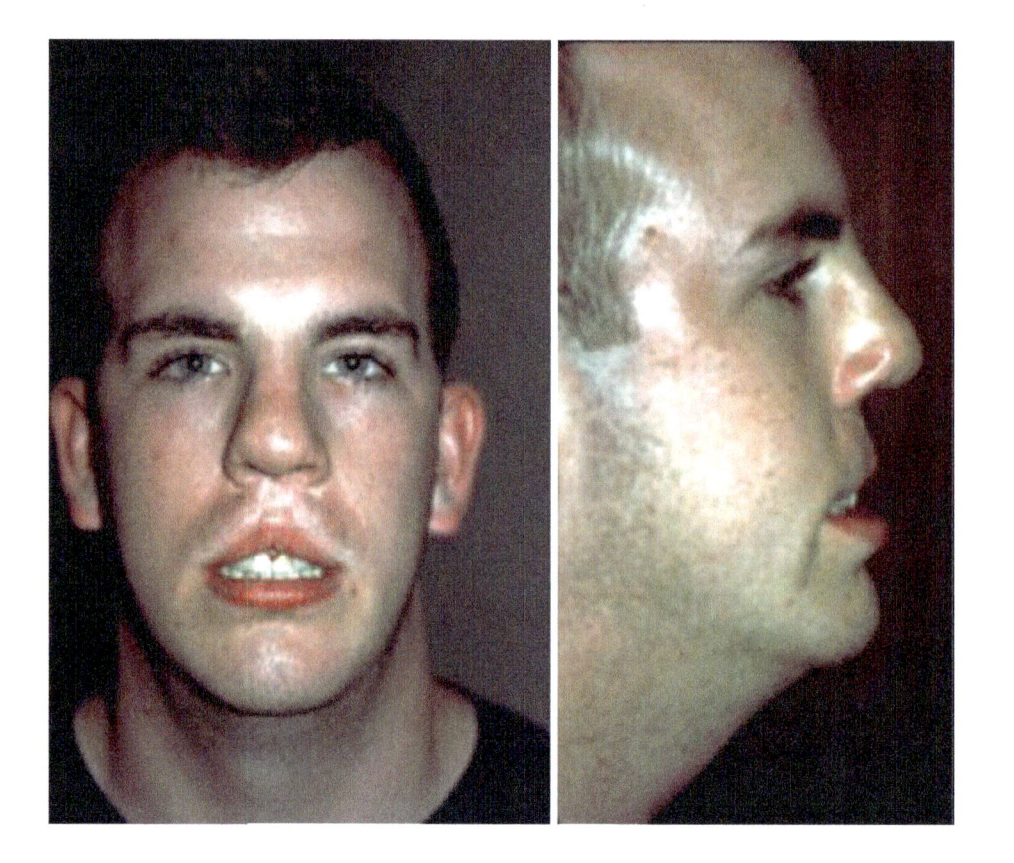

20 years

## 11.24 Recessed Mid-face With Concave Facial Profile After Surgery

Spontaneous reduction in the degree of premaxillary protrusion with good facial growth

Good overbite and overjet

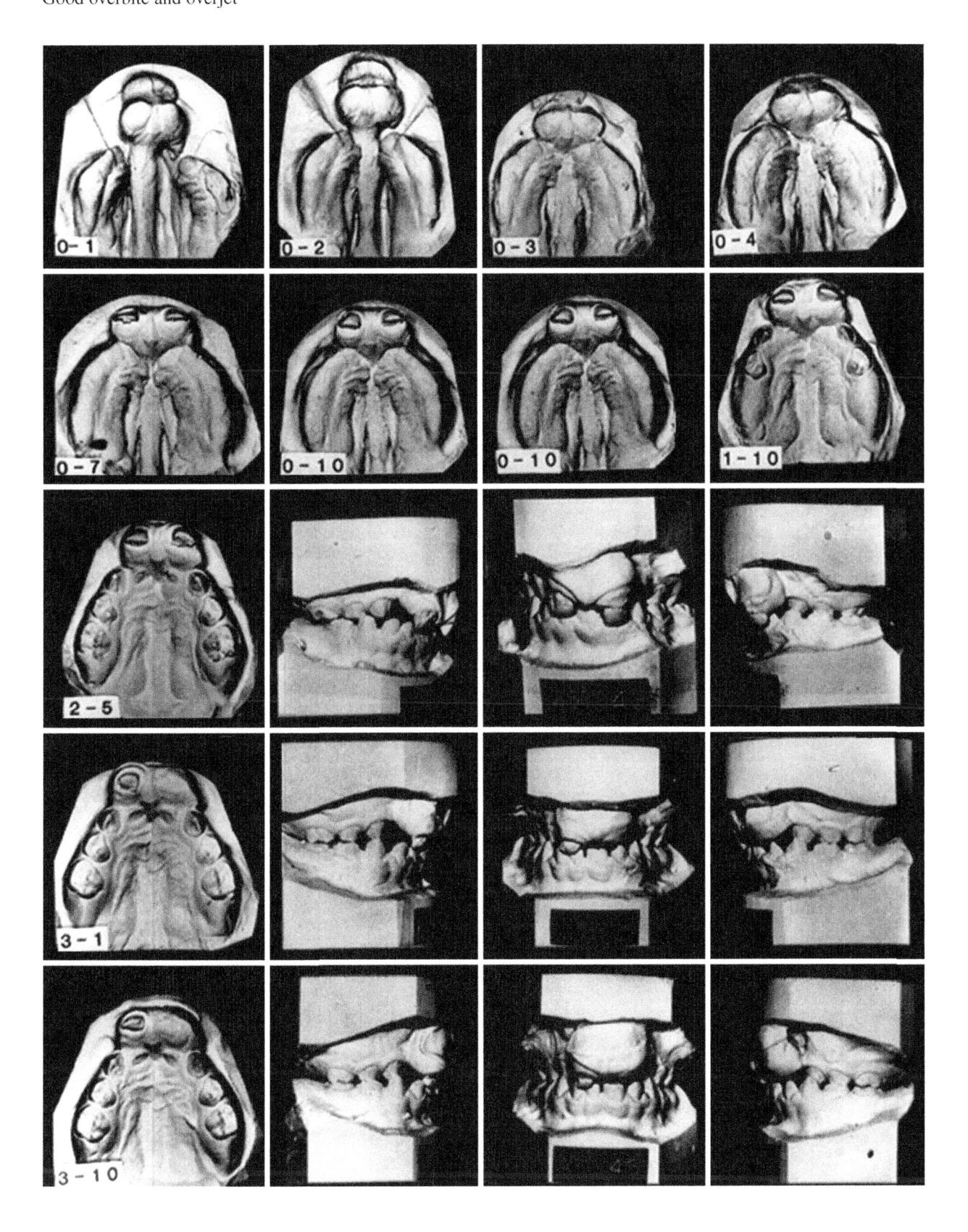

222   11 Presurgical Orthopedics with Lip Adhesion and Periosteoplasty (POPLA)

Beginning of the anterior crossbite
Unable to correct crossbite orthodontically. The use of a protraction facial mask was unsuccessful.

Anterior occlusion prior to midfacial surgical advancement
Final occlusion.
Note room for 4 anterior teeth.

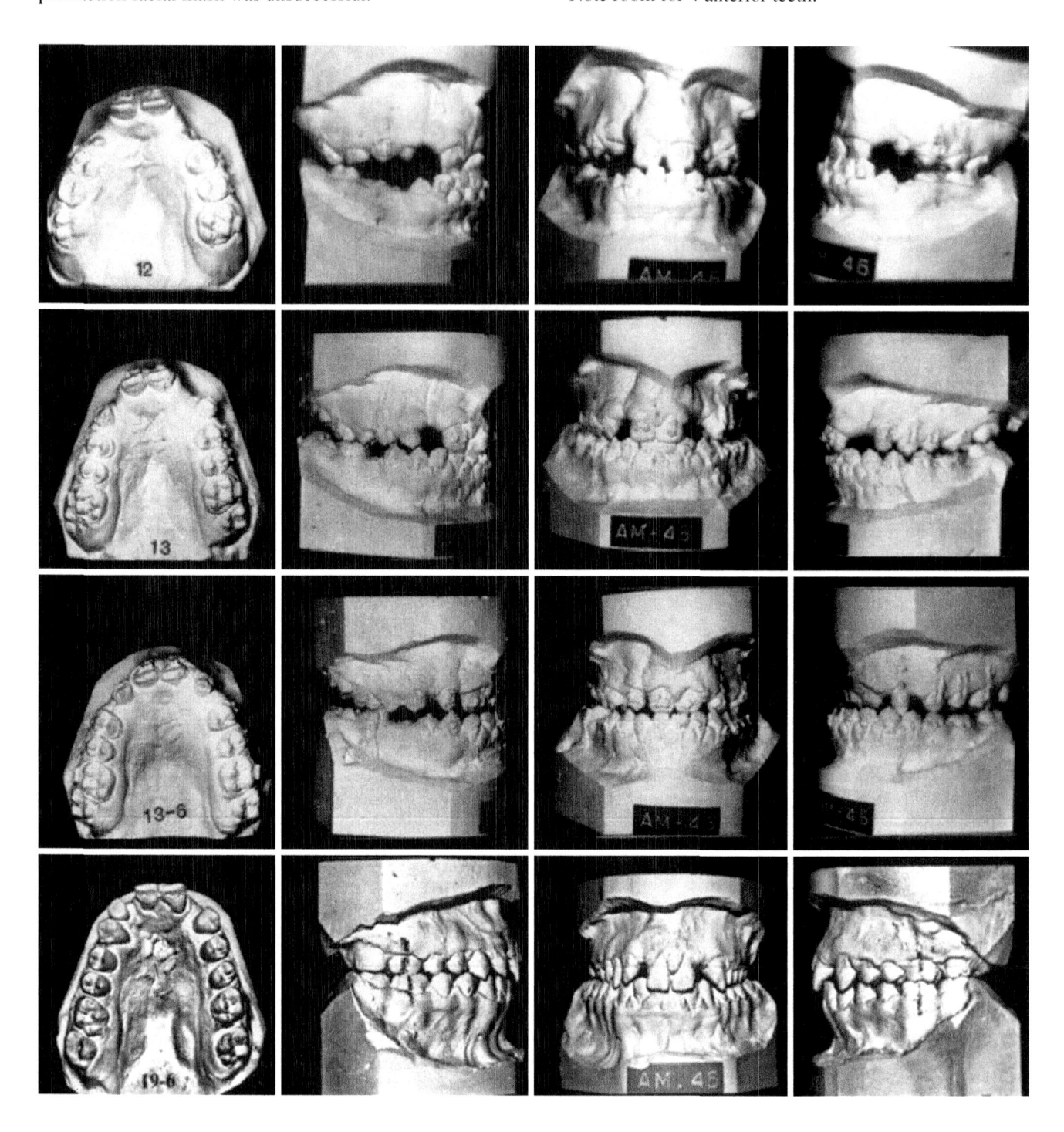

## 11.24 Recessed Midface with Concave Facial Profile After Surgery

This series of cast images is typical of most CBCLP cases. The lateral palatal segments come together behind the premaxilla. After palatal expansion, the premaxilla "falls" into proper alignment within the arch.

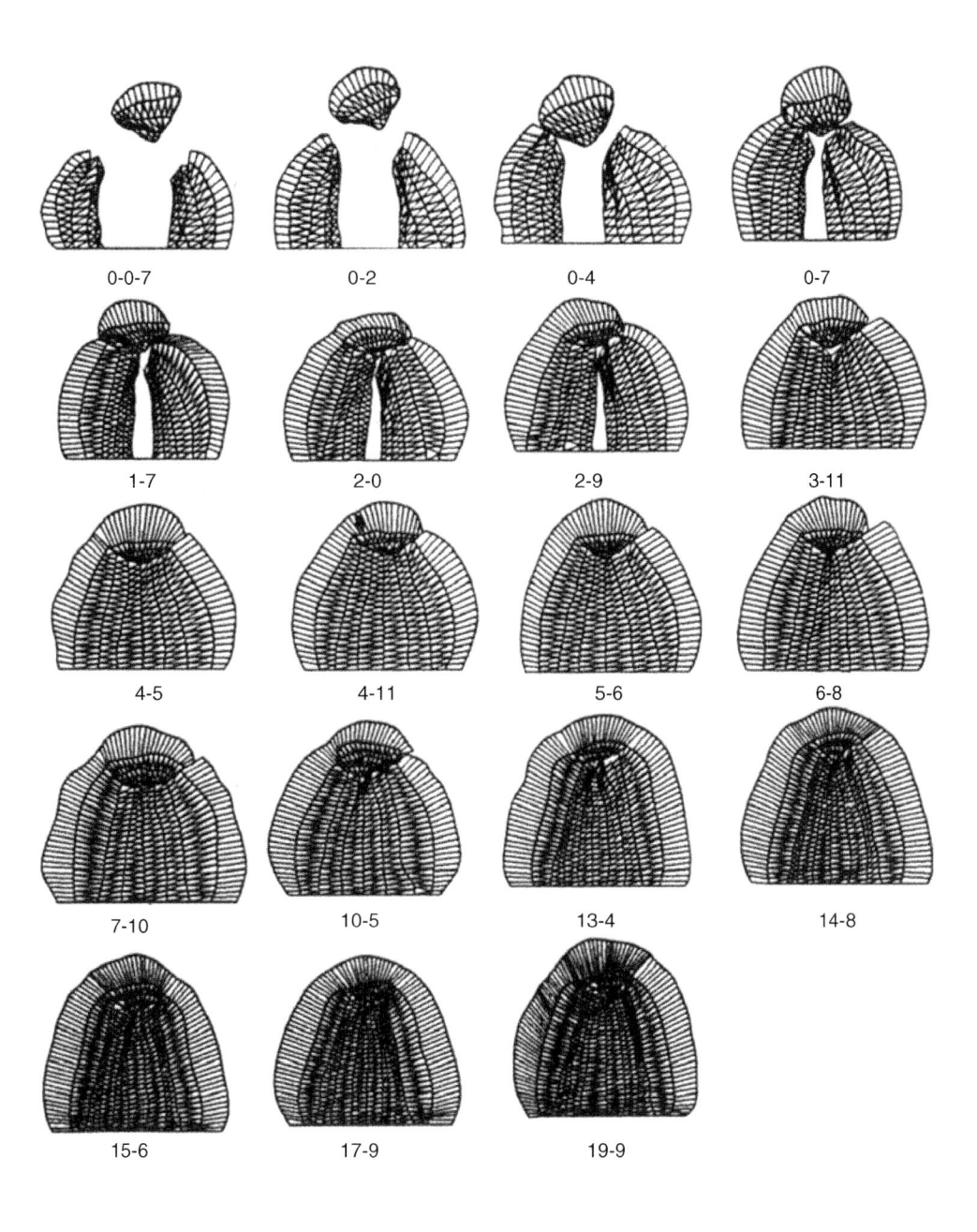

0-0-7    0-2    0-4    0-7

1-7    2-0    2-9    3-11

4-5    4-11    5-6    6-8

7-10    10-5    13-4    14-8

15-6    17-9    19-9

## 11.25 The Result of the Early Surgical Setback of the Premaxilla

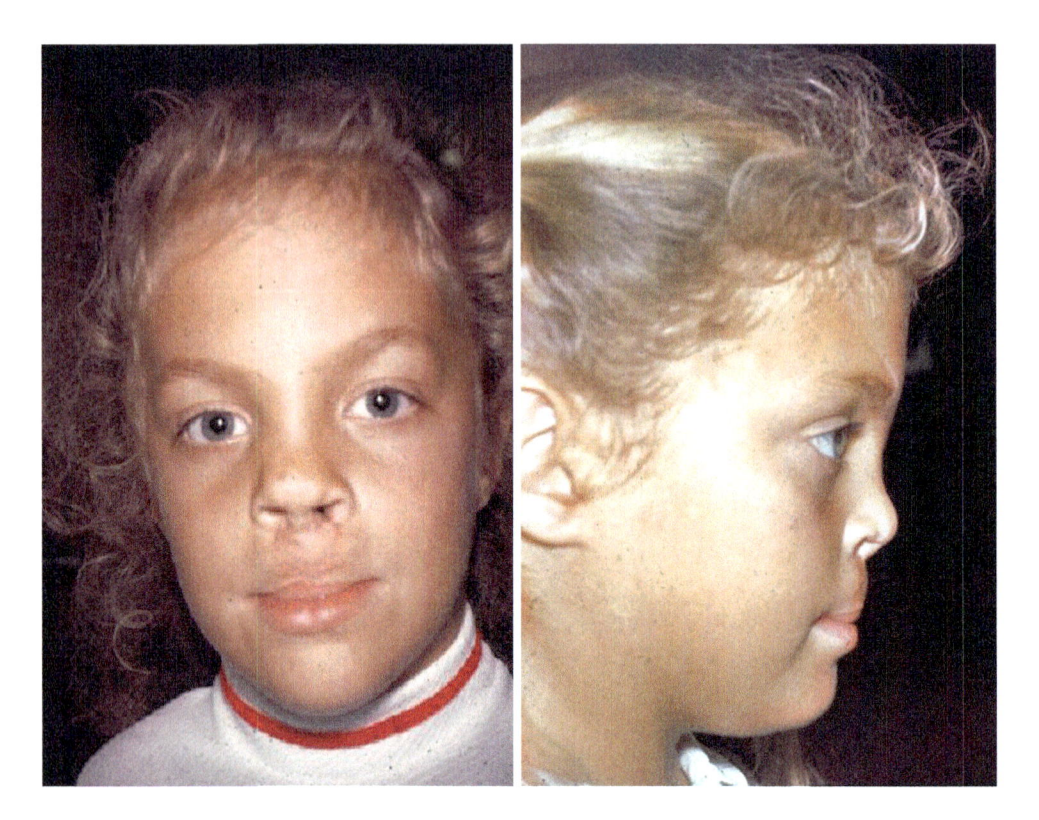

A long type upper lip due to the lateral elements being brought together beneath the prolabium.

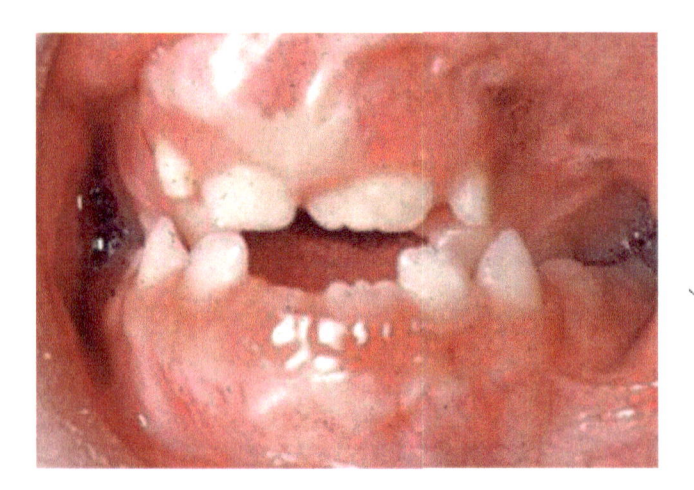

Note the premaxilla did not descend with the palate creating an anterior open bite.

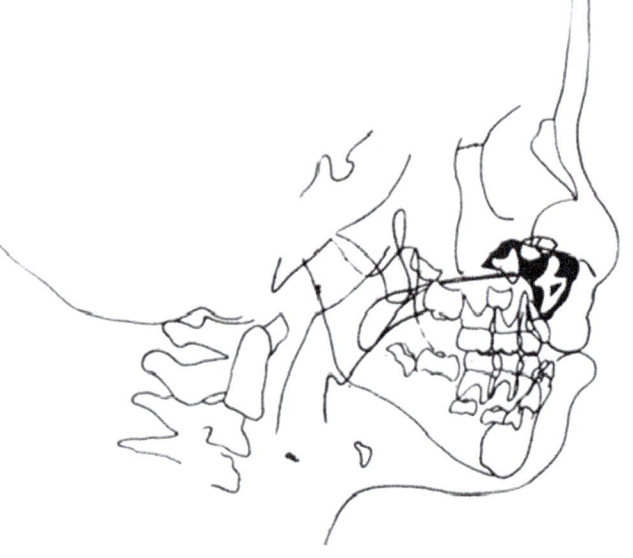

## 11.26 Orthodontic Treatment to Reduce the Anterior Openbite

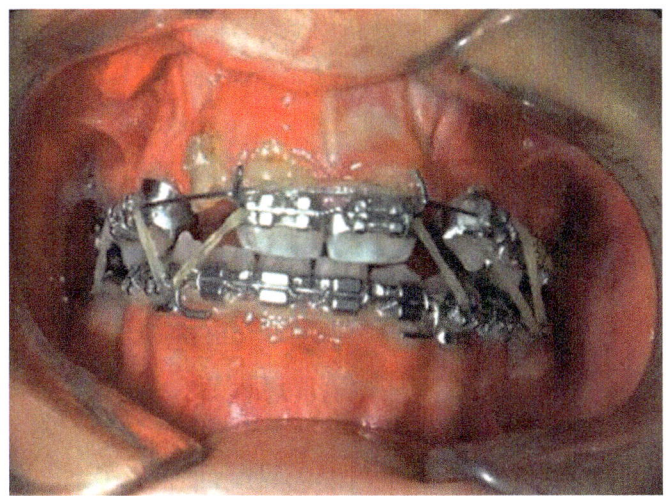

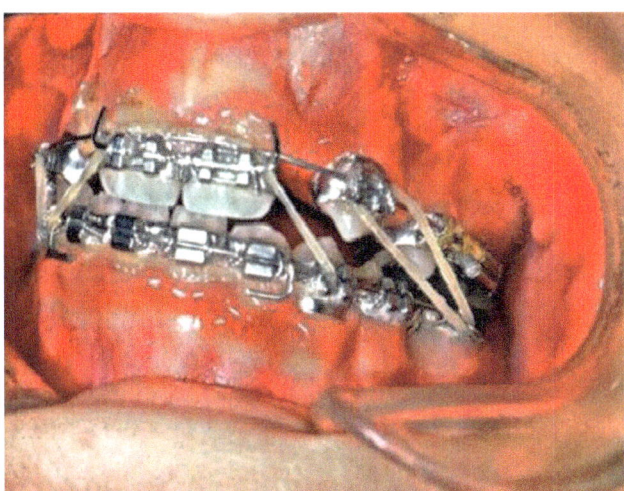

## 11.26.1 Will the Premaxilla Descend or Will the Teeth Extrude?

The detached premaxilla has failed to descend with the palatal plane.

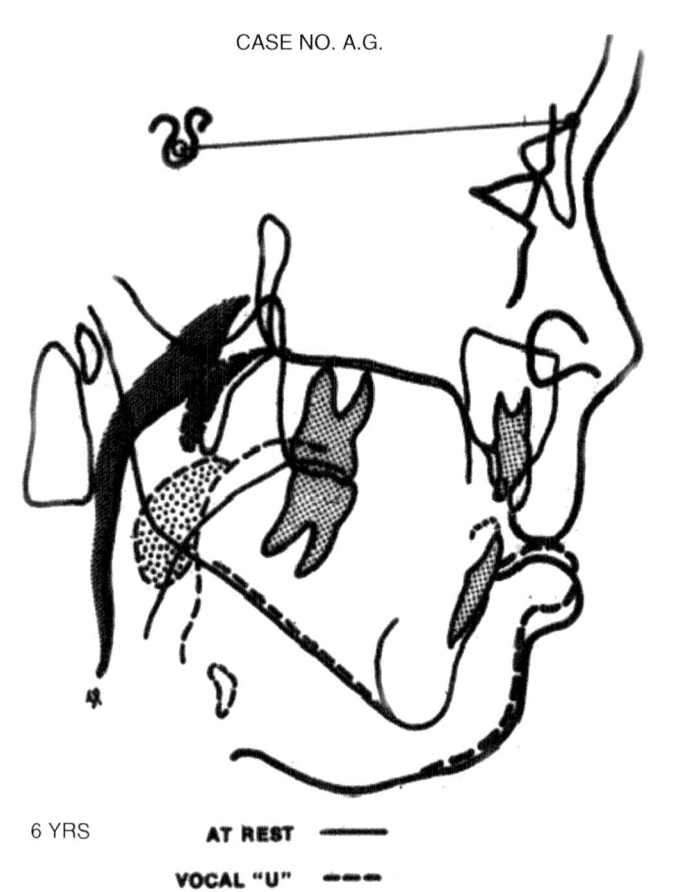

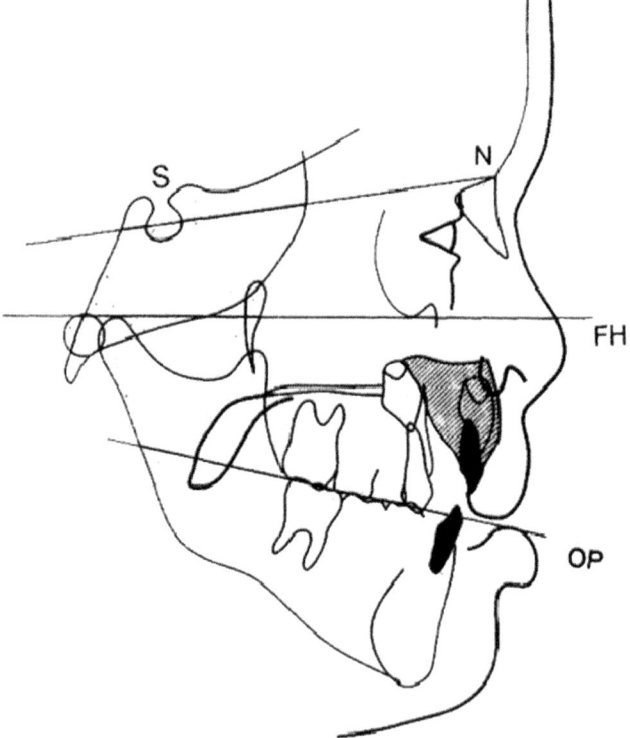

CASE NO. A.G.

6 YRS AT REST ———
VOCAL "U" ‐ ‐ ‐

With growth the palate continues to descend, however, the premaxilla only rotated

After orthodontics, the premaxilla did not change its position relative to the palatal plane, but the upper incisors were extruded.

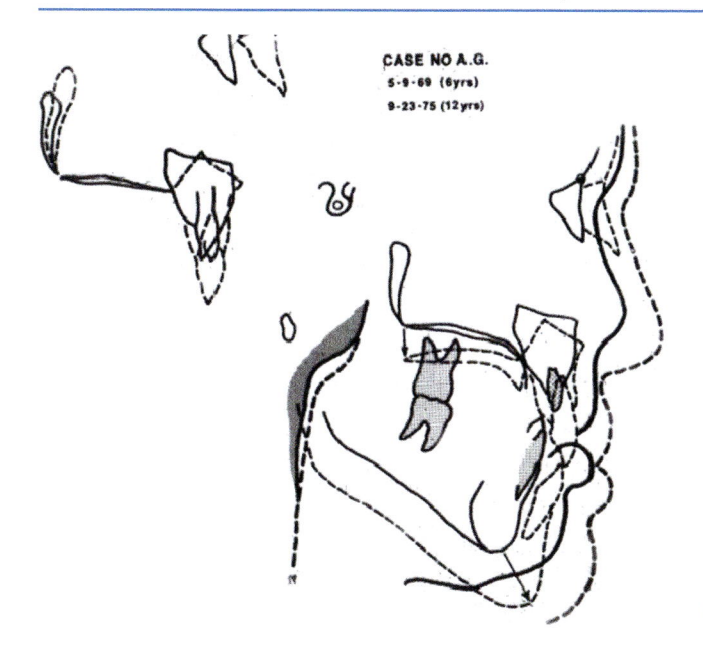

11.26  Orthodontic Treatment to Reduce the Anterior Openbite

The central incisors were extruded eliminating the open bite.

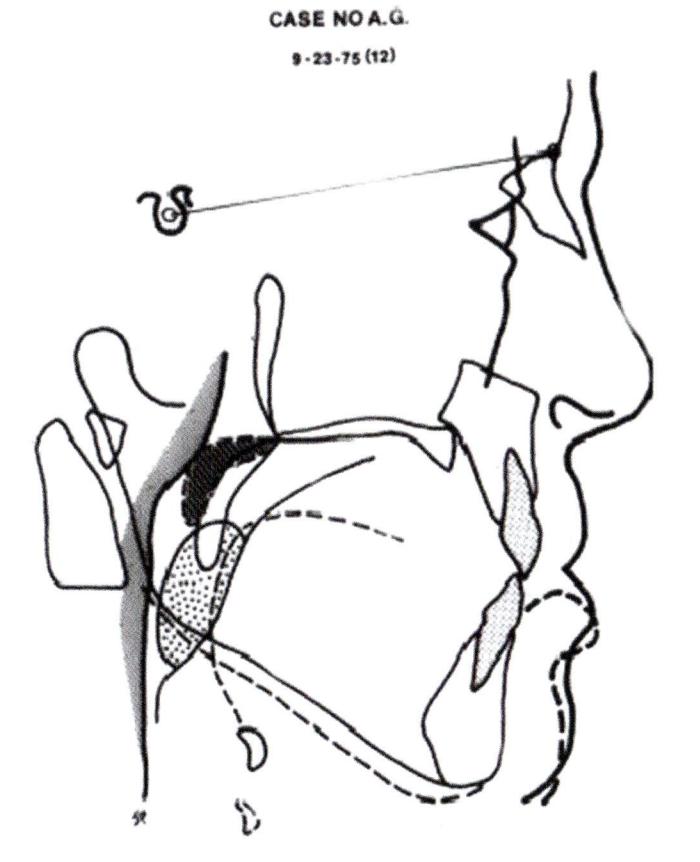

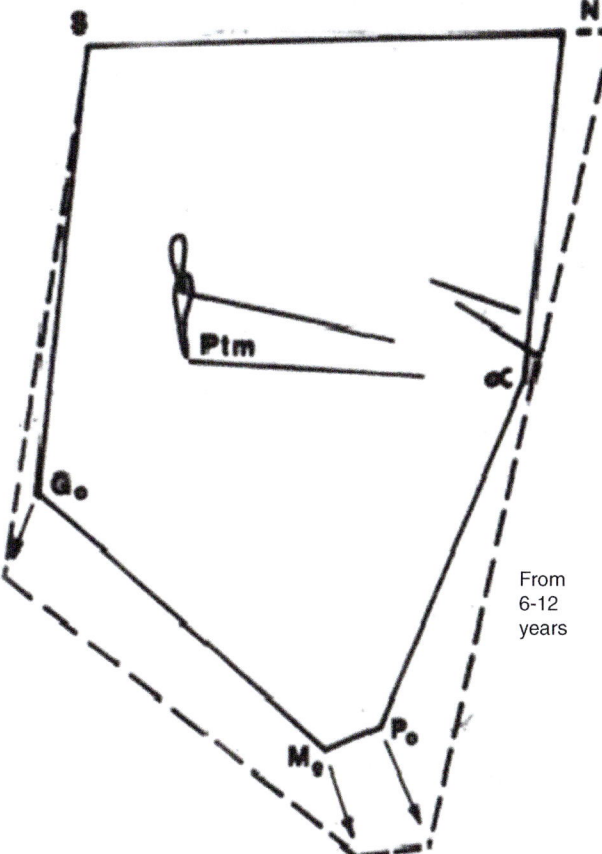

From 6-12 years

Serial casts demonstrating changes in the occlusion

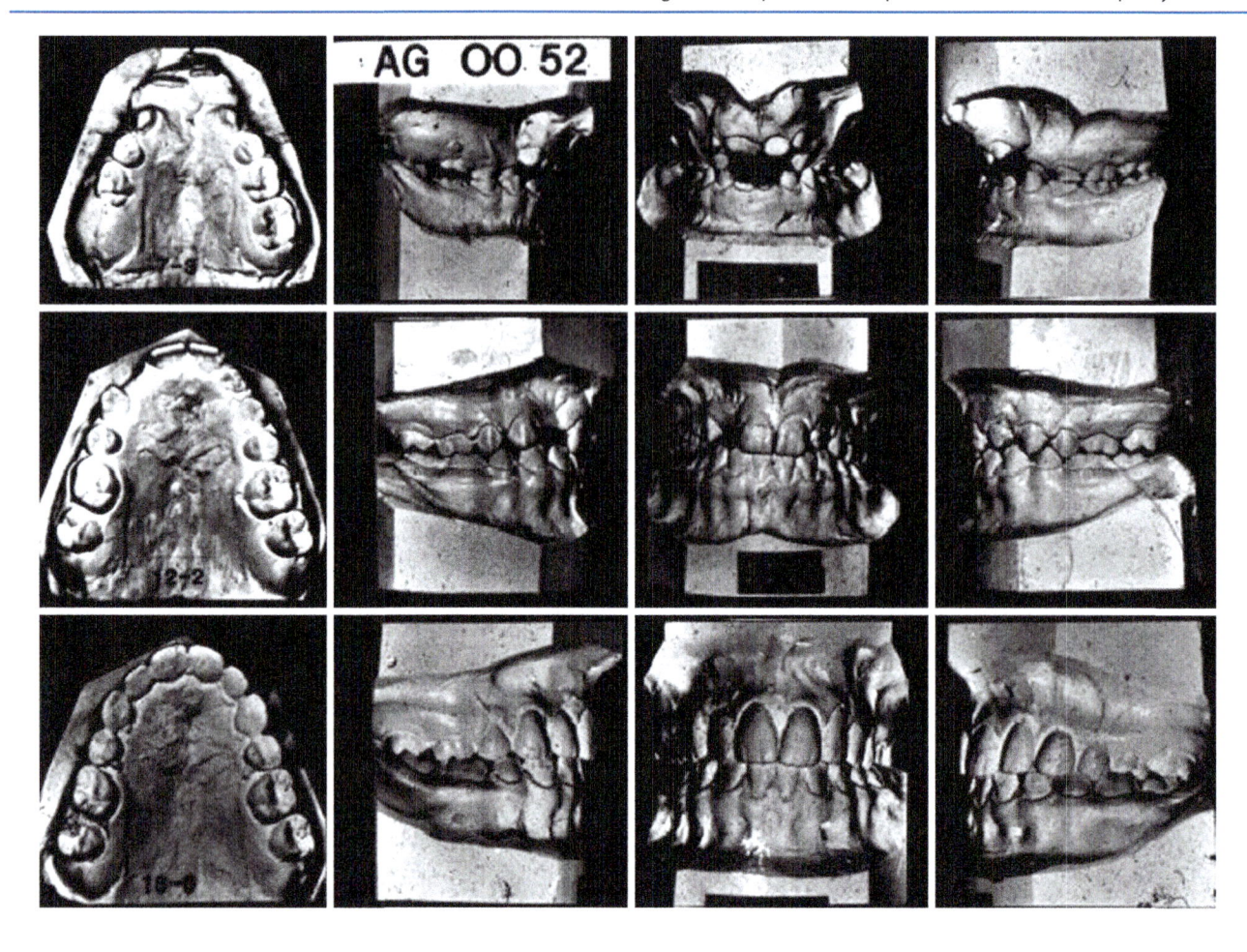

A missing lateral incisor was replaced with an anterior fixed bridge.

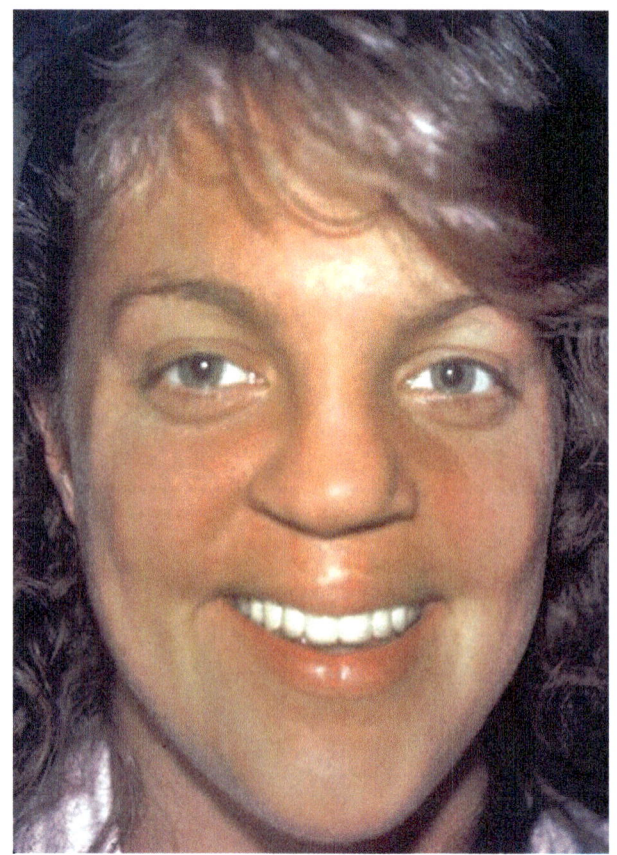

# Serial Palatal Growth Studies: Outcomes Analysis

Analyses of the initial state prior to palatal surgery (end of first period) suggest that under certain conditions surgical repair of the palate is feasible quite early, while in other instances, optimal conditions for repair will not be present until a later age. In our experience, a selected number of cases with relatively small cleft spaces underwent palatal repair at or before one year of age without detriment to midface growth. On the other hand, there are cases where the cleft space is too large when compared to the amount of available soft tissue, so surgery needs to be postponed to avoid creating growth inhibiting scar tissue. This is an example of individualized differential diagnosis and treatment planning.

If we assume that qualified surgeons within a given institution or region, practicing a specific series of techniques over a given period of time, represent a constant, the differences in success or failure should reside in the initial state (the size relationship of the palatal segments displacement). Of course, the sample must separate cases subjected or not subjected to presurgical maxillary orthopedics, as well as cases utilizing various cleft closure procedures since these variables can influence the subsequent state. This has been done in this study. Of the three components, the maneuver presented the greatest number of confounding variables. Difference between surgeons, variances in the performance by the same surgeon from day to day and over the course of several years, and differences in techniques which are difficult to identify and compare, complicate the analysis but our biostatisticians still believe the research objective was reached. It is possible to statistically test and covary for effects due to differences between and with surgeons.

We believe that within certain defined limits, the success or failure of the surgical procedure depended more on the initial state than on the variables inherent within the maneuver. To put it another way, we expect that subtle differences among the patient will be prognostic of the subsequent state than differences between surgeons.

Serial facial and palatal growth studies starting at the newborn period have shown that too many factors were operating in relation to the patients under study to permit the formulation of simple, all-inclusive rules, such as any suggestion regarding the age at which clefts of the palate should be repaired.

Serial palatal growth studies to date have led us to believe that size and geometric relationship of the palatal segments relative to the size of cleft space prior to surgery, coupled with the surgical procedure utilized, may influence the palate's arch form and size. If it did, then the surgical skill or procedure is not solely responsible for the different outcomes. This might explain why different surgical procedures can be equally successful and conversely, why the same surgical procedure can cause a different result especially if extensive scarring has been produced.

## 12.1 Molding Complications

- There are few serious complications associated with nasoalveolar molding. The most common is irritation of the oral mucosal or gingival tissue. Intraoral tissues may ulcerate from pressure or rubbing. Common areas of breakdown are the frenum attachments, the anterior premaxilla, or the posterior fauces as the molding plate is retracted.
- The intranasal lining of the nasal tip can become inflamed if too much force is applied by the upper lobe of the nasal stent. Notching along the alar rim can occur if the lower lobe is not positioned or shaped correctly. The area under the horizontal prolabium band can become ulcerated if the band is too tight.
- The most common area of tissue irritation is the cheeks. It must be emphasized that the tapes should be removed slowly and carefully so as to avoid skin irritation. The use of tape removal solvents or warm water can facilitate removal of tapes. If the tissue remains irritated, a skin barrier such as Duoderm™ or Tegaderm™ can be used as a base on which the tape-elastic retraction system can be

attached. It is sometimes recommended that aloe vera gel be applied to the cheeks when changing tapes.
- Poor compliance by the parents can cause loss of valuable treatment time.
- There is a small risk that molding plate will become dislodged and obstruct the airway. Taping the arms too horizontally or with inadequate activation will increase the possibility that the posterior border of the molding plate will drop down onto the tongue. There is only one reported incidence in which this happened, causing a temporary airway obstruction. They place a 5mm diameter hole in the center of the molding plate at fabrication to provide for passage of air in the event that the molding plate drops down from the palate onto the tongue. In the unlikely event that this occurs, the hole, centrally located on the palatal portion of the molding plate, can provide adequate airflow.

## 12.2 Latham Presurgical Orthopedic Procedure

Complete unilateral cleft lip and palate, 3 years ± 6 months

| Case # | Class I Right | Class I Left | Class II Right | Class II Left | Class III Right | Class III Left | Anterior Crossbite Right | Anterior Crossbite Left | Buccal Crossbite Right | Buccal Crossbite Left | Tip to Tip Right | Tip to Tip Left |
|---|---|---|---|---|---|---|---|---|---|---|---|---|
| AZ41 | X | X | | | | | | | | | | |
| AZ91 | X | X | | | | | AB | A | | | C | |
| BA97 | | | | | | | | | | | CDE | |
| BD31 b | X | X | | | | | | | | | A | |
| BD83 | X | X | | | | | | | | | | |
| BD89 | X | X | | | | | A | | | | | |
| BD40 | | X | X | | | | A | A | CD | | C | |
| BD54 | X | X | | | | | | | | | | |
| BD12 | | | | | | | | A | | | C | |
| BF59 c | X | X | | | | | AB | A | | | C | |
| BF70 | X | X | | | | | | B | | | C | |
| BG76 | X | X | | | | | AB | A | C | | C | |
| BG85 | | | X | X | | | A | A | | | | |
| BG86 | X | | | X | | | | | | | | |
| B127 | X | X | | | | | | | | | | |

a—4 years 5 months; b—years; 2 years 5 months; d—3 years 7 months; e—2 years 2 months; &—alveolar bone in crossbite although teeth are missing

## 12.3 Latham Presurgical Orthopedic Procedure

Complete unilateral cleft lip and palate, 12 years ± 6 months

| Case # | Class I Right | Class I Left | Class II Right | Class II Left | Class III Right | Class III Left | Anterior Crossbite Right | Anterior Crossbite Left | Buccal Crossbite Right | Buccal Crossbite Left | Tip to Tip Right | Tip to Tip Left |
|---|---|---|---|---|---|---|---|---|---|---|---|---|
| AW18 a | X | X | | | | | 1 | | 3 | | | |
| AY27 b | X | X | | | | | 1 | 1 | | 3 | | |
| AZ41 c T | X | X | | | | | | | | | | |
| AZ91 d | X | X | | | | | 12 | 1 | 4 | 4 | | |
| BA32 | X | X | | | | | | | | | | |
| BD31 e | X | X | | | | | | | | | | 2 |
| BD83 | X | X | | | | | | | | | | |
| BD40 | | X | X | | | | 1 | 1 | E4 | C | | 4 |
| BD54 | X | X | | | | | | | | | | 5 |
| BD59 f | X | X | | | | | 12 | 12 | C | C | | |
| BF70 g T | X | X | | | | | | | | | | |
| BF85 h | X | X | | | | | | | | | | |
| BF86 T | X | X | | | | | 1 | 1 | | | 3 | 3 |
| BI90 i T | X | X | | | | | 1 | 12 | 3456 | 3567 | | |
| BK 83 T | X | X | | | | | | | | | E | |
| BL63 i | X | X | | | | | 1 | 12 | | | | |

a—12 years 9 months; b—11 years; c—11 years; d—11 years; e—13 years; f—10 years; g—11 years; h—11 years; i—11 years 4 months; j—10 years 3 months; k—10 years 3 months; I—11 years; &—alveolar bone in crossbite although teeth are missing; T—under treatment

## 12.4 Northwestern: Rosenstein and Kernahan

Presurgical Orthopedics in CUCLP and CBCLP

(a) CUCLP: An appliance is fabricated and inserted at the posterior half of the palate. Lip adhesion molds the anterior half of the segments into butt contact. Primary bone graft using the Kernahan procedure.

Should the palatal segments overlap, an expansion appliance is used to allow for proper molding of the palatal segments prior to the placement of the primary bone graft.

(b) CBCLP: The appliance will hold the lateral alveolar segments apart until the premaxilla has been placed in close approximation within the palatal segments.

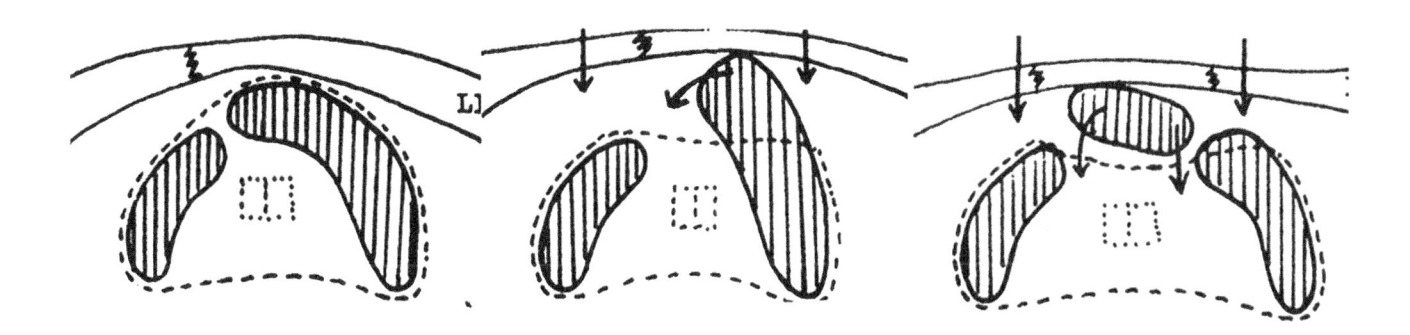

## 12.5 Serial Palatal Growth Changes After Various Forms of Treatment

**Normal Palate**

**No Presurgical Orthopedics**

*Premaxilla remains in the same place within the palate.*

Superimposed serial casts of non-cleft and CBCLP and CUCLP casts.

**The CBCLP**: The premaxilla is not retruded but ventroflexed. It then remains constant in the same relationship to the lateral segments as the palate grows in width and in length. The premaxilla remains in the same spatial relationship in all successfully treated cases. This holds true in complete **CUCLP** cases as well. The A-P palatal length increases posteriorly to permit the eruption of the permanent molars.

# A Multicenter Retrospective International 3D Study of Serial CUCLP and CBCLP Casts: To Determine When to Close the Palatal Cleft Space and the Need for Stages of Treatment as the Palate Grows

## 13.1 Study Design

Multicenter comparisons of surgical-orthodontic treatment outcomes using prospective and retrospective methods are the most efficient way of testing the effectiveness of various treatment philosophies and surgical techniques. Differences among surgeons, variances in performance by the same surgeon over the years, and differences in technique are difficult to identify and compare in isolation; however, in multicenter clinical studies, difference in clinical procedures among operators can, within certain defined limits, be compared and evaluated.

Because many of the participating institutions have continually used the same procedure even when using different surgeons, this helped answer such important questions such as: which variables previously listed are clinically the most significant? Why varying procedures might yield the same results even when performed by different surgeons. And, what are the significant factors that make these outcomes possible? Our biostatisticians believed the variabilities could still be examined.

Each of the subsamples of cleft children was compared to each other and to the age appropriate control samples. A variety of complex hypotheses concerning difference in means, treatment effects, and predictive relationships among variables were tested using multivariate statistical tests and longitudinal analysis models. Recent methods for separating out treatment from growth effects and regression effects were also applied.

## 13.2 3D Palatal Cast Velocity and Surface Area Growth Changes

Angular measurements derived from lateral cephalograms do not characterize adequately the three-dimensional nature of palatal growth. Virtually all studies of CLP using longitudinal samples have suffered from naïve statistical analyses. None have described or contrasted growth curves using appropriate longitudinal models.

Consistency in treatment strategies within each of these centers minimized the number of confounding variables while retaining a good overall sample size:

(a) Velocity—All growth changes show diminished growth by 18–24 months of age, sometimes earlier or later, when measured from successfully treated cases.
(b) Palatal soft tissue growth changes measured laterally from the alveolar ridge to the edge of the cleft space showed an average of 10% diminished growth between 18 and 24 months in all cases.
(c) 2D measurements taken from x-rays of casts showed a 5% decrease of the average growth measurements when compared to 3D measurements plus or minus 3 months is acceptable.

It is essential to know whether bone surrounding the cleft space can increase in dimensions and if it does to what degree and for how long incremental change (catch-up-growth) will take place. Such information could influence decisions as the best time to close the cleft space surgically. Berkowitz (15) has suggested that the surgeon should consider the possibility that growth at the cleft border can reduce the cleft space size and should in some instances delay the surgical procedures accordingly. Thus, the timing of palatal surgery should not be based on the patient's age alone. In some instances, when the cleft space is narrow, it can be closed early; however, when the cleft space is very wide, in Berkowitz's view, it would perhaps be wiser to wait for additional growth of the palatal processes to occur.

The great differences in opinion on all aspects of the nature of cleft palate highlights the need to measure palatal dimensions accurately and to determine where and what changes might occur with time. Only then will there be a better understanding of the influences of all aspects of treatment on palatal and occlusal development.

## 13.3 The Need for Three-Dimensional Measuring Techniques

Quantitative information relative to the normal palate is noticeably sparse because of measuring limitations inherence in using various forms of calipers and rulers. Some linear dimensional studies on the form of the newborn arch were performed by Ashley-Montague (33), Sillman (34), (35), Richardson (36), and Brash (37).

Unfortunately, there is no information regarding surface area and form changes that can be utilized for comparative studies of the cleft population.

Xerographic (2D) studies of casts were an advance over previous measuring systems, since they permitted a more accurate description of two-dimensional changes in surface area. Huddart (37), (38) concluded from these measurements that in complete unilateral clefts of the lip and/or palate (CUCL/P) the palatal surface area is deficient by age 16 when compared with a normal population of the same age. Huddart suggested that presurgical orthopedics may hinder palatal growth.

In 1971, Mazaheri et al. (39) and coworkers reported on changes in arch form and dimensions associated with unilateral clefts of lip and palate and cleft palate. They found a significant pattern of anteroposterior and lateral growth retardation immediately after surgical treatment.

Stockli (40) was very critical of his own research approach and reported that there are great limitations in the use of xerography for the study of cleft palate casts. He emphasized that arch form must be considered in the treatment of an infant with complete cleft of the lip and palate, and recognized that three-dimensional measurements would be more appropriate for longitudinal and comparative studies.

# Questions to Be Answered

- Why do US and European speech specialists differ on the timing of palatal closure?
- Does vomer flap surgery performed at 2–3 years of age interfere with palatal growth?
- Does palatal scarring interfere with palatal growth?
- Why is the timing of palatal closure based on the age and not on the extent of the palatal defect (cleft space) relative to palatal mucosal surface medial to the alveolar ridges?
- Does presurgical orthopedics stimulate palatal development?
- Why should there be a priority of goals—speech-language pathologists say 1st speech, 2nd aesthetics, 3rd dental function? Surgeons say 1st should be facial aesthetics.
- Are not all goals attainable?
- Is it necessary to postpone palatal closure until 5–9 years of age in order to obtain the smallest cleft space at the time of surgery? Is this necessary for maximum palatal growth?
- Using late (5–9 years) cleft palatal closure cases as the standard for comparison:

Do cases closed between 18 and 24 months of age grow as well?
Can their faces be equally as aesthetic and have good dental function as well as excellent facial aesthetics?

## 14.1 To Determine When to Close the Palatal Cleft Space

A three-dimensional palatal growth study from birth to adolescence was performed with the achievement of a research grant of $500,000.

This was made possible by the creation of a three-dimensional measuring machine made for the program by the United States *National Aeronautical Space Association* (*NASA*).

Serial casts were sent to the *Miami Craniofacial Anomalies Foundation* lab from select European cleft palate centers.

# Making of 3D Measurements of Serial Cleft Palate Casts

It demonstrates images in segmental palatal position and the changes in size over time:

(a) In CUCLP: only that of the right and left segments and the cleft space.
(b) In CBCLP: all 3 segments. It demonstrates that the bodily retruded premaxilla is retarded in anterior growth but this does not happen with the ventroflexed premaxilla which stays in its original anterior-posterior position.

Occlusal and periapical films of the premaxilla and lateral palatal segments: the close contact of the deciduous central incisors and rotated unerupted central incisors reflect a deficiency of premaxillary bone growth at the mid palatal suture area.

240  15 Making of 3D Measurements of Serial Cleft Palate Casts

## 15.1 Palatal Landmarks

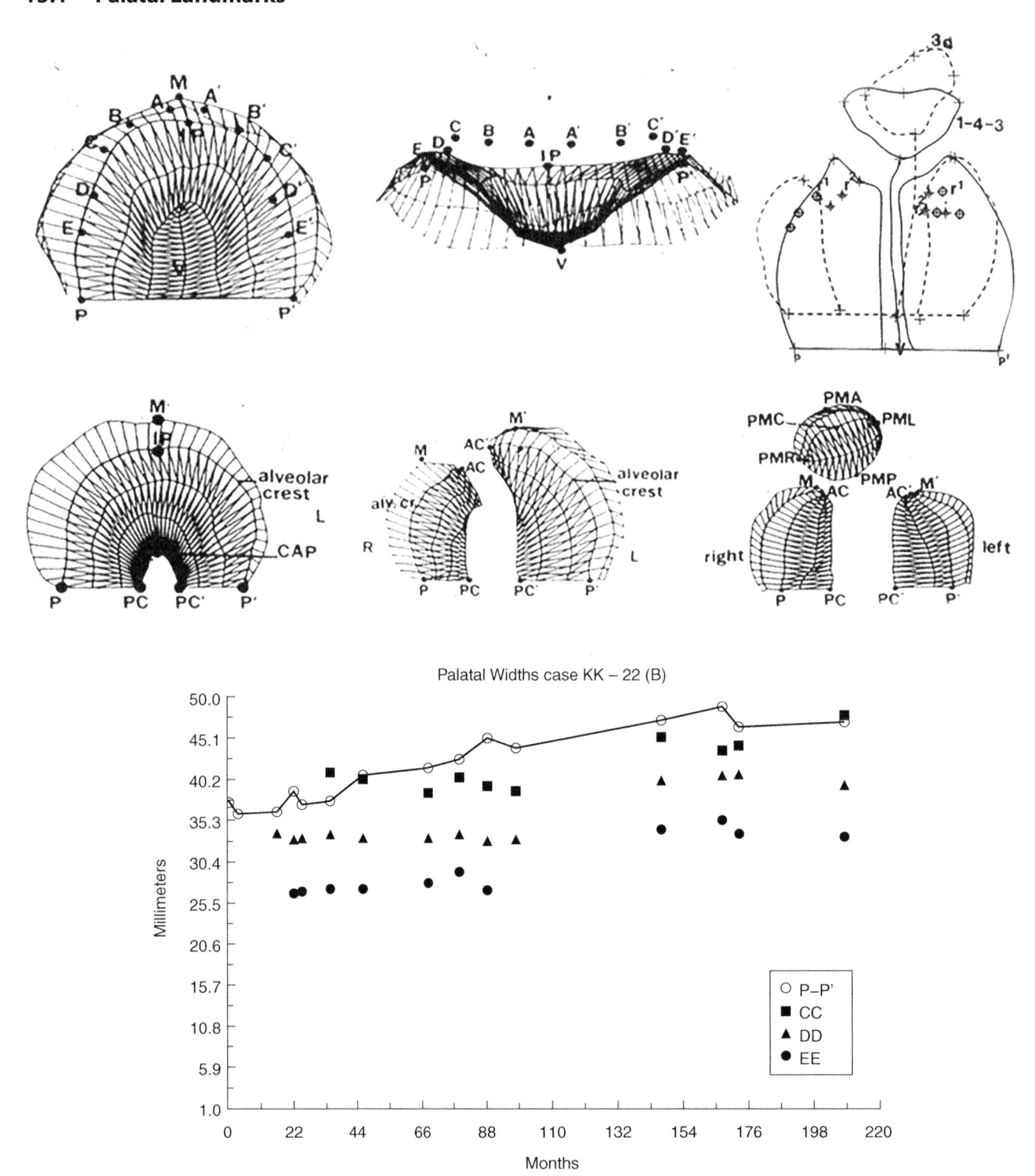

## 15.1 Palatal Landmarks

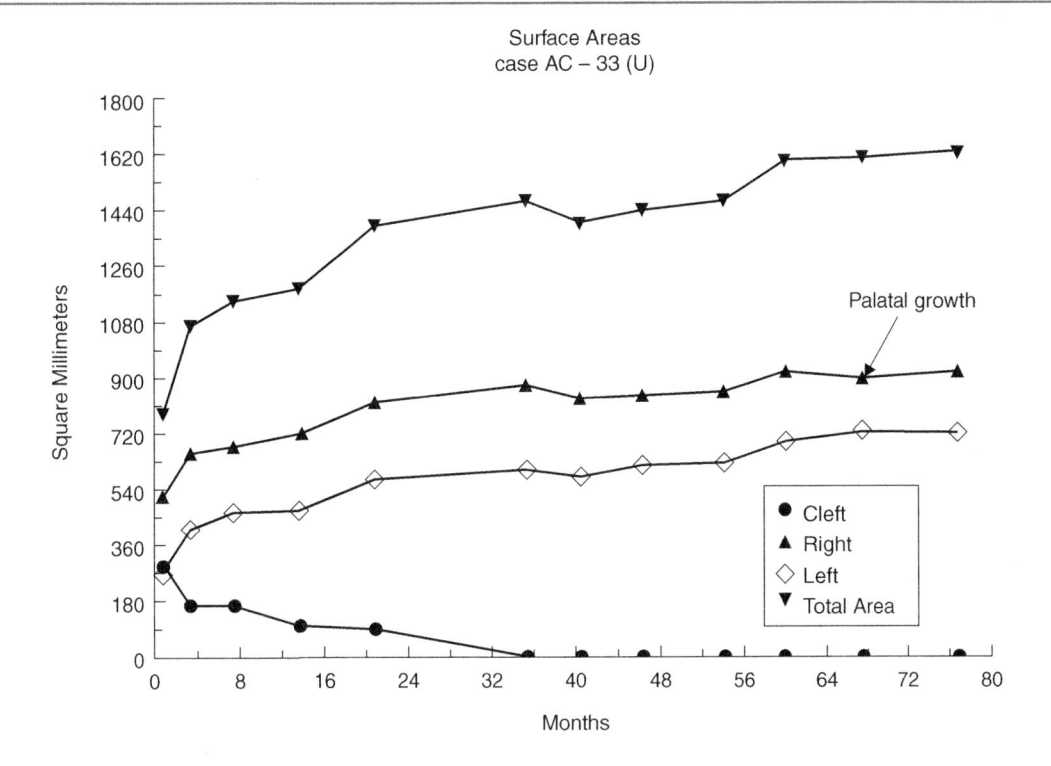

Surface Areas
case AC – 33 (U)

Palatal growth

- ● Cleft
- ▲ Right
- ◇ Left
- ▼ Total Area

## 15.2 Rapid Palatal Growth the First Year

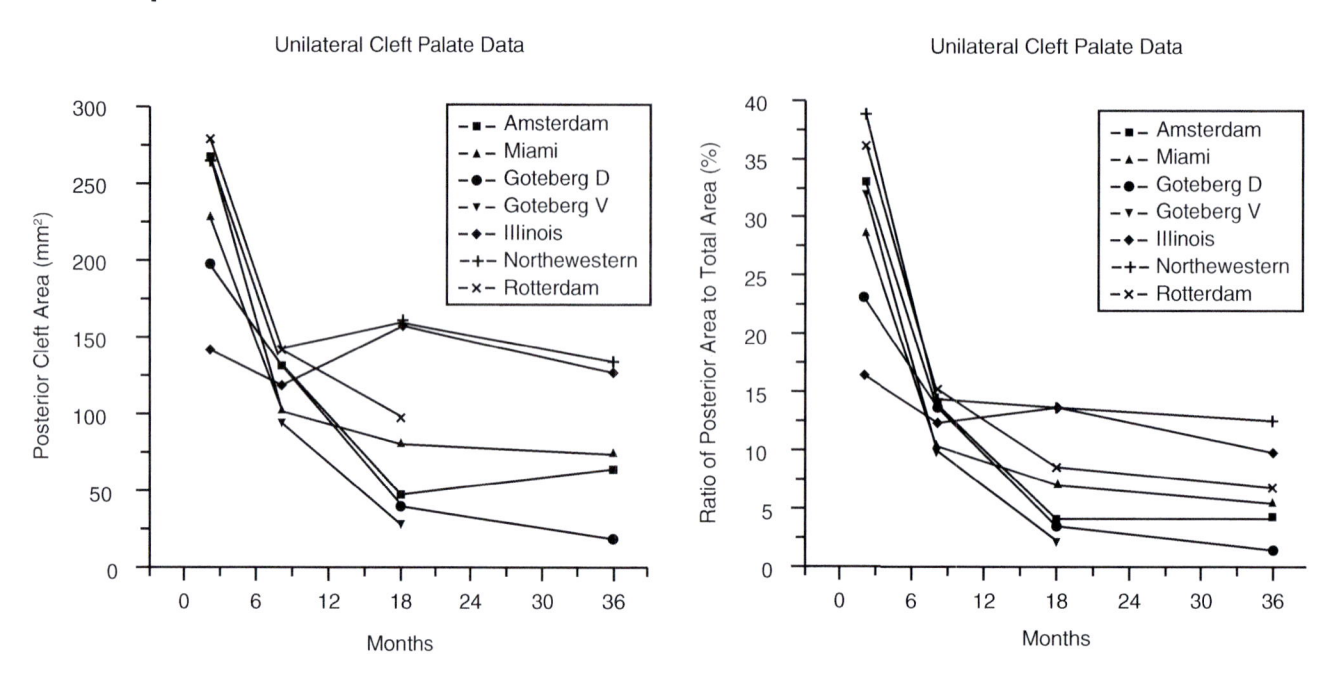

Posterior palatal growth is mostly rapid for the first 18 months. The ratio of cleft space to palatal size medial to the alveolar ridges averages at 10% at 18 months.

## 15.2 Rapid Palatal Growth the First Year

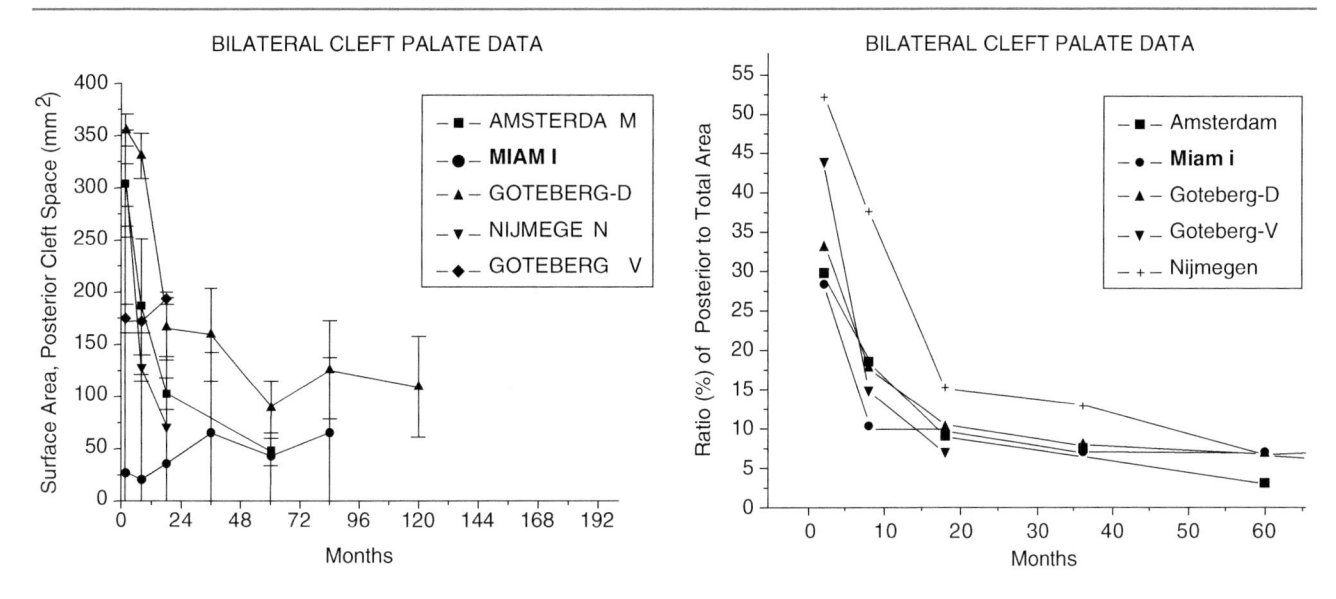

- Those cases that were treated with PSO had a larger cleft space at 24 months.
- The ratio of cleft space to total surface area in practically all cases was the same between 10 and 20 months.

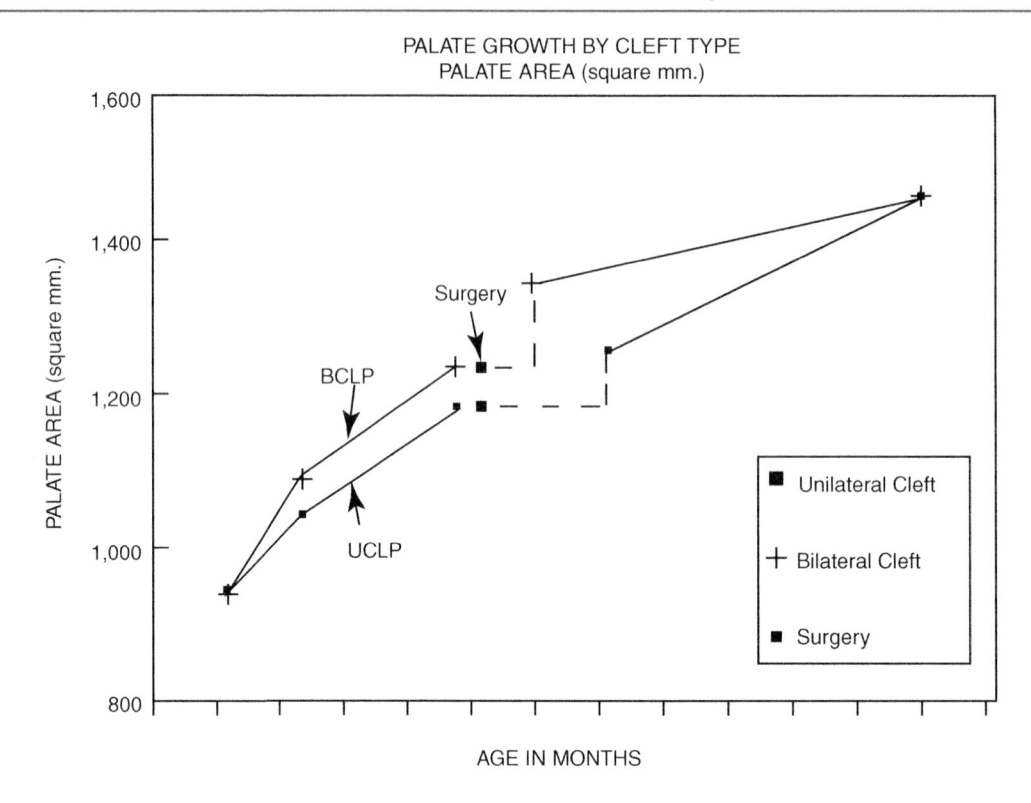

PALATE GROWTH BY CLEFT TYPE
PALATE AREA (square mm.)

## 15.2 Rapid Palatal Growth the First Year

### BILATERAL CLEFT PALATE DATA

Total Palatal Surface Area (mm2)

- Amsterdam
- Miami
- Controls
- Goteberg (D)
- Goteberg (V)
- Nijmegen

### BILATERAL CLEFT PALATE DATA

Total Surface Area (mm$^2$)

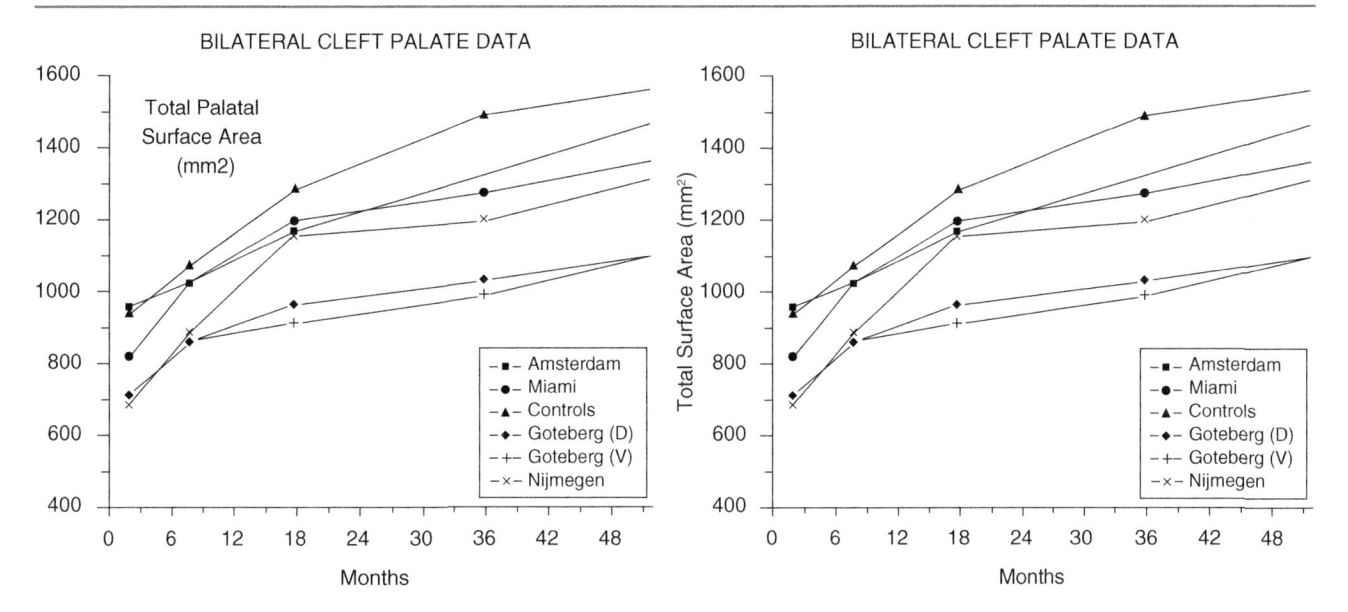

- Amsterdam
- Miami
- Controls
- Goteberg (D)
- Goteberg (V)
- Nijmegen

### Early Growth Velocity by Group and Time

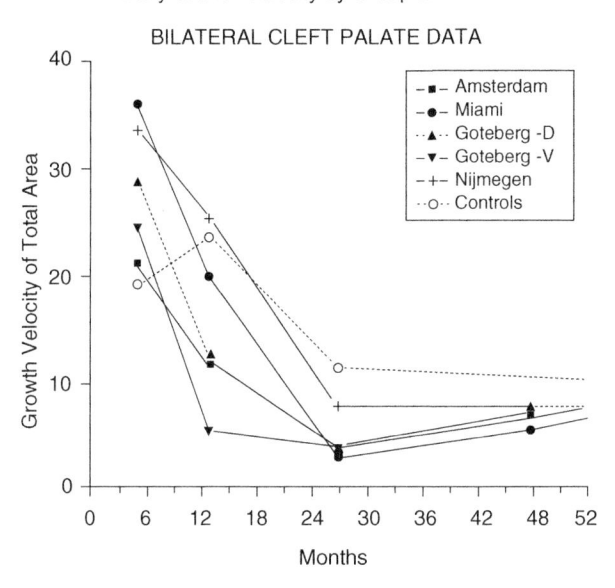

#### BILATERAL CLEFT PALATE DATA

Growth Velocity of Total Area

- Amsterdam
- Miami
- Goteberg -D
- Goteberg -V
- Nijmegen
- Controls

# Surgery Conclusions

- Vomer flap surgery, when modified and when compared to other procedures, does not inhibit palatal growth.
- Von Langenbeck with a modified vomer flap palatal surgery when preformed at 18–24 months of age allows for normal palatal growth and vault form.
- Non-physiological palatal surgery creating severe scarring can inhibit palatal growth. This occurs when performed prior to 18 months.
- The non-palatal cleft control series shows a greater degree of palatal growth.
- Presurgical orthopedics does not stimulate palatal growth.
- Goteborg: Surgery at 5–9 years.
  – Miami: Surgery at 18–24 months.
  – Amsterdam and Rotterdam: No closure surgery until 48 months.
  – All show similar palatal growth rates and same degree of total growth.

## 16.1 Berkowitz Best Time Ratio (BBTR) for Performing Cleft Palate Surgery

Ratio of the area of the cleft space to the area of palatal surface bordered by the alveolar ridge should be less than 10% at 18–24 months of age. In rare instances, closure should be at a later age to allow for more palatal tissue.

In order to determine the best surgical/orthodontic treatment plan for the complete unilateral and bilateral cleft lip and palate patient to achieve all treatment goals of facial aesthetics, speech, dental function, and psychosocial development, I reviewed 50 years of serial CUCLP and CBCLP dental casts and photographs starting at birth and continuing through adolescence with serial cephs starting at 4 years of age. Also the results of a Multicenter International 3D Study of serial palatal casts of patients starting at birth and extending into adolescence who developed good speech and facial growth.

This study proved that the latest presurgical orthopedic procedure introduced and accepted by many surgeons was Naso Alveolar Molding and Gingivoperioplasty (NAM + GPP), which had no proven longitudinal benefits. The procedure was found to bodily retrude the protrusive premaxilla by "telescoping" it backward. To do so causes a synostosis and growth retarding bone formation at the premaxillary vomerine suture (PVS). Therefore, in most instances, the resulting midfacial recessiveness with an anterior dental crossbite can only be corrected either by midfacial orthodontic protraction or by a LeFort I surgery. This study highlights that palatal cleft closure should be performed between 18 and 24 months of age when the growth velocity plateaus.

Staged orthodontic/surgical treatment limiting retraction forces to the protruding premaxilla is best performed by lip adhesion or forces that cause only premaxillary ventroflexion. The palatal cleft should be closed between 18 and 24 months when the ratio of the cleft to the palatal size medial to the alveolar ridge is at least 10%. The protruding premaxilla should only be ventroflexed but never bodily retruded. The facial growth pattern and degree of palatal bone deficiency is the main problem to be considered in treatment decision making during the first two years. One treatment plan for all cases with the same cleft type is un-physiological and will lead to anatomic problems.

# The Facial Growth Pattern and the Amount of Palatal Bone Deficiency Relative to Cleft Size Should Be Considered in Treatment Planning

## Abstract

**Background**

The aim of this study is to determine the best surgical/orthodontic treatment plan for the complete bilateral and unilateral cleft lip and palate patient to achieve all treatment goals of facial aesthetics, speech, dental function, and psychosocial development.

**Methods**

Review of 40 years of serial complete bilateral cleft lip and palate and complete unilateral cleft lip and palate dental casts and photographs from birth to adolescence, with serial cephs starting at 4 years. This was part of a multicenter international 3-dimensional palatal growth study of serial dental casts of patients who developed good speech, occlusion, and facial growth.

**Results**

Nasoalveolar molding and gingivoperiosteoplasty were introduced without proven longitudinal benefits. The procedure bodily retruded the premaxilla, which "telescoped" backward causing synostosis at the premaxillary vomerine suture. The resulting midfacial recessiveness with an anterior dental crossbite can only be corrected by midfacial protraction or a Le Fort I surgery.

**Conclusions**

Staged orthodontic/surgical treatment limiting premaxillary retraction forces to lip adhesion or forces that cause only premaxillary ventroflexion produce the best results. The palatal cleft should be closed between 18 and 24 months when the ratio of the cleft to the palatal size medial to the alveolar ridge is at least 10%. The protruding premaxilla should only be ventroflexed but never bodily retruded. The facial growth pattern and degree of palatal bone deficiency are the main items to be considered in treatment planning.

All facial skeletal surgery in growing or nongrowing patients can be regarded as an investigation of craniofacial growth, form, and function. Because facial skeletal surgery in growing children often affects craniofacial growth and function, informed decisions should be made concerning which structures need to be repositioned and reformed. Based on these decisions, a treatment plan is then formulated and a working hypothesis for successful treatment is established. The three following points need to be made at this juncture. First, remembering the value of failures as learning opportunities: clinicians cannot afford to forget them; rather, they must take ceph and dental cast records to thoroughly analyze results so that they are not repeated. Second, clinical investigators must be able to explain why some surgical procedures are successful and others fail. Third, clinicians must be able to fit the proper procedure to each individual problem and be willing to work with the consequences of their choices. Faces and clefts of the lip and/or palate within the same cleft type are not alike when considering possible physical growth changes [1] (Figs. A.1, A.2, and A.3).

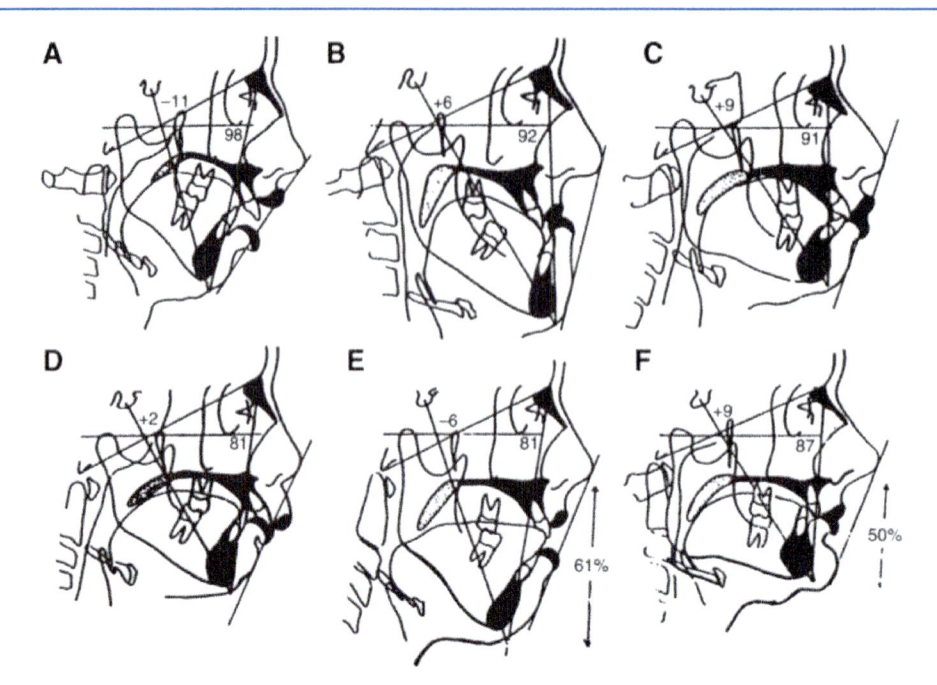

**Fig. A.1** Not all faces are the same; therefore, treatment must vary according to the facial growth pattern. Various types of facial patterns. (**a**) Retrognathic mandible with steep mandibular plane angle. Severe overbite and overjet. Chronic mouth breather. (**b**) Prognathic mandible with recessive maxilla. (**c**) Brachyfacial type with dental protrusion. (**d**) Slightly retrognathic type with protrusive maxillary denture and severe deep bite. (**e**) Long shallow face with severe tongue problems, extremely wide open bite and an inability to close the lips. (**f**) Extremely closed bite with short denture height. (Courtesy of R. Ricketts. The Biology of Occlusion and the Temporomandibular Joint in Modern Man, 1957. Reprinted with permission by Springer Science + Business Media from Berkowitz S, ed. Cleft Lip and Palate: Diagnosis and Management. 3rd ed. Heidelberg, Berlin, New York: Springer Verlag; 2013)

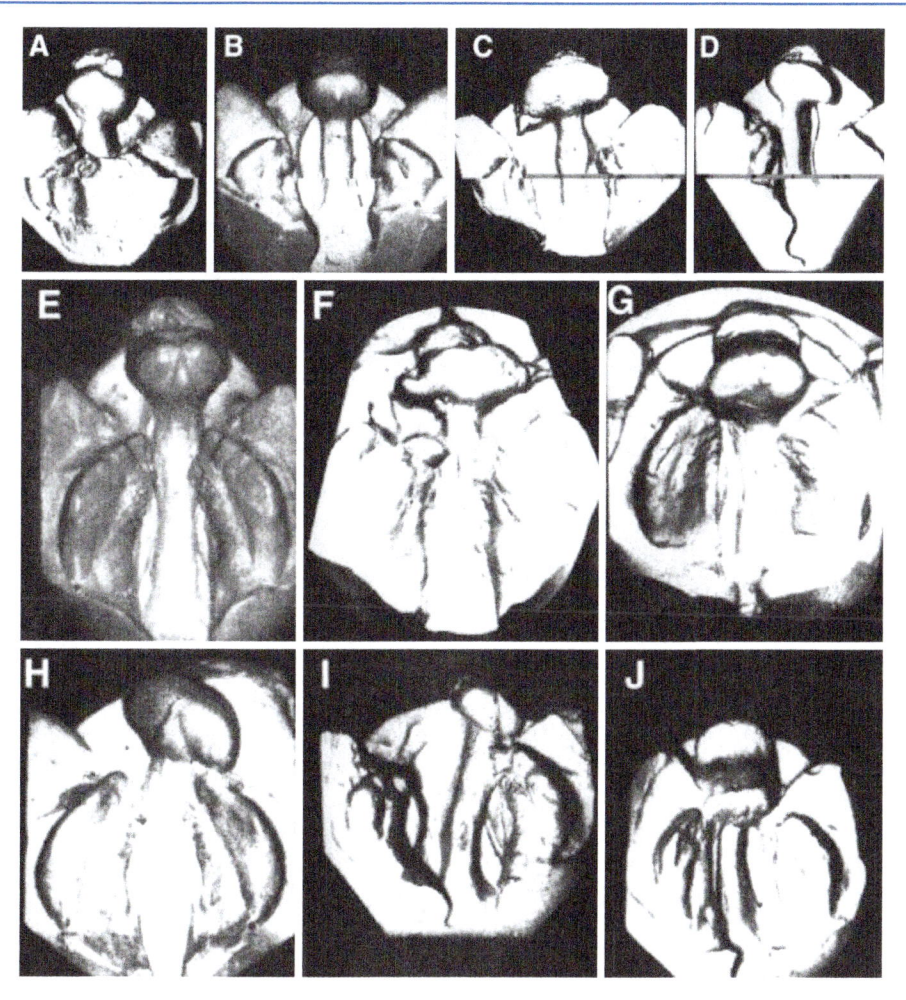

**Fig. A.2** (**a–j**) Variations in bilateral cleft lip and palate. The size of the premaxilla varies with the number of teeth it contains. Classification is dependent on the completeness of clefting of the lip and alveolus and whether there is a cleft of the hard and soft palate. Yet one or both sides of the hard palate may or may not be attached to the vomer. If it is attached to the vomer, it is classified as being incomplete. Even in complete clefts of the lip and alveolus, the extent of premaxillary protrusion will vary. (**a**) Incomplete bilateral cleft lip and palate. Complete cleft lip and palate (left side). Incomplete cleft lip and palate (right side). (**b**) Complete bilateral cleft lip and palate. Complete cleft palate (both sides). (**c**) Incomplete bilateral cleft lip and palate. Incomplete palatal clefts (both sides). (**d**) Complete bilateral cleft of lip and palate. Incomplete right and complete left palate. (**e**) Incomplete bilateral cleft lip and palate. Incomplete left palate and complete right palate. (**f**) Complete bilateral cleft of the lip and palate. Incomplete right and left palatal segments. (**g**) Complete bilateral cleft of the lip and palate. Incomplete left palate and complete right palatal segment. (**h**) Complete bilateral cleft lip and palate. Incomplete left palate and complete right palate. (**i**) Incomplete bilateral cleft lip and alveolus. (**j**) Complete bilateral cleft lip and palate (left side)

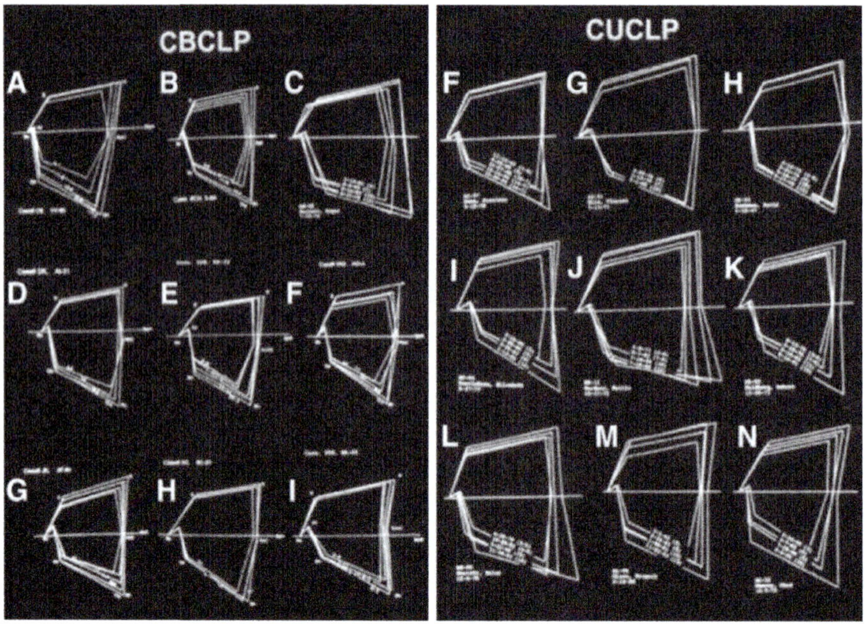

**Fig. A.3** Variations in facial growth patterns shown in cephalometric tracings when superimposed using basion horizontal analyses by Coben [2] in both CBCLP and complete unilateral cleft lip and palate. The facial growth pattern determines the final facial profile. It shows very clearly that midfacial growth is retarded, while the upper and lower facial growths proceed forward, resulting in a flattening of the facial profile convexity. These changes are greater in the bilateral cases because of the reduced gradual protrusion of the premaxilla. (Reprinted with permission from Berkowitz S., www.cleftlippalateaudiovisuallecture.org. © 2013)

The collected serial casts and cephalometric radiographs, beginning with those of the unoperated infant and continuing through adolescence, provide a view of the wide spectrum of variations encountered within each cleft type in its untreated state and a record of the changes that occurred thereafter resulting from natural growth or specific therapeutic procedures (Figs. A.4 and A.5). Clinical experience points out one important fundamental fact: all clefts cannot be lumped together as a single phenomenon (Fig. A.2). Within each type of cleft patient, there are great individual differences in the palatal geometry and size relative to the extent of the cleft defect, and these differences are clinically significant. The first line in the first article to emerge from Pruzansky's [3] research stated "Not all congenital clefts of the lip and palate are alike." This statement was to become the leitmotif of his and my subsequent research [4–11].

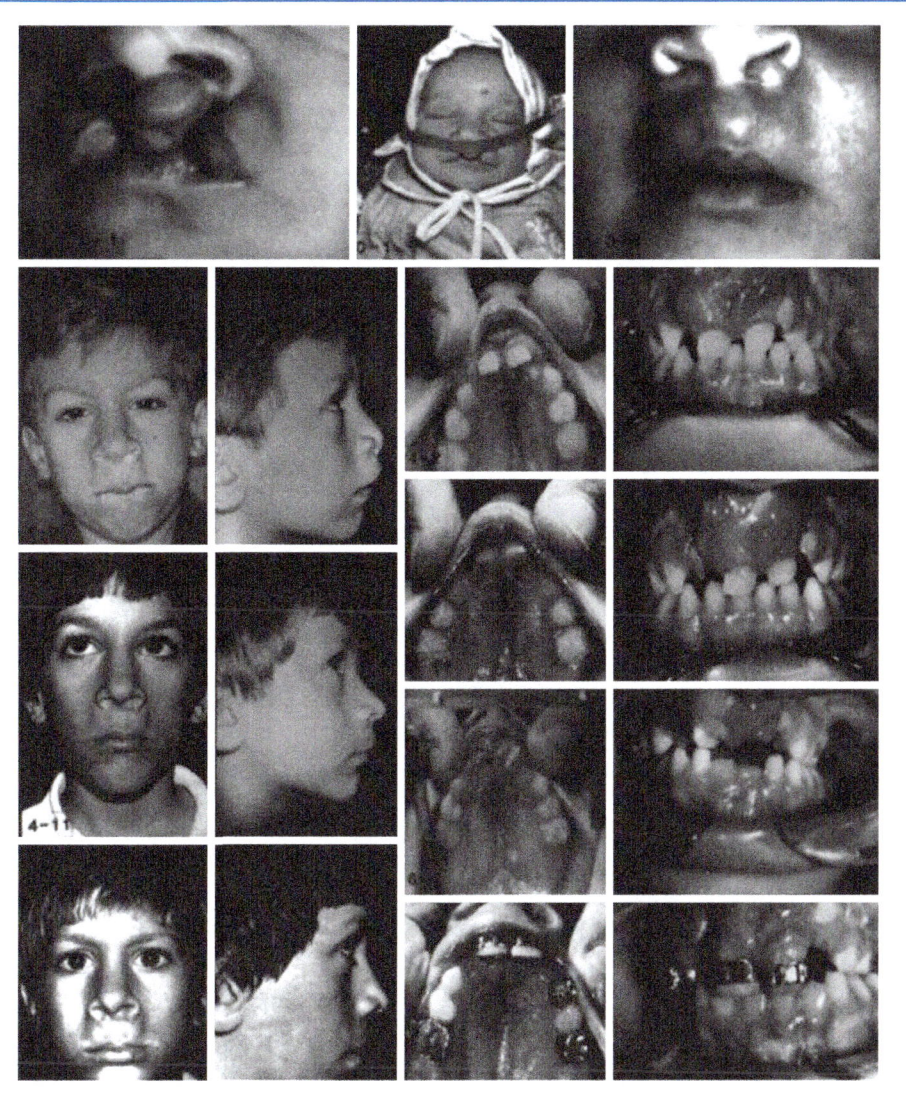

**Fig. A.4** Conservative CBCLP treatment surgery: Head bonnet with facial strap to ventroflex the protruding premaxilla. Lip adhesion at 3 months followed by a lip revision (rotation advancement) at 6 months. Palatal cleft closure at 18 months using a von Langenbeck with a modified Vomer Flap to maintain the vault space for tongue accommodation. First row: Head bonnet with facial elastic against the protruding premaxilla. Second row: The ventroflexed premaxilla bends at the premaxillary vomerine suture. The palatal segments are in a slight anterior and posterior crossbite. The molded positioned palatal segments cover a small fistula. Cleft closure at 18 months when the palatal segments were already medially positioned by external forces. Third row: Fixed palatal expander–corrected posterior and anterior crossbites exposing the small palatal fistula. In complete unilateral cleft lip and palate, the retracted anterior alveolar portion of the noncleft segment was brought laterally by opening the lateral incisor space. The medial molding of both palatal segments created an anterior crossbite either by an appliance or by lip adhesion. The teeth became more noticeable when the deciduous teeth were lost, and the permanent incisor erupted. The "thin" boney alveolar bridge created by the periosteoplasty permitted the right and the left palatal segments to be moved later, and the lateral incisor space opened. Opening of the lateral incisor space is dependent on the thickness of the boney bridge created by the periosteoplasty. A lower incisor was extracted, and the incisors were retracted to create an incisor overbite and overjet. The correction of the alignment of the upper incisor teeth was not stable even though an upper retainer was worn. Occlusal stability is dependent on the position of the basal bone, distorted nostrils, and lip because of aberrant muscle pull. Lip adhesion surgery reduces nasal and lip distortion. Rotation advancement surgery is used to improve aesthetics. Note that the vertical facial growth pattern creates an elongated anterofacial height. As a result, the midface does not appear to be retrusive. A facial protraction mask was utilized with an intraoral palatal expander to advance the maxillary incisors. Even though there was crowding of the maxillary anterior segments, the vertical facial growth pattern neutralized the obtaining of midfacial recessiveness. Lip/nose revisions were excellent in creating symmetry

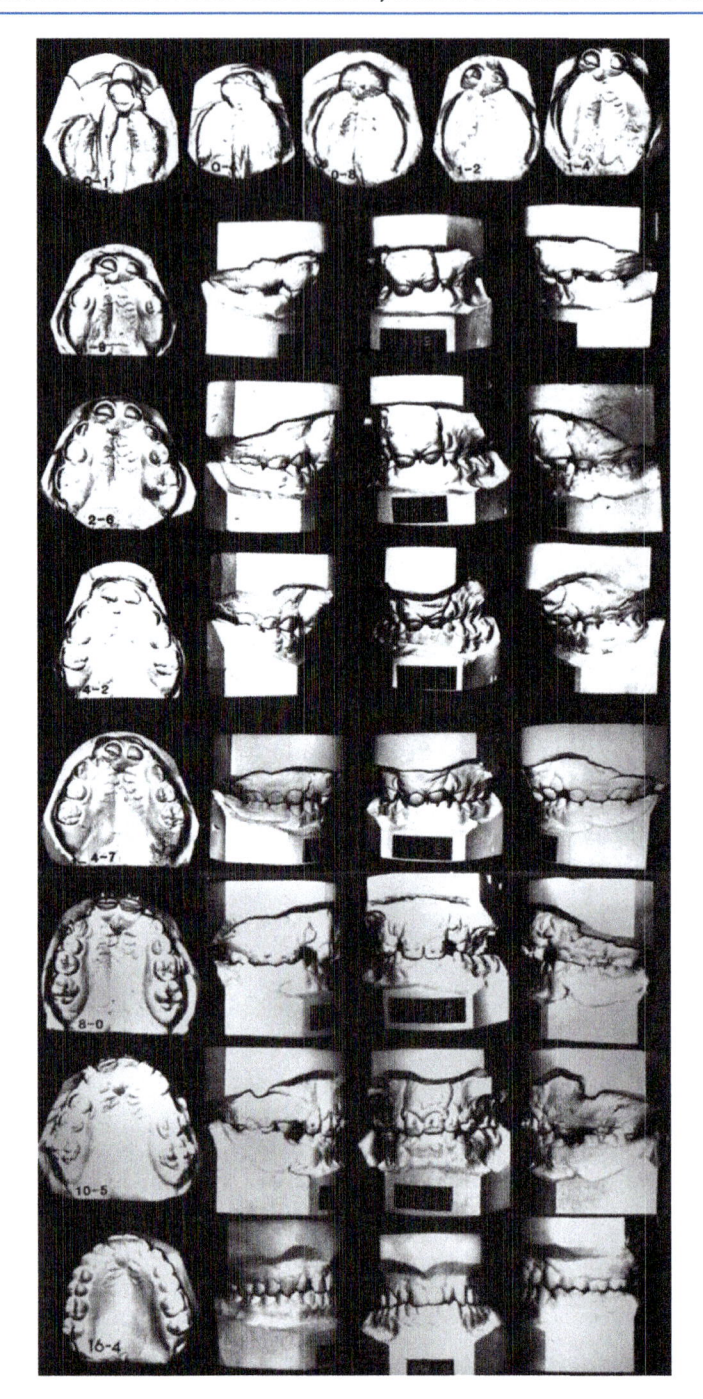

**Fig. A.5** Serial dental casts: The ventroflexed premaxilla is making contact with both lateral palatal segments resulting in anterior and posterior crossbites. Fixed palatal expander placed at 4 years corrected the crossbites. The premaxillary overjet decreased with growth. This is highlighted in Fig. A.6. (Reprinted with permission by Springer Science + Business Media from Berkowitz S, ed. *Cleft Lip and Palate: Diagnosis and Management*. 3rd ed. Heidelberg, Berlin, New York: Springer Verlag; 2013)

### 1.1.1 Surgical Treatment Modification and Remodification but with No Outcome Reports

Millard [12], in his lengthy and excellent book *Cleft Craft, Volume 3*, describes the contributions of many plastic surgeons involved in treating children with clefts. Many of the listed surgeons have used a modification of an earlier failed palatal surgical procedure. In many of the cases, the initial repositioned jaw relationship looked good but soon after additional growth, facial deformities became apparent. For example, the surgeon is confronted with the following options when faced with a protruding premaxilla at birth:

Uniting the lip over the protruding premaxilla and considering later surgical setback and other surgical options.
External elastics attached to a head bonnet or elastic tape to the cheeks to ventroflex the premaxilla (Figs. A.4 and A.5).
Early surgical premaxillary setback.
Complete removal (excision of the premaxilla).
Early lip surgery or presurgical orthopedic treatment with or without primary bone grafting or periosteoplasty (Figs. A.4, A.5, and A.6).
Lip adhesion followed by definitive lip surgery at a later age (Figs. A.4, A.5, and A.6).

After a number of poor treatment outcomes, a new surgical modification of a previous modification was made. An example of this is Brophy [13], who decided that the surgical setback of the protruding premaxilla was not successful and decided to use elastics off a facial mask to set the premaxilla posteriorly. He believed that because all palatal segments were of normal size, early neonatal palatal and alveolar cleft closure was beneficial. This procedure soon became popular even though no supporting outcome studies were published. Like many other procedures that were introduced earlier, it was later found to be unsuccessful and discontinued.

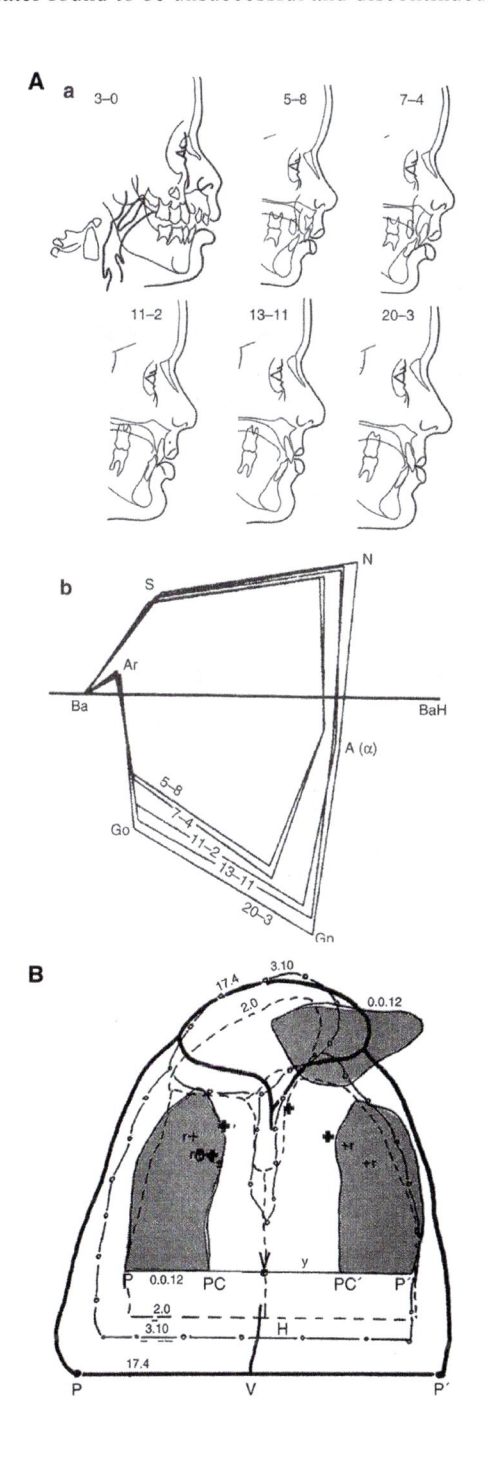

**Fig. A.6** Conservative CBCLP cases. **A** (**a**), Cephalometric serial tracings of the skeletal and soft tissue profile show marked reduction of the midfacial protrusion. **A** (**b**), Superimposed serial tracings using Coben's Basion Horizontal method show an excellent facial growth pattern, which flattens the skeletal profile. There is very little midfacial forward growth between 11 and 20 years of age. During the same time period, growth at the anterior cranial base and the mandible contributed to flattening of the facial profile. (**B**) Palatal outlines were superimposed using the palatal rugae and vomer imprint for registration. This series shows that the premaxilla's position within the maxillary complex at 17 years of age is similar to that seen at birth. Excellent growth occurs in all dimensions and is similar to the growth pattern seen in noncleft patients. Increased posterior palatal growth is necessary to accommodate the developing molars. Alveolar bone growth with tooth eruption increases midfacial height. The position of the anterior premaxilla relative to the anterior cranial base (nasion) to the anterior position of the mandibular symposium (pogonion) shows the same relative facial position from birth to 17 years of age. This study confirms that midfacial growth is retarded as the face grows at all other points. (Reprinted with permission by Springer Science + Business Media from Berkowitz S, ed. *Cleft Lip and Palate: Diagnosis and Management*. 3rd ed. Heidelberg, Berlin, New York: Springer Verlag; 2013)

From 1960 to 1980, Millard and I successfully used a conservative nonpresurgical palatal orthopedic treatment with a facial strap from a head bonnet to ventroflex the protruding premaxilla (Figs. A.4, A.5, and A.6). Lip adhesion was performed at 3 months and lip revision, called rotation advancement surgery, at 6–8 months. A von Langenbeck with a vomer flap palatal cleft closure procedure was used in most cases. Cleft closure was performed between 18 and 24 months of age and an alveolar bone graft at 7–8 years. It was hoped that performing palatal cleft closure at 18–24 months, additional palatal bone growth would prevent growth inhibiting scarring without disturbing good speech development (Figs. A.5, A.6, A.7, A.8, A.9, A.10, and A.11) [14]. In the latter 1970s, even after achieving good results at 7–8 years, Millard changed his procedure and believed that cleft lip and palate (CLP) staged treatment was not necessary and the same successful results could be attained by 2 years of age and adopted the use of presurgical orthopedics developed and introduced by Latham [15] (Figs. A.9 and A.10 [2]).

Latham, working with the anatomist James Scott in England, went to Ontario, Canada, to become an orthodontist and be involved in cleft treatment. He soon developed a presurgical orthopedic appliance held in place by pins into the palate. Its mechanics were very efficient and quickly

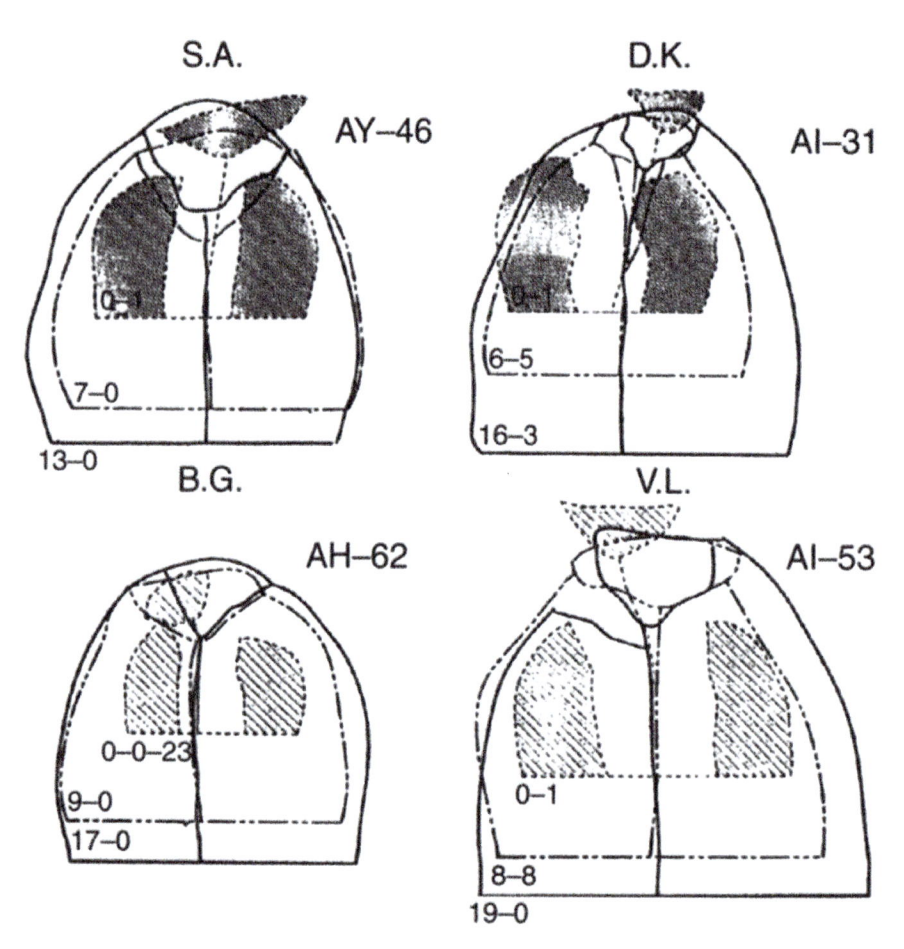

**Fig. A.7** Use of premaxillary orthopedics to retract the protruding premaxilla in the CBCLP neonatal period versus no presurgical orthopedics. In recent years, serial documentation of the natural evolution of postnatal facial and palatal development of children with complete bilateral and unilateral cleft lip and palate has yielded important objective data that help explain the dynamics of facial skeletal and palatal growth under the influence of various surgical and mechanical procedures. Superimposed palatal cast tracings of the premaxilla and the hard palate of four patients were acquired using a 3-dimensional electromechanical digitizer. In each tracing, the alveolar ridge is the lateral border of the measured surface area. The tracings are superimposed horizontally using the vomer impression and the rugae for anterior–posterior registration. In conservatively treated CBCLP cases, it shows very limited anterior alveolar growth changes but extensive posterior palatal growth to accommodate the developing molars. In conservative CBCLP treatment, the premaxilla is initially ventroflexed and ultimately needs to be elevated to open the lateral incisor spaces. The palate's anterior–posterior position remains in the same position within the face. The premaxilla's forward growth is retarded by forces generated by the lip repair. Upper and lower facial growth meanwhile reduces the facial convexity. These studies highlight that the protruding premaxilla should not be brought posteriorly at the neonatal stage. To do so will cause the premaxilla to be repositioned in the mixed dentition creating an anterior crossbite. These cases will need either orthodontic orthopedic and/or surgical treatment to improve aesthetics and the occlusion. (Reprinted with permission by Springer Science + Business Media from Berkowitz S, ed. *Cleft Lip and Palate: Diagnosis and Management*. 3rd ed. Heidelberg, Berlin, New York: Springer Verlag; 2013)

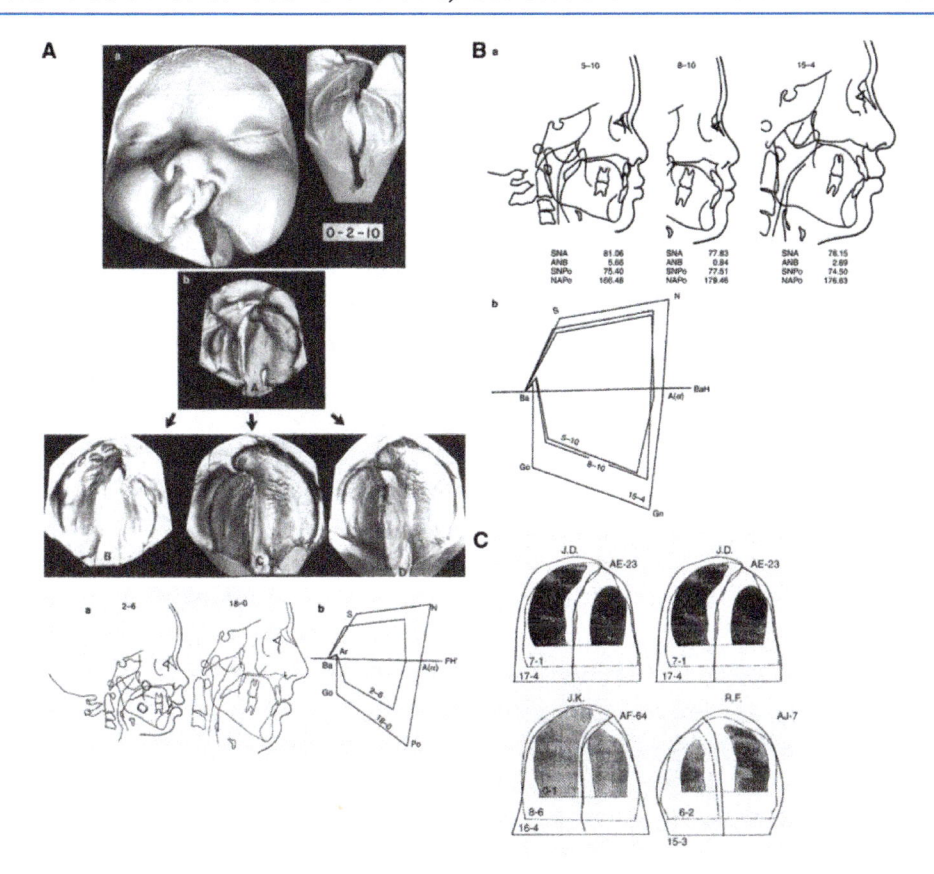

**Fig. A.8** (**A**) Complete unilateral cleft lip and palate (CUCLP)—early repair. (**a**) CUCLP. (**b**) Facial and palate casts. Complete unilateral cleft lip (CUCLP) before (**A**) and after (**B**) lip surgery. With the establishment of muscle continuity, the lesser segment moves medially, whereas the premaxillary portion of the larger segment moves medioinferiorly, both acting to reduce the cleft width. Any of the following segmental relationships can result. (**B**) No contact between segments. The inferior turbinate on the cleft side makes premature contact with the bowed nasal septum. (**C**) The premaxillary portion of the larger segment overlaps the smaller segment. (**D**) The segments form a butt joint showing good approximation. Aduss and Pruzansky's serial cast records have shown that there is no correlation between the original cleft width and the resultant arch form. Wider clefts seemed to demonstrate less of a tendency toward collapse than did the narrower clefts [14]. It must be understood that it is best for the patient that all the goals to be achieved should be postponed until approximately 6–7 years of age. To concentrate on having the child's treatment goals completed before 2 years of age is basically treating the parents and not the child. In time things that look good, that is facial aesthetics, will look satisfactory within the first year, but as growth occurs, it can negatively affect the various structures of the face. So it is best to think in terms of obtaining all the goals of good speech, facial aesthetics, dental occlusion, and just as significantly, the psychosocial development. There should be no priority of one goal versus another. With that in mind one is treating the patient and the parents should be educated to believe that time is an ally and they will be satisfied with the result at a later age. (**B**) Serial growth of the palatal segments in CUCLP. Lateral ceph computer-generated images of serial CUCLP casts superimposed on the rugae and registered on the vomer. The alveolar ridge is the outer limits of the palatal surface area. Surgery: Lip adhesion at approximately 3 months, definitive lip surgery at approximately 6 months, and hard and soft palate closure between 18 and 24 months using a von Langenbeck procedure with a Vomer Flap. No presurgical orthopedics. Results: The four illustrations show the result of molding and growth. Although the least growth occurs anteriorly, most of the growth occurs posteriorly to accommodate the developing deciduous and permanent molars. The palatal mucoperiosteum covering the cleft space led to increase in size. Because the most rapid period of growth occurs between 18 and 24 months when differentiated cells are most active, it is best to postpone palatal surgery to permit normal growth. (**C**) Serial growth of the palatal segments in CUCLP. Computer-generated images if serial CUCLP casts superimposed on the rugae and registered on the vomer AP line. The alveolar ridge is the outer limits of the palatal surface area. Surgery: Lip adhesion at approximately 3 months, definitive lip surgery at approximately 6 months, and hard and soft palate closure at 18–24 months using a von Langenbeck procedure with a Vomer Flap. No presurgical orthopedics. Results: The four illustrations show the result of molding and growth. Although the least growth occurs anteriorly, most of the growth occurs posteriorly to accommodate the developing deciduous and permanent molars. The palatal mucoperiosteum covering the cleft space led to increase in size. Because the most rapid period of growth occurs between 18 and 24 months when differentiated cells are most active, it is best to postpone palatal surgery to permit normal growth. (Reprinted with permission by Springer Science + Business Media from Berkowitz S, ed. *Cleft Lip and Palate: Diagnosis and Management*. 3rd ed. Heidelberg, Berlin, New York: Springer Verlag; 2013)

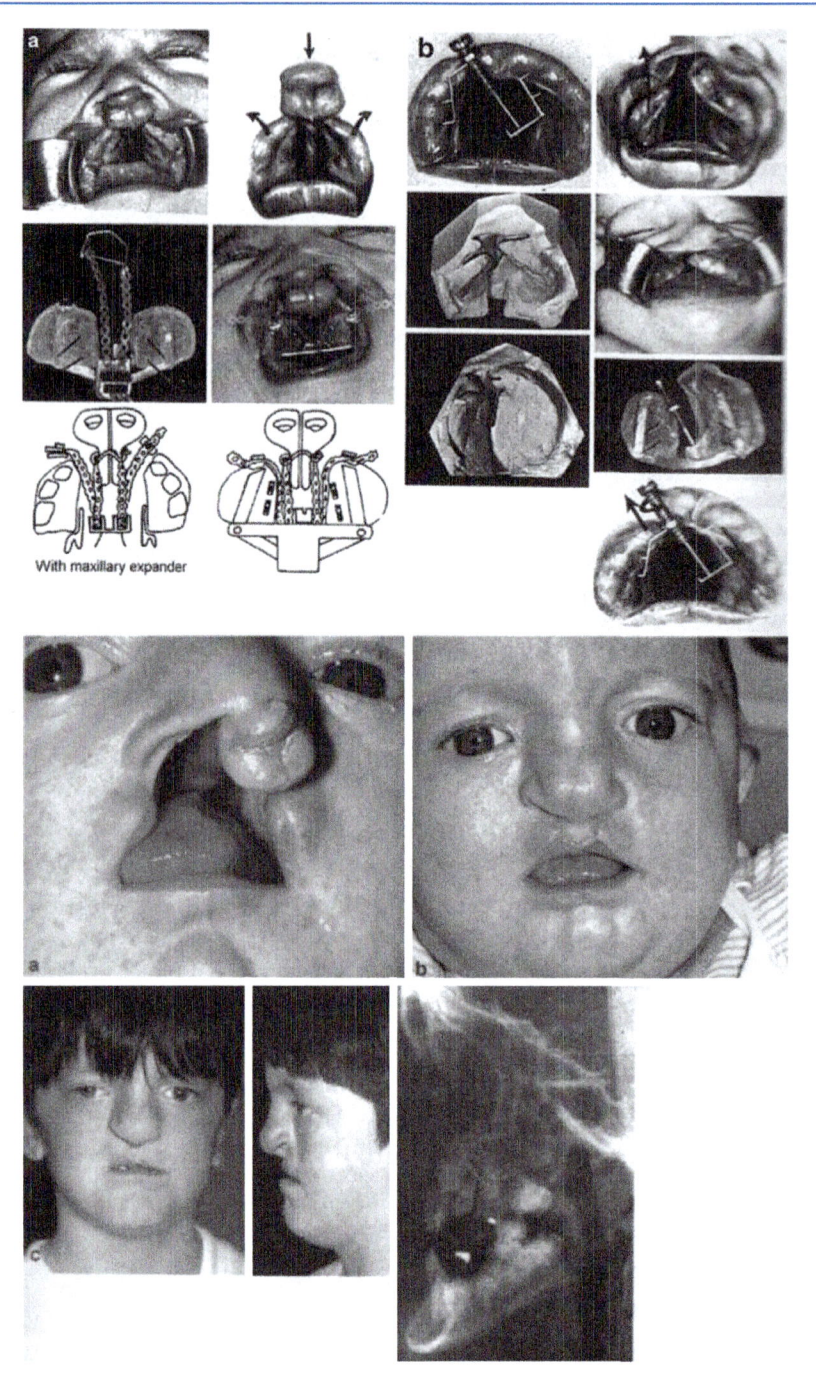

**Fig. A.9** The Millard-Latham presurgical orthopedics, periosteoplasty then lip adhesion (POPLA). These complete unilateral and bilateral cleft lip and palate appliances are pinned to both the palatal segments soon after birth. In the bilateral case, the palatal segments are first expanded to widen the intracuspid space, and then the premaxilla is bodily retracted creating ideal arch form and facial aesthetics. The periosteoplasty hopefully will replace the missing lateral incisor bone and stabilize the corrected arch. The bodily retruded premaxilla ultimately results in midfacial recessiveness with an anterior crossbite. The synostosis of the premaxillary vomerine suture is because of the "bodily" retraction, but not from united lip forces. The closure of the lateral incisors space(s) with new bone prevents the premaxilla from being advanced and the crossbite and recessiveness corrected. Additional comment: nasoalveolar molding + gingivoperiosteoplasty usage is similar in its action to the Latham-Millard (POPLA), in that it bodily retrudes the premaxilla. (Reprinted with permission by Springer Science + Business Media from Berkowitz S, ed. *Cleft Lip and Palate: Diagnosis and Management*. 3rd ed. Heidelberg, Berlin, New York: Springer Verlag; 2013)

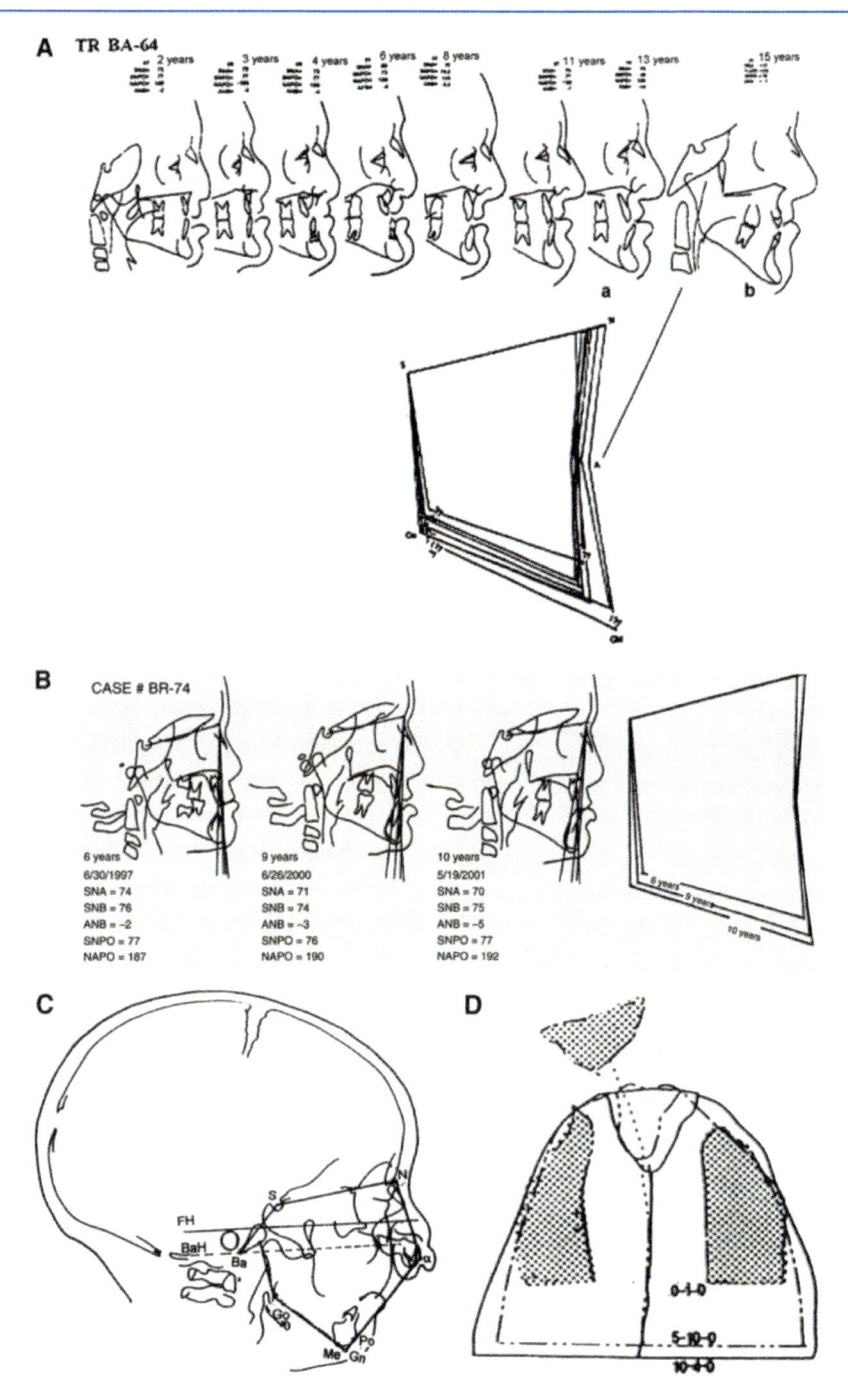

**Fig. A.10** POPLA. **A** (**a**), Serial cephalometric tracings showing the stability of the midfacial recessiveness even after the use of a protraction facial mask. There was no change in the class I buccal occlusion because the orthopedic forces were directed to only advance the retruded premaxilla. **A** (**b**) Postmaxillary distraction osteogenesis. Because of severe hypernasality, maxilla advancement was discontinued. (**B**) Complete unilateral cleft lip and palate. Severe anterior crossbite with crowding of the maxillary incisor teeth as a result of retracting the premaxillary portion of the larger segment. This created a concave facial profile (cephalometric analysis). (**C**) Basion Horizontal facial polygon (Coben) [2]. The method of superimposing tracings graphically reflects the overall concept of facial growth. A plane at the level of the anterior border of foramen magnum (basion) parallel to Frankfort horizontal where basion is the point of differential reference for the analyses of craniofacial growth. (**D**) Because the conservative CBCLP cases show that the stability of the premaxilla's position within the face with growth, it is, therefore, obvious that the retruded premaxilla will not be able to be advanced out of anterior dental crossbite to correct the midfacial recessiveness and the occlusion. This is because of the synostosis of the premaxillary vomerine suture: this change in position is also inhibited by the periosteoplasty connecting all the palatal segments so that the lateral cleft spaces cannot be recovered. The only successful correction treatment is maxillary surgery. (Reprinted with permission by Springer Science + Business Media from Berkowitz S, ed. *Cleft Lip and Palate: Diagnosis and Management.* 3rd ed. Heidelberg, Berlin, New York: Springer Verlag; 2013)

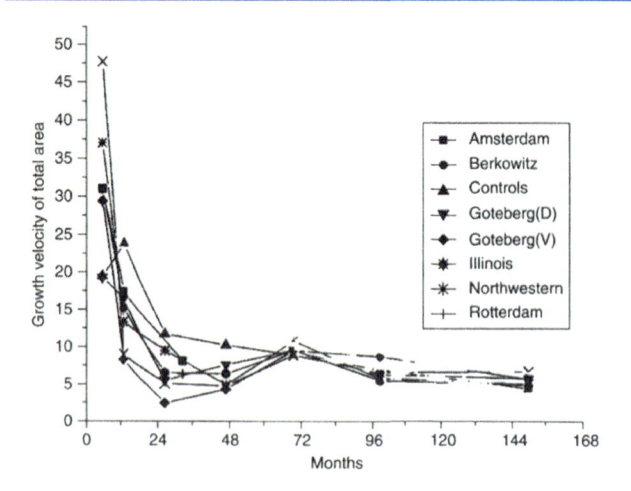

**Fig. A.11** Velocity curve: 3-dimensional study of palatal closure after various palatal procedures. All surface growth studies were calculated from the alveolar ridge medially extending posteriorly to the end of the hard palate (pterygopalatine fissure) and medially to the cleft space. All cases examined were complete unilateral cleft lip and palate. The delayed treatment series are from Goteborg, Sweden. Berkowitz cases are from Miami (closure between 18 and 24 months). This graph shows a rapid growth between 18 and 24 months no matter what procedure was utilized and then a plateauing of the growth curve. The results show that Berkowitz's cases have grown very well for the entire investigation, but the controls (no cleft) grew to a larger size, so whatever cleft treatment procedure was utilized, it had reduced palatal growth. The vomer flap treatment grew the worst. The study also shows that all velocity curves are very similar: palatal growth is very rapid in the first 18–24 months and then slows down before plateauing. They grew the most amount at approximately 50 months. Good growth was maintained even after the adolescent period. (Reprinted with permission by Springer Science + Business Media from Berkowitz S, ed. *Cleft Lip and Palate: Diagnosis and Management*. 3rd ed. Heidelberg, Berlin, New York: Springer Verlag; 2013)

moved the laterally distorted palatal segments into a normal anatomic relationship. He continued his procedure at Duke University [16] and then went to Miami to work with D. Ralph Millard, Jr. at the University of Miami School of Medicine. Millard started with lip adhesion followed by the Latham appliance and added an alveolar periosteoplasty hoping to replace the need for a secondary alveolar bone graft. Although there were no outcome studies from Canada or Duke, Millard still wished all cleft surgery to be completed earlier than was previously done. The new treatment plan with presurgical orthopedics, periosteoplasty, and lip adhesion (POPLA) [17] was used for 20 years.

Because of my reluctance to use the untested procedure, another orthodontist in Miami performed the manipulation of the palatal segments, whereas I took extensive serial records of casts, cephs, and photographs as well as performing the later orthodontia for 20 years. A comparative study by Berkowitz et al. [17] followed to compare it with the conservative protocol previously described. The results clearly showed that POPLA led to severe facial and occlusal distortions. In both complete unilateral cleft lip and palate and complete bilateral cleft lip and palate (CBCLP), the resulting midface recessiveness with an anterior crossbite became more severe over time. Computerized tomography scans and periapical films of CBCLP cases showed a synostatic premaxillary vomerine suture changes with solid bone uniting the retruded premaxilla to the vomer. The closed alveolar cleft space became occupied with the solid bone preventing the opening of the lateral incisor space. This outcome study was the only comparative POPLA longitudinal treatment study published on the use of neonatal premaxillary orthopedics in complete unilateral cleft lip and palate and CBCLP cases. Unfortunately other surgeons, both Mulliken and Cutting, who had also used POPLA for many years, have failed to perform their own facial and occlusal outcome studies as well.

After 15 years, Cutting discontinued POPLA's use and joined with Grayson, an orthodontist at NYU, to introduce a modification of POPLA calling it nasoalveolar molding (NAM) with a removable appliance and a gingivoperiosteoplasty (GPP) [18, 19]. The removable palatal appliance carried an extended stent to contact the premaxilla hoping to stimulate columella size. Their palatal appliance was found to accomplish one of its goals of bodily retracting the premaxilla to create an aesthetic lip and nose during the neonatal period. They only reported aesthetic lip/nose results avoiding any developing occlusal comments but fortunately a serial cephaloradiographic study of the NAM + GPP procedure from Taiwan reported severe midfacial recessiveness. No similar comparative cast, ceph, or photographic study has been published by Cutting and Grayson since its inception. Unfortunately, none of the surgeons who adopted the NAM + GPP treatment procedure reported their occlusal/profile outcome studies either.

### 1.1.2 What We Learned

My 40-year serial clinical records of more than 400 patients from birth through adolescence of all cleft types with conservative treatment have shown that varied surgical staged treatment procedures were necessary to achieve good treatment results with all treatment goals to be reached at least by 7–8 years of age.

Current treatment, i.e., closing the lip cleft in two stages: the first year and the palate at a later age usually between 18 and 24 months [9] or sometimes earlier, or even later, depending on the 15–20% ratio of cleft to palate size. Doing so offers a more encouraging prognosis than that of the surgeons who closed the palatal cleft before 1 year, a practice that has prevailed for the last 50 years. This finding was determined by a Multicenter International serial cast study from the South Florida Cleft Palate Clinic, the University of Illinois College of Dentistry Cleft-Craniofacial Clinic and Northwestern University Craniofacial Clinic in the United States, the University of Goteborg in Sweden, the University of Amsterdam, and the University of Nijmegen in the Netherlands. The age of the patient and the type of surgery to be applied are the two variables needed in determining the long-term effect of surgery on facial growth. Quantitative and qualitative characteristics of the cleft defect, plus the general health and genotype (facial growth pattern) of the individual patient, are additional determining factors that affect outcome results. Under certain conditions, surgical repair of the palate is feasible quite early, at about 1 year of age, when the cleft space is very small with good posterior occlusion. In others, as already stated, optimal conditions for repair will not become evident until a later age to reduce cleft size and encourage good palatal growth (Fig. A.11).

### 1.1.3 Discussion

The pattern of progress in dealing with the sequence of scientific advances with the evolution of diagnosis and therapy in cleft lip and palate is excellent. Although the literature on facial clefts can be traced back to several centuries, it is principally concerned with surgical and prosthetic rehabilitation. Furthermore, such therapy in the recent past was based largely on empiricism and reflected no real understanding of the morphology and pathophysiology. Reconstructive procedures were rarely founded on an intimate knowledge of the embryology and comparative anatomy of the region involved.

These criticisms do not imply that surgery for cleft lip and palate is in a state of chaotic disorganization. As in all branches of surgery, plastic reconstruction of the face has benefited from advances in all of the sciences. Indeed, plastic repair of the face reflects some of our most imaginative and skillful surgery and has produced remarkable cosmetic and functional results. Nevertheless, it is only in recent years that we have noted attempts to classify and delineate clinical entities among the large variety of anomalies that comprise the complex of cleft lip and palate, and only recently we have begun to make full use of the new radiographic techniques, cephs, and dental casts to study palate size, position, and function in the oropharyngeal region. The accumulation of longitudinal data to describe the natural history of facial anomalies during postnatal development and the effects of various modes of therapy is still in progress. Our understanding of the developmental processes in the formation of the face is adequate to explain the variety of problems encountered and their varying patterns of postnatal development.

As the relationship between speech, facial growth, the timing of palatal surgery, and the use of presurgical orthopedics to bodily retract the premaxilla, the reliance on clinical insight and upon case reports that lack independent documentation of results, still prevails. On the one hand, one must commend the continuing and indeed zealous pursuit of this critical question: Are serial records necessary? On the other hand, we must ask whether there is a way to increase the relative proportion of reliable, valid data and decrease the dependence on undocumented opinion.

A bilateral cleft of the lip and palate can be complete or incomplete on one or both sides. Any number of variations can exist in all cleft types, and the size and shape of the premaxilla is dependent on the number of tooth buds and their distribution making it symmetrical or asymmetrical. Because clefts of the lip/alveolus and the hard and soft palate come from different embryological sources, the cleft may involve the lip and alveolus with or without involving the hard and soft palate.

A critical review of the literature on the clinical management of the cleft lip and cleft palate, together with an evaluation of the cumulative palatal and cleft size data from longitudinal palatal growth studies, has led most orthodontists to the following hypothesis: conservative lip and palatal surgery facilitates rather than inhibiting growth in both the maxillofacial skeletal complex and the soft tissue of the labio-facial complex. In the cleft palate cases, operative intervention that involved bone growth potential will guide maxillofacial growth in the individual in such a way that postoperative "catch-up" growth of the palate will result in acceptably normal development (Fig. A.12).

Most facial and palatal-skeletal malformations in cleft patients are the result of surgical procedures that cause some growth retardation or there are osteogenic deficiencies that

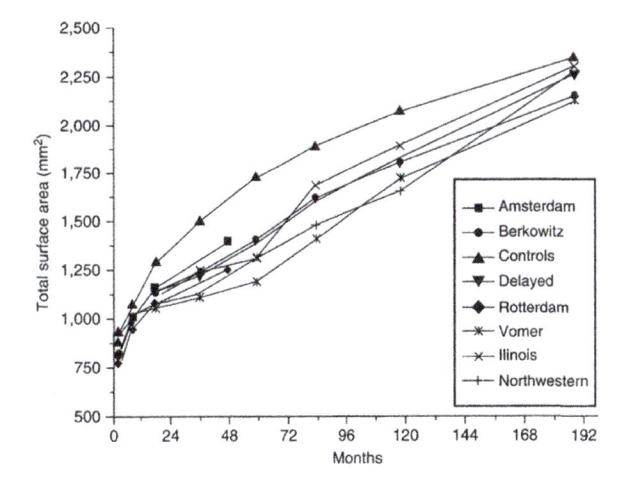

**Fig. A.12** International study—total surface area measurements from birth to mixed dentition. The control groups are cases from Amsterdam, who have had no surgery or orthopedics. They were part of a clinical trial study to determine the effectiveness of presurgical orthopedics. The other cases represent various good treatment programs. The delayed treatment and vomer flap treatment cases are from Goteborg, Sweden. They clearly show that vomer flap surgery has interfered with the palatal growth. Other cases using various surgical procedures have similar effects on the palatal growth; however, in each case, there was a retardation in growth when compared with the control series. This study highlights that the Berkowitz's (Miami) timing of surgery, between 18 and 24 months, had the least negative effect on growth. (Reprinted with permission by Springer Science + Business Media from Berkowitz S, ed. *Cleft Lip and Palate: Diagnosis and Management*. 3rd ed. Heidelberg, Berlin, New York: Springer Verlag; 2013)

lead to maxillary hypoplasia. All maxillary discrepancies are 3 dimensional, and bone size relative to cleft size at the time of surgery is crucial.

Differences between surgeons, variance in the performance by the same surgeon from day to day, and during the course of several years, and differences in techniques that are difficult to identify and compare, complicate the analysis. However, the research objectives to test the influence of presurgical orthopedic treatment and the relationship of cleft palate space to surgical outcome can be reached. It is possible to statistically test and covary for effects because of difference between and within surgeons.

### 1.1.4 Results

The facial and palatal natural history of children with clefts and those with specific syndromes demonstrates that some improve over time, some grow worse, and others remain unchanged despite the surgical effort. Presurgical orthopedics to bodily retrude the premaxilla by "telescoping" it, except for the use of a facial elastic to ventroflex the premaxilla to aid the surgeon before uniting the lip, have no long-term utility. Primary bone grafting at the neonatal period also has a deleterious effect on future palatal and facial growth.

### 1.1.5 Conclusions

These findings show that within certain defined limits, the success or failure of the surgical procedure depends on the initial state and the variables inherent in the maneuver. Subtle differences among patients will be prognostic of the subsequent state and the differences between surgeons. No matter what type of treatment surgeons have favored, they have not been able to explain why their surgical method of choice, when performed on similar clefts at the same age, often yielded different results. Why some cases appear to show "catch-up growth" resulting in good facial and palatal form and functional dental occlusion, whereas others show poor facial and palatal development?

If we assume that qualified surgeons within a given institution or region practicing a specific series of techniques over a given period of time represent a constant, the differences in success or failure should reside in (1) the initial state (the geometric and size relationship of the palatal segments to the size and shape of the cleft space, which reflects the degree of palatal-skeletal deficiency and palatal segment displacement) and (2) the facial growth pattern. Of course, the sample must separate cases, subjected to or not subjected to presurgical maxillary orthopedics, as well as cases utilizing various cleft closure procedures, because these variables can influence the subsequent state.

Cleft palate surgery is best performed between 18 and 24 months or later if the ratio of the cleft space to the palatal soft tissue medial to the alveolar ridges is greater than 15% [8].

### References

1. The biology of the occlusion and the temporomandibular joint in the modern man. Angle Orthod. 1957;27(1).
2. Georgiade NG, Latham RA. Maxillary arch alignment in the bilateral cleft lip and palate infant, using pinned coaxial screw appliance. Plast Reconstr Surg. 1975;56:52–60 . [PubMed].
3. Pruzansky S. Not all dwarfed mandibles are alike. Proceedings of 1st conference on clinical delineation of birth defects. Part 2. Malformation syndromes. In: Bergsma D, editor. Birth defects. Original article series. Vol 2. New York: The National Foundation; 1969. pp. 120–129.
4. Berkowitz S, Krischer J, Pruzansky S. Quantitative analysis of cleft palate casts. A geometric study. Cleft Palate J 1974;11:134–161 . [PubMed].
5. Berkowitz S. A comparison of treatment results in complete bilateral cleft lip and palate using a conservative approach versus Millard-Latham PSOT procedure. In: Sadowsky PL, editor. Cleft lip and palate. Philadelphia: Saunders Co; 1996. pp. 169–184 . [PubMed].
6. Millard DR, Berkowitz S, Latham RA, Wolfe SA. A discussion of presurgical orthodontics in patients with clefts. Cleft Pal J 1998;25:4 . [PubMed].
7. Lestrel PE, Berkowitz S, Takahashi O. Shape changes in the cleft palate maxilla: a longitudinal study. Cleft Palate Craniofac J 1999;76:292–230 . [PubMed].
8. Berkowitz S, Mejia M, Bystrik A. A comparison of the effects of the Latham-Millard procedure with those of a conservative treatment approach for dental occlusion and facial aesthetics in unilateral and bilateral complete cleft lip and palate: part I. Dental occlusion. Plast Reconstr Surg 2004;113:1–18 . [PubMed].
9. Berkowitz S, Duncan R, Evans C, et al. Timing of cleft palate closure should be based on the ratio of the area of the cleft to that of the palatal segments and not on age alone. Plast Reconstr Surg 2005;115:1483–1499 . [PubMed].
10. Berkowitz S. Ch. 17: Timing of cleft palate closure should be based on the ratio of the area of the cleft to that of the palatal segments and not on age alone. In: Berkowitz S, editor. Cleft lip and palate: diagnosis and management. 2nd ed. Heidelberg: Springer; 2006 . [PubMed].
11. Berkowitz S. Cleft lip and palate: diagnosis and management. 3rd ed. Heidelberg: Springer; 2013.
12. Millard DR., Jr Cleft craft. The evolution of its surgery: alveolar and palatal deformities. Vol. III. Boston: Little Brown; 1980
13. Brophy TW. Cleft lip and palate. Philadelphia, PA: Blakiston's; 1923.
14. Aduss H, Pruzansky S. The nasal cavity in complete unilateral cleft lip and palate. Arch Otolaryngol 1967;85:53–61 . [PubMed].
15. Latham RA. Orthopedic advancement of the cleft maxillary segment: a preliminary report. Cleft Palate J 1980;17:227–233 . [PubMed].
16. Millard DR, Jr, Latham RA. Improved primary surgical and dental treatment of clefts. Plast Reconstr Surg 1990;86:856–871 . [PubMed].
17. Berkowitz S, Mejia M, Bystrik A. A comparison of the effects of the Latham-Millard procedure with those of a conservative treatment approach for dental occlusion and facial aesthetics in unilateral and

bilateral complete cleft lip and palate. Part 1. Plast Reconstr Surg 2004;115:1483–1499 . [PubMed].
18. Grayson BH, Cutting CB. Presurgical nasoalveolar orthopedic molding in primary correction of the nose, lip, and alveolus of infants born with unilateral and bilateral clefts. Cleft Palate Craniofac J 2001;38:193–198 . [PubMed].
19. Hsin-Yi Hsieh C, Wen-Ching Ko E, Kuo-Ting Chin P, Chiung-Shinget H. The effect of gingivoperiosteoplasty on facial growth in patients with complete unilateral cleft lip and palate. Cleft Pal Craniofac J 2010;47:439–446 . [PubMed].
20. Grayson B, Cutting C. Presurgical nasoalveolar orthopedic molding in primary correction of the nose, lip and alveolus of infants born with unilateral and bilateral clefts. Cleft Pal Craniofac J 2000;37:528–532 . [PubMed].

Printed in Great Britain
by Amazon